Mental Health for All Nations

Culture and Psychiatry

Edited by Neil Aggarwal

'Aṣfūriyyeh: A History of Madness, Modernity, and War in the Middle East by Joelle M. Abi-Rached

Mad by the Millions: Mental Disorders in the Age of World Citizenship, Experts, and Technology by Harry Yi-Jui Wu

Families on the Edge: Experiences of Homelessness and Care in Rural New England by Elizabeth Carpenter-Song

Mental Health for All Nations by Dinesh Bhugra

Mental Health for All Nations

Dinesh Bhugra

The MIT Press
Cambridge, Massachusetts
London, England

The MIT Press
Massachusetts Institute of Technology
77 Massachusetts Avenue
Cambridge, MA 02139
mitpress.mit.edu

The MIT Press would like to thank the anonymous peer reviewers who provided comments on drafts of this book. The generous work of academic experts is essential for establishing the authority and quality of our publications. We acknowledge with gratitude the contributions of these otherwise uncredited readers.

This book was set in Stone Serif and Stone Sans by Westchester Publishing Services. Printed and bound in the United States of America.

Library of Congress Cataloging-in-Publication Data

Names: Bhugra, Dinesh author
Title: Mental health for all nations / Dinesh Bhugra.
Description: Cambridge, Massachusetts : The MIT Press, [2026] |
Series: Culture and psychiatry | Includes bibliographical references and index.
Identifiers: LCCN 2025028952 (print) | LCCN 2025028953 (ebook) |
ISBN 9780262045247 paperback | ISBN 9780262362139 epub |
ISBN 9780262053860 pdf
Subjects: LCSH: Mental health services | Mental health promotion |
Community psychology | Mental health services—Standards
Classification: LCC RA790.5 .B48 2026 (print) | LCC RA790.5 (ebook)
LC record available at https://lccn.loc.gov/2025028952
LC ebook record available at https://lccn.loc.gov/2025028953

EU Authorised Representative: Easy Access System Europe, Mustamäe tee 50, 10621 Tallinn, Estonia | Email: gpsr.requests@easproject.com

For Michael Thacker
For all that you do and mean to me, with love

Contents

Foreword

It is a pleasure to recommend this book to readers within the fields of mental health and psychiatry and to those who, by choice or circumstances, are not directly concerned with it or avoid it.

The reasons for saying this are three. First, the book avoids the notion of global mental health recognizing that the vast sociocultural, economic, and historic differences among countries make it necessary to accept that—while respecting basic ethical principles (e.g., helping disadvantaged members of societies)—countries and parts of countries have and will have mental health programs that differ in the routes chosen to make progress.

The difference between international and global psychiatry is important because it challenges the notion that there is someone (or a group of people) who will define how all the psychiatrists and mental health programs in the world will organize services, deliver treatment, promote health, and prevent mental illness. Mental health programs can learn from those in other parts of the world that are making progress, and they can inspire others working in the field in their own country. This should happen by learning about the work of others rather than by following prescribed global instruction. Professor Bhugra offers a menu of strategies and approaches as pieces of a mosaic that allow readers to learn about possibilities and compose their own mental health program adjusted to their past, their culture and their income.

The second reason for liking the book and recommending it is the breadth of the field it covers. It defines the components of mental health programs and provides definitions of strategies and options for action. The strivings of public health and the useful strategies it can offer to mental health programs are particularly welcome in this comprehensive assembly.

The third reason for recommending the book to psychiatrists, psychologists, and other mental health workers, as well as those active in the field of public health, is the author's style, which makes reading easy and provides a vast amount of useful information in a simple and straightforward manner.

Norman Sartorius

President, Association for the Improvement
of Mental Health Programmes (AMH)

Acknowledgments

I am grateful to Dr. Susham Gupta, Dr. Antonio Ventriglio, Professor Allan Young, Ms. Caroline Loveland, Dr. Iona Heath, Professors Sir Graham Thornicroft, Norman Sartorius, Sir David Goldberg, Dr. Soumitra Pathare, Dr. Keshav Desiraju, Sir Anand Satyanand, Albert Persaud, Dr. Sarah Wollaston, Sir Norman Lamb, Dr. Adrian James, Dr. Saul Levin, Professor Paul Summergrad, Sir Louis Appleby, and Professor Alistair Burn for sharing their thoughts, ideas and views over several months and indeed years. I am grateful to them for their diligence and advice. Thanks are also due to members of the group on geopsychiatry including Albert Persaud, Alexander Smith, Professors Neil K Aggarwal, Rachel Tribe, Joao Castaldelli-Maia, Julio Torales, Helena Maura, and Michael Liebrenz. The development of various ideas and discussion are mine, as are any omissions.

Thanks are also due to five anonymous reviewers who commented extensively on the first draft of the manuscript.

I am grateful to Professor Mauro Giovanni Carta and the University of Cagliari for their hospitality in hosting me for a month, which allowed me to revise the earlier draft extensively.

An earlier version of chapter 2 was published in a themed issue of the *International Review of Psychiatry* on "Mental Health for Nations" (Bhugra, 2016a, 342–374). Parts of that chapter were also published in Pathare et al. (2017) as "Discrimination in Urban Settings" in *Mental Health and Illness in the City. Mental Health and Illness Worldwide.* I have taken the liberty of using some of the material published elsewhere and am grateful for its use.

Sue Duncan provided initial support and administrative help. Thank you. Grateful thanks are due to Dr. Craig Taylor for his diligence and support along with his wonderful insights and an overview that really shaped the volume and helped me tidy it up. Thanks as well to Ralph Footring for all his hard work and support in earlier versions of the manuscript.

Grateful thanks to Matthew Browne from the MIT Press, who suggested and supported the idea of a book on the topic and gave ongoing assistance and unflinching support. Anne-Marie Bono provided helpful steer. My many thanks to you.

1 Introduction

Background

Over the past four decades that I have been practicing psychiatry, I have had the good fortune of meeting colleagues from all over the world in various roles and capacities. I have also visited many countries, from those categorized as very low income to those categorized as middle or high income, examining their services, examples of good practice, and the challenges they face. While the SARS-2 (COVID-19) pandemic illustrated that all countries are interconnected and that some of the health challenges they face are the same, cultural perceptions and explanations of mental disorders are very different around the world. Therefore, the idea that a single global mental health campaign is appropriate is nonsensical. There are geopolitical determinants that influence the social determinants of health, including mental health. Health—again, including mental health—is strongly affected by education, housing, employment, economic conditions, the justice system, and structural inequalities. It is essential, then, for all government policies to have a mental health impact assessment.

The idea for this book arose from discussions with numerous colleagues over the past decade. As president of the World Psychiatric Association from 2014 to 2017, I had the opportunity to discuss ideas as they emerged with multi-professional colleagues from around the globe and to observe and learn about local clinical services, their challenges, needs, and innovative solutions. What impressed me most is that, despite limited resources and the presence of stigma and discrimination, a vast majority of my colleagues around the world show enormous dedication, commitment, interest, and ability for innovation. Health care systems around the world range from completely public to the mostly private, although generally there is a combination of the two. Limited integration of physical and mental health services adds to the difficulties that patients, their caregivers, and families face in finding their way around the system amid their distress. Often there is rightly a loud clamor for more resources, be they financial or human. Yet there are excellent examples around the world of superb services being provided with limited resources by working collaboratively with the third sector—local communities, community and faith leaders, and teachers, among many others.

We who are passionate about improving the mental health of nations face significant challenges. Rates of various psychiatric disorders are on the increase, especially since the pandemic. There are several reasons for this. Obviously, there is better recognition both by clinicians and by the public, although some conditions are being overdiagnosed and often self-diagnosed online, and this feeds into what has been described as concept creep (Haslam, 2016; Haslam et al., 2020). Haslam et al. (2021), citing Frances (2013), suggest that "normal behaviors" are being squeezed out in favor of psychopathology. In addition, there may be a genuine increase in prevalence because of changes in causative factors such as the social determinants of mental health. These factors are related to economic factors, rapid urbanization, and industrialization around the globe and the resulting changes in family structures, cultures in transition, and changing social support. Moreover, political, geographical, and commercial determinants (Bhugra & Ventriglio, 2023a, 2023b, 2023c) influence social determinants and in many cases trump them as very often these are inter-national factors which lead to migration. Furthermore, factors like conflicts, droughts, famine, epidemics and pandemics, and climate change also influence health both directly and indirectly.

Finally, the role of the internet generally and social media specifically is a global experiment from which we are starting to see concerning signals about mental health. As discussed in chapter 8 (on school mental health) and in chapter 10 (telepsychiatry), the internet can be a force for good in improving access to information and connection, but it can also carry misinformation, negative social comparison, and simultaneous electronic hyper-connectedness and "real life" loneliness, all of which can affect our mental health in complex ways, and especially in younger people (Nagata et al., 2024; Wang & Zeng, 2024).

There are key components that must be considered when health policies are developed and discussed. These include, first and foremost, social context and analysis of epidemiological data, mental health care needs, demands, and explanatory models of illness. Second, it is crucial that entire services are considered rather than solely focusing on mental health services, as models of illness and disease will vary across cultures. Accordingly, workforce development needs to be prioritized, and recruitment and retention must be at the top of the agenda. Thereafter, partnerships with communities and other healers must be encouraged and developed, and appropriate resources must be allocated, while allowing room for local innovations to be encouraged.

As people globally are generally living longer, multiple complex comorbidities between physical and mental disorders are coming to the fore, making it even more urgent to plan for the integration of mental and physical health. In many cultures, this integration is already the case, and people use these comorbidities in their explanatory models. This Cartesian mind-body split in allopathic medicine has led to services being split and mental health services often being underfunded and difficult to access due to institutional stigma. Mental health must be the top priority for the citizens of any country for several reasons, including the burden on health and social care services and quality of life. Integration of physical and mental health, primary and secondary care, and social and health care is crucial for ensuring well-rounded care for individuals with mental illnesses. Similarly, public mental health, including the prevention of mental illnesses and the promotion of mental health, needs to be integrated with both primary and secondary health care delivery. These aims may be even more difficult to achieve in countries where the health care system is heavily privatized or insurance based. However, it is important for policymakers and health care professionals to be proactive and innovative in pulling these strands together.

Although mental health across all ages is at the heart of good social functioning for both individuals and society, it is also well known that three-quarters of psychiatric disorders in adulthood begin before the age of 24 and half start before the age of 15. Mental ill-health affects physical health; conversely, physical illness and poor physical health lead to poor mental health. Health care providers must recognize that no matter how rich the country, resources allocated to health care, especially mental health care, will often not be enough. They therefore need to think outside the box and learn from each other. Many examples of good clinical practice exist outside the formal systems, and some are presented in this book.

In the context of both physical and mental health care, care providers need to form partnerships and links with nongovernmental agencies, communities, faith leaders, folk healers, and informal carers and families because such links can be used to develop mutual learning, which will improve acceptance of and engagement in mental health care. Funding for mental health services and research funding must have equity with funding for physical health care based on population need. Hence, while working with stakeholders like patients, families, carers, and policymakers, providers need to focus on the effective and efficient use of resources. Furthermore, when a case is to be made for improved and increased funding, all stakeholders are an integral part of advocacy.

For a variety of historical reasons, research funding is not equitable between physical and mental health. This may reflect the separation of the two services, along with accompanying stigma, discrimination, and other factors. It is important to ensure that, wherever possible, there is clear and close integration and collaboration between physical and mental health services. This is probably easily achieved in primary care settings, although consultation liaison psychiatrists and secondary care services exist in many countries. It is of vital importance that these consultation liaison specialists are available in primary care settings where most patients with mental illnesses are likely to be seen. In many countries, psychiatrists also carry a heavy workload of neurological disorders, such as epilepsy, as well as physical disorders; the reverse, though, is often not true. Wherever applicable, integration between psychiatric care and social care is important because different levels of funding and separate services can create difficulties in providing optimal care as well as artificial boundaries and competition for resources. Equally importantly, primary care services and secondary care services for people with psychiatric disorders need to be permeable. Ideally, mental health services should be integrated with physical health services, but with protected funding, because in times of economic stress in particular, cancer, heart disease, and other acute conditions tend to attract the resources while psychiatric or mental health services tend to lose out (Hilton, 2016).

Principles for mental health care of nations must be focused on the individual who is distressed and needs help and those who care about them. The target of interventions may be the patient, but other factors, such as employment, housing, and finance, must be considered. In many cultures, people live in sociocentric societies where family and community can and often do play a big role in the daily lives of people with mental illnesses. Family and community are considered as positive factors for recovery. Mental health services must be not only geographically accessible but also emotionally and culturally sensitive and appropriate. These characteristics will encourage people who need them to use services according to their needs. Not every health care system will have enough personnel to have psychiatric multidisciplinary teams. A fully inclusive psychiatric team might include professionals such as psychiatric nurses, psychologists, social workers, occupational therapists, and physiotherapists but also religious healers/leaders, culture mediators, culture brokers, representatives from voluntary agencies, teachers, and others, depending on resources and the local population's needs.

Explanatory models play a significant role in how mental illness is perceived by the individual and their carers and where intervention is sought. Therefore, governments and policymakers must ensure that services are designed to consider these factors so that they are more likely to be used. When individuals begin to experience what could be termed psychiatric symptoms, they often consult family and friends initially to make sense of what they are feeling and may follow self-treatment advice to save both money and time. If the health care system is free or affordable, people may well seek help there, but if services are costly, they may try to get better without any medical or psychiatric intervention. Thus, interventions must be seen first to operate at the personal, folk, or social level. The second level is primary care. The third level focuses on secondary specialist care, and the fourth level is tertiary superspecialist care. Services and support are needed not only for individuals with mental illnesses but also for their carers and their families. Additional services and resources will require attention to the delivery of public mental health, which as mentioned above, focuses on prevention of mental illnesses as well as promotion of mental health.

Mental health should be seen at three levels: the population as a whole; vulnerable individuals; and those who develop mental illnesses. The factors affecting mental health are summarized in box 1.1. The responsibilities at the three levels for mental health are summarized in boxes 1.2, 1.3, and 1.4.

The prevention of mental and physical ill-health is crucial. The promotion of good mental health must be part of overall health care delivery,

Box 1.1
Factors Affecting Mental Health

a. Fixed factors: genetics, gender, age, and aging at the individual level
b. Political factors: political ideology of the governing party that will affect economic status, allocate funding and determine the focus on, for example, detention and compulsory medication
c. Socioeconomic factors: poverty, employment, and social exclusion
d. Environmental factors: social environment, poor housing
e. Lifestyle factors: alcohol intake, smoking, physical activity, sexual behavior, drugs and so on.
f. Access to services: health care systems, but also public transport and so on

Box 1.2
Individual Responsibilities for Mental Health

Individuals can take responsibility for their health by

- controlling smoking and alcohol consumption
- eating healthy food and getting proper sleep
- increasing physical activity
- having social interactions with friends and family members
- improving parenting skills (identifying stress and coping skills, in particular)

Box 1.3
Community and Local Responsibilities for Mental Health

Communities can work in partnership with stakeholders to provide high-quality support and services, green spaces, and easy access to public transport and public education. These can help reduce loneliness.

Box 1.4
National Responsibilities for Mental Health

National governments are often best positioned to provide leadership and must do so with a clear vision and the resources needed to design, develop, and deliver mental health services that are accessible and appropriate.

Mental health must become an important consideration and responsibility not only of governmental health departments but also of other ministries, notably employment, justice, education, and transport.

National governments need to work collaboratively with international partners and local agencies, and examples of good practice must be shared widely.

National stakeholders should provide educational information, ascertain acceptable risk levels, and regulate and legislate, as necessary.

Tackling the root causes of mental ill-health is the responsibility of national governments through their efforts to reduce poverty, unemployment, and economic disparity as well as improve the conditions in which people live, work, and play. National governments cannot work in isolation and should partner with local authorities, nongovernmental organizations (NGOs), and international agencies, where possible, to improve individuals' mental health.

with prevention, treatment, and habilitation (including rehabilitation) at its core. Individual members of society, no matter where they live in the world, must take responsibility for their own health, but to succeed, they need clear and accurate information and education and support from various sources, including the government. A proper balance between individual and governmental responsibility must be recognized. As part of the social contract, governments have a moral responsibility and indeed an ethical duty to provide individuals with accurate and balanced information, in a language they can understand, so that they can be encouraged to take responsibility for their health. The network of participants in the venture must include non-statutory or voluntary agencies (often called the third sector in many countries and terms will be used interchangeably in this volume), health professionals, community leaders, and others. People can look after their health if they have the right information and receive the right amount and the right level of support.

These observations were confirmed in the WPA-Lancet Psychiatry Commission on the future of psychiatry (Bhugra et al., 2017). A series of questions on the topic were asked of psychiatrists from around the globe. Of 2,383 respondents, 1,925 answered every question. Of these, 1,230 were from Europe (53 percent), including 186 from Spain, 178 from Italy, 155 from the UK, 82 from Ireland, 69 from Belgium, 65 from Denmark, and 32 from Greece. Another 296 were from Australasia (13 percent), including 249 from Australia and 46 from New Zealand; 291 were from South America (12 percent), including 114 from Argentina, 93 from Brazil, 33 from Colombia; 287 were from Asia (12 percent), including 101 from India; 49 were from Israel; 125 were from North America (5 percent), including 90 from the US; and 100 were from Africa (4 percent), including 60 from South Africa. Several key themes emerged from the survey. Interventions should be based on research evidence and professional experience (of equal importance in decision-making). Psychiatrists were seen as crucial in providing treatments for organic causes of mental illness.

Although this may be seen as self-evident as psychiatrists were asked these questions, their skills and knowledge must still be considered. More emphasis was recommended on primary prevention, with a preference for using the recovery model rather than the disease model. There was broad agreement that psychiatrists should actively collaborate with other professionals and enable and empower others to be trained in task-sharing. There was significant support for anti-stigma campaigns and public engagement but also for lobbying for fair, effective mental health and public health legislation and increased funding for mental health services and antidiscrimination laws. There was support for a globally agreed-on length of training with standardized content and a globally standardized examination and qualification method, which must include all psychiatric disorders along with biological, social, cultural, and spiritual aspects of mental illness. Research should focus on the lifespan, taking into account the different cultural variations evident around the world. There was overwhelming support for patients being involved in decisions not only about their own care but also in designing mental health services, actively participating in educating professionals about mental health, and conducting research and peer support.

As societies continue evolving, the patient population of the future will reflect general demographic shifts toward older, more urban, and migrant populations (Wu et al., 2023). Even with technical advances such as the development of biomarkers that may potentially alter diagnosis and treatments and digital technology that facilitates the assessment of remote populations, the human elements of practice—such as cultural sensitivity and the ability to form a strong therapeutic alliance with the patient—will continue to remain central in therapeutic engagements and outcomes. Delivering mental health services to those who need them may well require reform of the traditional structure of services. These reforms should consider stepped care, increased use of multidisciplinary teamwork, a greater emphasis on a public health approach, and the integration of mental and physical health care. These services must fit into the cultural and economic framework of a nation and be offered in a diverse range of settings where those who need these services are gathered.

Mental Illness and Mental Health Promotion

"Mental illness is a syndrome characterized by clinically significant disturbance in an individual's cognitive, emotion, regulation or behavior that reflects dysfunction in the psychological, biological or development process underlying mental functioning"—this definition is from the fifth edition of the *Diagnostic and Statistical Manual (DSM)* (American Psychiatric Association [APA], 2013). Mental illnesses also include substance use disorders and personality disorders. A serious or persistent mental illness is defined as a mental, behavioral, or emotional disorder that is diagnosable within the past year, is chronic or long lasting, and results in a significant impairment in social occupational or other important areas of functioning. The manual goes on to emphasize that an expectable or culturally approved responses to a common stressor or loss is not considered a mental disorder. Similarly, socially deviant behavior and conflicts between the individual and society are not mental disorders unless the deviance or conflict results from a mental dysfunction in the individual.

The promotion of mental health and the prevention of mental illness should target the whole population as well as individuals, especially those who are vulnerable. Depending on the health care system and available resources, the services—both directly and indirectly—should promote mental health for all, working with individuals, their families, NGOs, and other partners, including employers, schools, universities, teachers, and community and religious leaders.

A major aspect of population mental health is social inclusion and the elimination of social discrimination against individuals with mental illness.

Embedded within mental health promotion is the need to target vulnerable groups and populations, such as children, women, ethnic minorities, the elderly, those with intellectual or learning disability, migrants, refugees and asylum seekers, and lesbian, gay, bisexual, transgender, and queer (LGBTQ+) groups (see chapter 2).

It should be possible in every nation to not only agree on minimum standards of care that should be available to its citizens but also to establish systems that help deliver these standards. Services should be equitable and nondiscriminatory, especially for those with psychiatric disorders, so that people do not feel stigmatized. It is essential that policymakers and governments work with people with mental illness, their families and caregivers, psychiatrists and other mental health professionals, and researchers to design, develop, and deliver services. Patients can provide both expertise through lived experience and peer support and education, thus facilitating the sharing of what works best (and what does not) in a particular service. Mental health care policies may be decided at national level, but delivery must be local, with appropriate funding. Public mental health should be an integral part of the services and should include not only mental health promotion and prevention of mental ill-health but also psychological first aid and mental health first aid. In addition, school mental health and workplace mental health are essential parts of a national mental health service plan, as is public mental health. These services should be inculcated across the lifespan of the individual starting at an early age, ideally from prenatal onward.

Scope of the Book

This book presents some of the core principles and key components of a good psychiatric and mental health care system for any country. The intention is to summarize the evidence required to promote good mental health, prevent poor mental health, and treat mental disorders, globally and equitably. This book covers general principles potentially applicable to all nations and has focused on what the author considers examples of good practice from both developing and developed nations.

Chapter 2 sets out the broad principles of mental health care and services, and chapter 3 addresses the geopolitical and social determinants of mental health. Chapter 4 considers the issue of stigma, discrimination, and the human rights of people who have a mental disorder.

Chapter 5 examines the epidemiology of psychiatric disorders around the globe and chapter 6 the arrangements made for public mental health in a wide range of countries. Chapter 7 looks at community care. The more specific aspects of school mental health and mental health in the workplace are covered in chapters 8 and 9.

The emergence and role of tele-mental health and e-mental health are discussed in chapter 10.

The global spread of COVID-19 made the relevance of mental health issues in the times of pandemic all too evident, and this is the subject of chapter 11. Finally, the role of social prescribing is discussed in chapter 12.

The appendices outline minimum standards for mental health services and various psychiatric conditions, core competencies for mental health practitioners, the roles and responsibilities of psychiatrists, and examples of good practice in the workplace and in task-shifting.

This book has many limitations. It cannot hope to cover every country in the world and their cultures, economics, mental health needs and health care services. It is inevitable that there will be some overlap of ideas, given the centrality and intersectoral nature of mental health to nearly every component of human life. Moreover, there will be omissions, given the vast amount of ever-increasing knowledge, for simple reasons of global focus and brevity. Each country and region must decide on how relevant and appropriate the examples are for them. This book is written through the lens of a psychiatrist who grew up in the East and trained and worked in the Western medical model. Finally, the range of psychiatric treatments is vast and ever evolving. Treatment alone would be several volumes and is outside the scope of this book. The interested reader is encouraged to peruse each section's recommended reading and references for more detail.

2 Principles of Mental Health for All Nations

Introduction

Optimal mental health across all ages of the human lifespan is central to the effective social functioning of individuals as active members of society. Every civil society needs to ensure that its members are well looked after in terms of education, health, and employment so that they can perform to their best ability. These factors, along with the broader geopolitical and social determinants of health (see chapter 3), play a significant role in staying physically and mentally healthy. Consequently, the mental health of the whole population and individuals should be a significant priority for any government. It is also critical that once any individual develops a mental or physical illness, they receive the best evidence-based and appropriate care needed for them to recover to their optimal functional ability.

Mental ill-health is seen across all cultures and all societies, even though rates of various psychiatric disorders differ (see chapter 5). The way individuals present with their experiences of mental ill-health will depend on their educational and socioeconomic status and the explanatory models they use in understanding their symptoms and distress. The symptom content may differ because it is likely to be strongly influenced by cultures and cultural values. Often mental illness is seen as a single entity, which most certainly it is not, hence wherever possible, the term *mental illnesses* is used in this book.

All governments, irrespective of their political leanings, have a moral duty to develop and deliver mental health prevention and treatment services that are accessible, appropriate, and nondiscriminatory. These services should include a wide range of options to meet the needs of the population. In most countries, funding for mental health services (as well as research) lags way behind that of physical health services (and research). Equity in funding is critical to address the treatment gaps between the prevalence of mental illnesses (chapter 5) and available services (this chapter and chapters 6 and 7). Across nations, the quality as well as accessibility and availability of mental health services vary dramatically. It is critical that services are equitable and nondiscriminatory. National policies must set national standards, but with local delivery and adequate funding. Services must be easily available and both emotionally and geographically accessible. In this context, primary care services, which are often the most accessible, have a major role to play. Training for all mental health professionals needs to be an integral part of service planning and delivery.

It is therefore crucial that every effort is made to keep the population mentally as well as physically healthy and that people who develop mental illness have access to evidence-based treatment at the earliest possible opportunity. Two key requirements, then, are

1. to improve the mental health of the population as part of total health and well-being
2. to improve the mental health of vulnerable individuals in society and narrow the health gap.

The aim of this chapter is to set the scene by highlighting principles that are essential to ensure that populations remain healthy and function well. Starting with definitions of (mental) health and illness, the principles for services, mental health policy, and treatment gaps are discussed. The compelling economic case for investing in mental health is made. The needs of specific groups with higher than average vulnerability to mental illness and usually higher barriers to care are reviewed. Key basic components of primary care and psychiatric services and minimum standards of service are described. Mental health research and service development, along with relevant information systems and training of mental health professionals, are all considered.

Mental Health—What Does It Mean?

Definition of Health

Almost 80 years ago, the World Health Organization (WHO, 1946) in its constitution defined health as a state of complete physical, mental, and social well-being and not merely the absence of disease or infirmity. The WHO constitution notes that the enjoyment of the highest attainable standard of health is one of the fundamental rights of every human being irrespective of race, religion, political belief, and economic or social condition. The latter should also include sexual orientation, age, intellectual ability, and legal status along with other protected characteristics. Health can also be seen as the absence of disease and infirmity, or the focus can be on full functioning or a sense of balance between one's physical and social environment (Sartorius, 2002). The WHO constitution notes that the health of all people is fundamental to the attainment of peace and security. The protection of health and its promotion by the state are important, and unequal development influences communicable and noncommunicable diseases, including mental health. The health of the population depends not only on governments, which have a duty to provide adequate health and social measures, but also on the population itself. A nation's health is a shared responsibility across key stakeholders.

Definition of Mental Health

Mental health may be seen as a state of equipoise where individuals are at peace with themselves, able to function effectively socially, and able to look after their own basic and higher needs (Bhugra et al., 2013). A state of good mental health means that the individual can form and maintain affectionate relationships with others, is able to carry out their expected social and cultural roles, and has the skills and ability to manage change. Those with good mental health are able to recognize, acknowledge, and communicate positive actions and thoughts as well as deal with difficult emotions such as anxiety and sadness (Bhugra et al., 2013). The Mental Health Foundation (MHF, 2008) defines mental health as how individuals think and feel about themselves and their lives, which affects how people cope with adversity.

As mental health frameworks evolve, they increasingly emphasize inclusivity and the recognition of human diversity, including neurodiversity. Neurodiversity acknowledges that variations in cognitive functioning, such as autism, ADHD, and dyslexia, are natural and valuable aspects of human diversity (Miranda-Ojeda et al., 2025). Neurodiversity approaches challenge deficit-based views and advocate for understanding these variations as contributing to individual strengths and unique ways of thinking (Armstrong, 2015; Baron-Cohen, 2000). This perspective, further defined by Baron-Cohen

(2000) particularly in relation to autism, advocates for a spectrum-based understanding rather than categorical diagnoses.

There is wide variation in definitions of mental health depending on culture, profession, and clinical or research diagnostic classificatory systems (Hwang et al., 2008; Moleiro, 2018). In the Indian context, for example, Thirunavurakasu et al. (2013) suggest that *manas* (equated with "mind") should be seen as an amalgamation of three components—mood, intellect, and thought. These authors argue that the range and degree of mental health are mentally healthy, mentally not healthy, mentally unhealthy, and mentally ill. (Limitations in defining and measuring mental illnesses are discussed further in chapter 5.) In many countries, the term mental illness(es) has been abandoned in favor of mental health issues or mental health concerns. A key problem with such an approach is that serious mental illnesses then get ignored. Terms such as mental ill-health or mental illnesses should be preferred.

Mental Well-Being

The term well-being is to be seen as a state of mental, physical, and social well-being, and all three domains are inextricably linked. Emotional and mental well-being are often used interchangeably. Mental well-being, as used in the London Faculty of Public Health and Mental Health Foundation (LFPH & MHF, 2016) report, encompasses the positive end of mental health, covering both feeling good and functioning well (called hedonic and eudemonic components, respectively, in the report). The authors go on to describe feeling good as a personal subjective experience, whereas functioning well embraces psychological well-being, which includes self-acceptance, personal growth, positive interpersonal relationships, autonomy, purpose in life, and environmental mastery (Ryff, 1989).

Resilience

It is important to note that not all people will develop mental ill-health even when they are exposed to similar stressors. A major protective process against developing mental illness, despite risk factors, is resilience, although we do not know conclusively why some people exposed to the same stressors appear more resilient than others. Resilience is defined as an ability to cope with the normal stresses and stressors of life and loving and the capacity and ability to bounce back from problems (Sisto et al., 2019). There is some considerable debate on the actual definition of resilience and its practice, which may well vary across cultures. People may feel able to cope with certain levels of stresses but not with others. However, resilience is important to well-being in that it can contribute to prevention of mental ill-health (Southwick & Charney, 2012). There is confusion, though, over whether resilience is a character trait, an outcome, or a process.

Despite these variations, as highlighted in a report by the National Scientific Council on the Developing Child (2015), there are common, defining features of resilience that illustrate how the concept has been used in research and intervention sciences:

1. The capacity of a dynamic system to adapt successfully to disturbances that threaten its function, viability, or development and to resume positive functioning after dealing with adverse circumstances
2. The ability to avoid deleterious behavioral and physiological changes in response to chronic stressors
3. A process to harness resources in order to sustain well-being, whether that is physical or mental or both
4. An understanding of the in-built vulnerability to stress and the ability to adapt successfully following trauma, stress, and other adversity (National Scientific Council on the Developing Child, 2015)

Whether considered an outcome, a process, or a capacity, the essence of resilience is a positive, adaptive response in the face of significant adversity. It is neither an immutable trait nor a resource that can be depleted. Biologically, resilience leads to healthy development because it protects the developing brain and other organs from the disruptions caused by excessive activation of stress response systems. Simply put, resilience transforms potentially toxic stress into manageable stress. Ultimately, resilience is rooted in both the physiology of adaptation and the experiences we provide for children.

Mental Health Policy for the Nation

Although it is now half a century since the WHO (1975) recommended that countries develop a national mental health policy (and create a unit within their ministry of health for such an activity) along with the provision of resources in their budgets for workforce development, essential drug procurement infrastructure development, data collection, and research, these actions have not been delivered in many countries, especially low- and middle-income countries. In 2017, fewer than half of Commonwealth countries had a mental health policy (Bhugra et al., 2017).

Every nation must establish a national mental health policy to guide planning and service delivery for individuals with mental illnesses. This policy must include training and education and encourage collaboration across different sectors, such as physical health, education, employment, and justice, ensuring that health is not seen in a silo. Policymakers should consider the impact of all their relevant policies on health, including mental health. The broader impact of factors such as climate change and disasters must be part of policy discussions, too. Though primarily the responsibility of the ministry of health, collaboration with other ministries such as education, social welfare, employment, and housing is crucial. Mental health is affected by biological, behavioral, and social determinants, and understanding these factors is essential for effective interventions. Clear policy objectives, outcomes, and targets must be defined for effective health care delivery.

A program promoting mental health at the national level should take account of the following:

- Promoting mental health and preventing mental illnesses
- Linking health, including mental health, with education, employment, and housing rather than seeing it in isolation
- Being aware of existing discrimination, resources, and levels of inequity
- Providing a range of services with a stepped-up approach, from community partnerships to inpatient care
- Offering evidence-based treatments with minimum acceptable standards
- Adopting a life course approach in policy, planning, and service delivery
- Empowering patients, carers, and their families, and including them as key stakeholders

As noted previously, all policies introduced by governments should undertake a mental health impact assessment. Persaud et al. (2018) developed an index—the CAPE Vulnerability Index—to measure levels of corruption within countries that receive foreign aid, allowing the donor countries to thus assess the impact of the aid on policies. They also argue that the mental health impact of policies must be considered; however, their context is related to aid-receiving countries, which brings certain ethical challenges.

There need to be certain minimum standards for services wherever in the world services are being delivered (described below and in appendix 1). Designers of services have an obligation to ensure that vulnerabilities and variations are identified in the population they serve, and they must be cognizant of the health care and social needs of the population. Mental health services, whether they are public or private to meet community needs, must be appropriate, evidence-based, affordable (financially for the government and the payers), and acceptable (culturally suitable and sensitive) to all those who are likely to use them and their carers and families. As mentioned in chapter 1, a knowledge of explanatory models of mental illness can help develop appropriate and suitable educational packages as well as therapeutic interventions. It needs to be emphasized that cultures are not homogeneous, and thus heterogeneity within cultures must also be recognized by clinicians, other health care workers, and policymakers.

It is worth emphasizing again that there may be community resources such as religious bodies and nongovernmental organizations (NGOs) that individuals with mental illnesses may prefer to use, so close links must be forged with them to provide seamless care. This is likely to reduce stigma and create opportunities for socially acceptable interventions.

For mental health services to be accessible, their planning, design, and delivery must include key stakeholders such as patients, their carers and families, and community organizations. This needs to be a serious and not a token engagement. Such approaches bring an investment by the community members, who become both contributors and consumers of the services and therefore more willing to use them. In some settings, primary care services will be well placed to provide initial assessments and suitable referral to secondary care. Tertiary specialist services may be needed for psychiatric conditions that may be rare and therefore may have to be established at regional or supra-regional levels. For example, offenders with serious mental illness(es) may require medium- or high-security units and intensive treatment, which may well be resource-intensive and therefore viable only at a tertiary level. Evaluation and planning of services and staff training (in some settings described as continuing professional development) are important components in the delivery of services that are up to date. In countries where the health care system is largely private, patients may refer themselves directly to specialists who will be influenced by the patient's ability to pay directly or indirectly through insurance companies. Most countries tend to have mental health services in the public domain, even though access to private therapies is available.

The demographic characteristics of local populations and communities, and therefore their health care needs, are likely to change regularly. People move in or out of communities, and there are other changes related to social determinants (see chapter 5 on epidemiology). Hence, services must take these factors into account, and not just keep pace with them but be proactive and flexible enough to develop additional services as the needs of the communities change. In many settings, flexibility to develop and deliver services is very helpful, as was seen in countries that developed services for long COVID. On the other hand, increasing demands for a particular service may not necessarily reflect actual need. It is often helpful to set and try to meet targets that may well be aspirational but are worth agreeing to and then prioritizing. Understanding and agreeing to outcomes can be helpful in designing and targeting services so that everyone working in these services is clear about expectations of those who need these services. A clear understanding between policymakers, health professionals, and the community is needed to prioritize the objectives and agree on the outcomes.

Mental Health Policy Objectives

The key policy objectives and underlying principles must identify the degree and the extent of the main mental health problems—for example, the rates of common mental disorders, psychosis, and alcohol and substance use disorders (see chapter 5 on epidemiology). In low-income countries, where often the priority is more visible conditions like communicable diseases and malnutrition, mental health is at risk of being overlooked. Health care policies must focus on the promotion of good mental health, habilitation, and rehabilitation as well as primordial, primary, secondary, tertiary, and quaternary prevention of mental illnesses. Integration of support from schools, colleges and universities (where appropriate), and employers (when and where suitable) should be encouraged. Training programs for mental health must be targeted at staff according to the populations they serve, including ethnic minority groups or sexual minorities. The aim is to provide training that is culturally appropriate and sensitive to local needs. Equally importantly, the public needs to be educated about mental health and well-being.

Public Education

An important component in any nation's mental health program is public education to help develop resilience, reduce distress, and combat stigma and discrimination. Such education campaigns may need to be targeted specifically at vulnerable groups such as the young, the disadvantaged, and minority ethnic groups, as they are much more likely to develop psychiatric disorders (see the section on education and training later in this chapter as well as chapter 6 on public mental health). Other stakeholders and partners may be better placed to develop specific and targeted messages for mental health promotion and prevention of mental ill-health focusing on specific groups. Public education and public health messages and interventions must be applied across the whole age span but need to have the capacity to be flexible and tailored according to local social, cultural, and ethnic groups and communities along with their needs.

Parents and schools need training in mental health care for effective support, as do workplaces. Parenting skills and education nurture children, fostering secure attachments. Early intervention for emotional issues is crucial, enhancing community ties and forming support networks against violence (WHO, 2013a, 2013b). These actions reduce stigma toward mental illness and caregivers. Additionally, educators and policymakers must consider generational differences in technology use and attitudes to life (and work-life) and adopt interventions accordingly (Bernstein & Bhugra, 2011).

Principles for Services

A clinical service is not the buildings but the institutional culture embedded in the people who work there, whether they are doctors, nurses, midwives, social workers, porters, cleaners, or others. For a service to work, at its core there must be competent, trained staff members who deliver the service based on shared values. However, for the services to be accepted and utilized, they must be accessible, affordable, and sensitive to the needs of the local communities. These requirements can be achieved through regular consultations with the community being served and the creation of partnerships. It can be extremely fruitful to work with patient groups, community and faith leaders, teachers, or other interested individuals and groups.

Principles for services are that they must be local and accessible, comprehensive, flexible, and patient-oriented, and they must be attended to by well-trained and competent staff and accountable to both patients and policymakers. They must offer a connected range of services, from admission to rehabilitation as needed, along with employment (sheltered or independent), housing, further education, and support. Therapeutic interventions must focus on the strengths and resilience of patients and their empowerment. Meeting the needs of the community—with clear principles of service and clear priorities—is a must. Such a model is set out in box 2.1. Services should also attempt to understand the resilience and strength not only of those who require services but also their formal and informal carers, families, and communities at large. Resilience depends on a number of factors, such as achievement orientation, role adaptability, spirituality, family and kinship bonds, resourcefulness, and community involvement.

Box 2.1
Model of Service Development

1. Clear, agreed-on professional definitions of mental ill-health
2. Community epidemiological data and needs assessment
3. Bottom-up information systems
4. Agreed components of the service and their function
5. Shared systems for priorities
6. Shared systems for resources
7. Patient and carer/family involvement
8. Clearly documented plans, policies, and strategies
9. Competent trained staff with ongoing training
10. Evaluation and understanding of outcomes

The Mental Health Treatment Gap

The concept of the mental health treatment gap—the disparity between individuals requiring mental health services and those receiving appropriate care—has been a subject of scholarly attention for several decades. This is expressed as a percentage and can be used as an outcome measure. The treatment gap depends on the prevalence of the specific psychiatric condition, including substance and alcohol use disorders, social attitudes toward mental health, and the availability of resources for treatment. One of the earliest comprehensive examinations was conducted by Kohn et al. (2004), who analyzed data from various global studies to assess the extent of untreated mental disorders. Their findings revealed significant treatment gaps across different conditions and regions, highlighting a critical public health concern.

Recent studies continue to highlight significant treatment gaps across various mental health disorders globally. For instance, a study in India reported a 12-month prevalence of common mental disorders at 5.52 percent, with a substantial treatment gap of 95 percent, indicating that only 5 out of 100 individuals with these disorders received treatment over the past year (Sagar et al., 2017). In the Americas, the weighted mean treatment gap for moderate to severe mental disorders was found to be 65.7 percent, with regional variations: North America at 53.2 percent, Latin America at 74.7 percent, Mesoamerica at 78.7 percent, and South America at 73.1 percent (Kohn, 2013). These findings underscore the persistent challenges in accessing mental health care, emphasizing the need for enhanced services and policies to bridge these gaps.

These selective headline figures raise important questions for service planners as well as pathways into care and help-seeking along with those who are providing services. Qin and Hsieh (2020) from China reported four barriers to help-seeking: costs, stigma, high out-of-pocket expenses with limited resources, and perceived low treatment benefit. They suggested four possible solutions: information campaigns, increased public investment in primary care, transforming integrated care, and capitalizing on e-technologies. In a study from South India, Weaver et al. (2023) noted that when compared with men, women were more aware of local psychiatric services and were able to guide others toward these services, yet they were reluctant to use the same services for themselves. Thus, it appears likely that information and educational campaigns coupled with sufficient resources can enable a reduction in treatment gap, certainly for some (if not all) conditions.

WHO (2006) recommended options for disease control. The development of the Mental Health Atlas (WHO, 2020a) was a key step in highlighting the discrepancy in resources allocated to mental health across nations and provides direct evidence that mental health services are generally woefully under-resourced. The median public expenditure on mental health per capita was 2.1 percent. The median number of mental health workers is 13 per 100,000 population, but this varies from 2 per 100,000 in low-income countries to over 60 per 100,000 in high-income countries. The median number of beds is below 2 per 100,000 population in low-income countries and over 25 per 100,000 in high-income countries. Additionally, there are significant discrepancies in outpatient services and welfare support. Some 75 percent of countries have a mental health policy and plan (an increase from 68 percent in 2014), while just over half (57 percent) possess a standalone mental health law. However, in only 39 percent of countries, these policies and laws fully align with human rights instruments; furthermore, implementation is weak, and patients, carers, and their families are often excluded from the planning process. Some of the data was collected as the pandemic began and should therefore be considered in that context. It appears that in the past six years, there has been some progress; however, this has not been substantial or consistent enough.

Different countries face distinct mental illness challenges and treatment gaps. For example, the UK Mental Health Foundation (MHF, 2015a) provides collated information on the burden of disease and prevalence of mental disorder. Common mental disorders are indeed common, and they include depression, generalized anxiety disorders, social anxiety disorders, panic disorder, obsessive compulsive disorder, and post-traumatic stress disorder (National Institute for Health and Care Excellence [NICE], 2011). Mental disorders are differentiated from mental health condition covering mental disorders, psychosocial disabilities along with other disturbances in functioning and distress, self-harm or mental stress (WHO, 2022f).

In an adult psychiatric morbidity survey, the one-week (prior to being surveyed) prevalence of generalized anxiety in England was 4.4 percent; for depression, it was 4–10 percent, and women had higher rates of both in comparison with men (McManus et al., 2009). UK data from the Mental Health Foundation (MHF, 2015b) highlights that perinatal and paternal mental health have often been ignored, and yet parental mental health is essential for a child's growth and development and early life journey.

Using lower-cost medication can help reduce treatment gaps. Chandra et al. (2006) showed that in treatment of epilepsy, using old-fashioned drugs can reduce the burden of disease and the treatment gap, which still exceeds 90 percent in many low-income countries. Thus, these examples can be deployed in treating certain psychiatric conditions to help reduce the burden of disease. They can also be used as illustrations to raise the profile of psychiatric disorders and develop advocacy roles.

Mental Health Advocacy

Raising the profile of mental health requires advocacy with local communities as well as policymakers and experts who can help set the health agenda. Those individuals in their leadership roles or personal capacity who recognize the importance of mental health must continuously engage with policymakers and the media to help make the voices of patient advocacy groups heard, with a clear emphasis on "Think National and Act Local." When clinicians work with such individuals, they help raise their profile as advocates. This advocacy must include patients, their care partners (both formal and informal), families, and community organizations, which will help change attitudes and consequent funding.

Health reform agendas by governments throughout the world should not only incorporate mental health but also highlight it positively. As alluded to earlier, national health policies must meet not only the needs of the individuals diagnosed with mental illnesses but promote good mental health in all citizens and push for equity between mental and physical health. Despite efforts to raise awareness of mental health, international charities remain few and often lack the resources to advocate effectively. Additionally, many mental illnesses lack obvious symptoms, making it harder to generate public empathy, while more attention-grabbing conditions overshadow them. Since funding often correlates with a cause's marketability, the absence of compelling imagery for mental illnesses hampers fundraising efforts for charities and NGOs (also see chapter 7).

The World Health Organization in its *Comprehensive Mental Health Action Plan* (WHO, 2013a) aims to promote mental well-being, prevent mental disorders, provide care and enhance recovery, promote human rights, and reduce the mortality, morbidity, and disability of persons with mental disorders. It has cross-cutting themes. In the *Mental Health Atlas* (WHO, 2020b) four objectives are identified: strengthen effective leadership; promote comprehensive integrated and responsive health and social care; strengthen strategies for mental illness prevention and mental health promotion; and strengthen administrative systems, evidence, and research. These worthy aims focus on public mental health. However, there needs to be a clear understanding between the government and the governed about what is expected of each other. This social compact or social contract is worth exploring because it may well vary across cultures and countries.

Investing in Mental Health

There is considerable agreement that the burden attributed to mental illness exceeds that of other major noncommunicable diseases (see chapter 5). The case for investing in mental health, therefore, can be seen in three different ways.

The Health Case

It has been known for decades that individuals with mental illnesses die 15 to 20 years younger than those who do not have psychiatric disorders (Harris & Barraclough, 1998; Walker et al., 2015; de Mooij et al., 2019; Office for Health Improvement and Disparities, 2023). Often, they also have worse physical health than those without mental illness. This variation is due to many causes, which include suicide (around 720,000 a year globally, though not all are attributable to underlying psychiatric disorders); worsening mental health problems that interfere with care and self-management of physical health problems like diabetes, heart disease, and lung disease; and poorer treatment of those problems by the health system. There is now compelling evidence that individuals with mental illnesses undergo fewer investigations and receive inferior clinical care for their physical well-being, alongside delays in diagnosis by physicians and other health care professionals (Thornicroft, 2011).

The Social and Economic Case

Social determinants of health include poverty, unemployment, overcrowding, lack of access to green spaces, and so on (Marmot, 2014, 2017; also see chapter 3 on geopolitical and social determinants of mental health). However, many of these social determinants are influenced by supranational-level geopolitical determinants that include political, geographical, commercial, economic, cultural, and other factors influenced by man-made and natural disasters, conflicts, and climate change, leading to internal and external migration. Geopolitical determinants affect social determinants directly and indirectly.

The Human Rights Case

People with mental illnesses are often subjected to serious abuses, such as being chained and physically abused in many countries, and they may be denied their fundamental basic human rights and protections through discriminatory laws (see chapter 3's section on discrimination). Discrimination can also lead to delays in help-seeking, thereby increasing duration of untreated illness which then leads to poorer prognosis.

The value of mental health must be seen at different levels: the personal level (ensuring that individuals function optimally); the family or kinship level (reducing the burden on individuals and turning them into productive members of society); and the community, societal, cultural, or national level. The value of mental health can also be seen at the economic and well-being levels and context, too. The ability to realize their own potential while managing stress and working fruitfully means that individuals can contribute significantly to the betterment of society and to economic prosperity. Barriers to investment in mental health are attitudinal as well as behavioral. These barriers include stigma, discrimination, lack of political will, and limited knowledge, among other factors. Equity in legal terms and integration of mental and physical health are important aspects of investing in mental health (box 2.2).

The Social Justice Case

Social justice entails equal access to liberties, rights, and opportunities, as well as care for the least advantaged members of society. Overlapping with the human rights case, the social justice case seeks to redress historical oppression and marginalization. Social justice requires nations to acknowledge their involvement in the shameful list of gross injustices committed by one group against another: slavery, colonialism, imperialism, segregation, white supremacy, apartheid, warfare, and so on; to recognize how they impact affected communities in the present day; and to seek correction of these imbalances. This requires both a legal and financial commitment to justice as well as developing prevention and clinical services to be culturally attuned and acceptable, empowering of individuals, and therapeutic for all who use such services.

Box 2.2
Reasons for Investing in Mental Health

1. Public mental health with prevention of mental illnesses
2. Economic well-being and better functioning
3. Economic growth and productivity
4. Equity in status
5. Social and cultural impact
6. Political impact

The World Health Organization (WHO, 2013a; 2020a) highlights that the current state of investment in mental health in many countries is woefully inadequate. It proposes that the basis for renewed investment in mental health systems lies in several contexts, including human rights protection; public (mental) health and burden of (mental) disease; cost and cost-effectiveness of treatments (for various psychiatric conditions); and equitable access and financial protection. Combining human rights protection with equitable access leads to the elimination of social discrimination. Planning and designing, developing, and delivering services for people with mental illness must be a joint endeavor between governments and mental health care professionals as well as other stakeholders, including patients, carers, families, communities, and community organizations.

The role that policymakers and governments can play in improving the mental health of their populations has to be addressed at two levels. First, and importantly, is investment in public mental health. The key aspects of public mental health must address investment in information at a very basic level, addressing all ages. Obviously, such actions will depend on existing health care systems. Second, all governments must address the easy accessibility and availability of mental health and psychiatric services for individuals with mental illnesses. Minimum standards of services for some of the main types of service provision are outlined in appendices 3 through 6. Equally relevant in any delivery of mental health care is the elimination of social discrimination. Such discrimination works at personal, social, economic, and political levels and must be eliminated using legal frameworks. Individuals with mental illness may require social and financial protection.

Mental Health Service Development

Policymakers as well as mental health professionals have an ethical duty to assess the state of health—including mental health—of the people they serve. They then have a responsibility to ensure that effective and collective action is taken to maintain good health and prevent and treat ill-health, including mental health, with adequate resources. They also need to ensure that support and care are available for those who are disabled, chronically ill, or dying. Finally, they must ensure the quality and effectiveness and efficacy of services and therapeutic interventions.

The basic aim for any politician (or other individual) responsible for health is to take all necessary and desirable steps to ensure the preparation, effective implementation, and coordination of measures conducive to the health of the people and populations. That includes ensuring access to correct diagnosis and treatment of ill-health (physical or mental) and illness prevention. The fundamental tasks of any ministry of health (anywhere in the world) are to assess the health needs of the population, monitor interventions, take suitable and appropriate action, and continue to monitor the impact in an ongoing manner with the basic aim of improving and protecting health. In addition, as mentioned before, given that mental ill-health is present in every sector of society, health ministries should make every effort to link up with other ministries such as justice, education, housing, and employment and monitor the impact of all government policies on the mental health and well-being of the population. Governments can and must take the lead but cannot by themselves secure the health of the population.

Any plan for action to improve the population's health relies on a national strategy and health plan and policy. The strategy must include not only the development of policies, plans, and legislation, but also clear implementation and direction in the field of physical *and* mental health. This must include plans for the prevention of mental illness and the promotion of mental health. These strategic initiatives must have clearly stated lines of responsibility and governance. These strategies need to have a clear outline for the preparation and implementation of programs for health promotion and prevention, encompassing both physical and mental health, in the areas of mental illness, substance misuse disorders, and developmental disorders.

As the Pan American Health Organization (2014) recommends, gender, equity, ethnicity, and human rights must feature across all themes. It is vital that policymakers take into consideration environmental, biological, socioeconomic, cultural, and health system dimensions. Broader geopolitical factors such as climate change and pollution reduction need to be at the forefront of health care planning and delivery.

Service design must include short-, medium-, and long-term vision and planning, and the delivery of services must be based on best practices with appropriate use of artificial intelligence (AI), telehealth, tele-mental health and e-mental health to improve clinical access and clinical information with proper knowledge and skills management. Wherever possible, multidisciplinary teams must be encouraged, developed, and supported. The services need to extend across specialties, geographical areas, and communities. Infrastructure must focus on ongoing audits, evaluations, and synthesis of the medical evidence with clear delineation of specific practice guidelines.

In setting up services, policymakers must accomplish the following:

1. Identify mental health needs of the entire population, of vulnerable and at-risk populations, and of those individuals who have developed mental illness.
2. Use standard, well-understood terms that are clearly defined.
3. Gain commitment to setting and achieving material standards as well as models of service delivery, through identification of needs and by engaging with stakeholders.
4. Engage with the private health care sector and with practitioners at similar levels.
5. Identify key players—individuals, groups, or agencies—and engage with them on a regular ongoing basis.
6. Identify a clear chain of command and responsibility in delivery once service plans have been agreed on and ensure that an implementation plan is accepted by the stakeholders.

The implementation plan must be handled at the local level, with a clear leadership structure and defined responsibilities. Members of the team must be aware of their roles and have the right level of support available as well as the skills necessary to ensure that the agreed-on plans are delivered.

Teams at the local level must assess existing mental health services against the standards and service models and develop priorities that align with the national strategy. These priorities include working partnerships; developing clinical governance; workforce planning; the design and delivery of education, training, and support; appropriate information technology systems; and monitoring and ongoing evaluation of services.

Patients, their caregivers, and their families must be involved in planning and evaluating services, with regular feedback. Appropriate and adequate funds must be made available for research into the prevalence and etiology of mental illness and for service development. Local gaps in service delivery must be identified and plugged appropriately. Long-term goals must be set and evaluated regularly. National mental health services planning must consider issues related to finances, workforce planning, education and training, research and development, and clinical decision-support and information systems.

In annual health care planning at the national level, equal importance and equitable funding should be allocated to mental health services. Various components of the mental health care system should be considered while distributing sufficient resources. Equity between physical and mental health must form the core principle.

A range of services must be provided and adequately resourced. No matter where in the world, these services should offer a variety of accommodations, from short-stay crisis homes to early intervention and long-stay supported accommodation, as well as sheltered employment, which can be expanded along with new skills development. Equity of access and safety must be paramount principles. Specialist services for children and adolescents, the elderly, those with intellectual disabilities, and other underserved populations, such as LGBTQA+ individuals, migrants, and prisoners, should form part of the fabric of mental health services. A clinical model called "accompaniment" is a process of "radical empathy" that involves listening, witnessing, and advocating with patients and attempting to minimize power imbalances, which is important in confronting mental health inequities (Shim & Vinson, 2021).

Strategies to improve access to mental health care for underserved populations include community-based interventions, telemedicine, culturally adapted services, and task-shifting. Task-shifting approaches, where trained lay health workers provide basic mental health support, have been successful in low-resource settings (Fernando et al, 2021; Patel et al., 2018; also see appendix 12 for examples of good practice in task-shifting from different countries). Telemedicine has helped bridge gaps in access, particularly during the COVID-19 pandemic (Witteveen et al., 2022). Culturally adapted mental health services, such as bilingual counseling and Indigenous healing practices, have improved treatment engagement (Kohrt et al., 2018). Technological advances including artificial intelligence may improve detection, diagnosis, care, and scaling of services (Gutierrez et al., 2024).

A vast majority of psychiatric problems are addressed in primary care, therefore training and support for primary care service providers—doctors, nurses, occupational therapists, and others—must be strengthened wherever necessary. Locally agreed-on models may be used—for example, shared liaison services or referral services. In countries where there are not enough primary care physicians, services must train community midwives, health visitors, nurses, and other health professionals; additionally, resources such as teachers, religious or spiritual leaders, and others may need to be tapped as well. Arrangements for specific referrals must be agreed on at the local level. Cost-effectiveness of interventions must form part of the overall planning and resulting funding. Every effort must be made to develop and deliver services that are evidence-based rather than simply based on ideology.

Quality of Care as a Basic Principle

As mentioned earlier, to deliver the best quality care, health and health care must be linked with education, employment, housing, finances, and justice. Clearly defined referral networks are required, supported by proper IT systems and taking into account local needs and the availability of access to digital services. Seamless coordination of care across conditions, specialties, and disciplines is fundamental to high-quality health care. Patient experience is significantly influenced by the knowledge and skills of health care professionals who provide care in a coordinated manner. Services need to be designed for common conditions, but it is equally important to be prepared for unusual and rare cases as well as emergencies. Systems must be established to prevent errors that are not concealed, and processes should be clear and easily accessible for learning from these mistakes. Whistleblowers must be heard and, if necessary, protected. Managing expectations and change is essential. Access to expert intervention should be straightforward. Professionals have a moral and ethical responsibility to ensure that care is of good quality, no matter what the setting, and that they themselves would be happy to receive it.

The quality of health care is often overlooked in terms of where, when, and how therapeutic interactions occur. The level of quality of available services is likely to influence early help-seeking, improve engagement, and consequently lead to better outcomes. Quality of care relies not only on structures but also on processes. These processes in mental health care depend on what transpires during the interaction between the patient and the clinician, as well as mutual understanding, rapport, and mutual respect.

Donabedian (1980) points out that quality of care can be evaluated based on structures, processes, and outcomes. Structures are physical, such as buildings, but quality of care is also about accessibility and capacity. Processes are interactions between patients, their caregivers, and formal carers, including frontline staff. Outcomes should focus on changes to patients' health status. Outcomes can be particularly important because patient expectations and those of the treating clinician may differ. An orthopedic surgeon may have fixed a fractured femur perfectly according to radiographic evidence, but the patient may still find it difficult to walk. In mental health, the distinction between *disease* (as understood by the clinician) and *illness* (as understood by the carer and the patient) may cause a dissonance of expectations. Such discrepancies have to be addressed through better and more effective education and organizational support services.

Schuster et al. (2001) assert that services must be safe, effective, patient-centered, timely, efficient, and equitable. Accessibility—both geographic and emotional—is crucial for individuals to seek help. While the focus in care delivery is on the patient, families and informal carers also play significant roles and may require support. The core principle of health care is the ongoing healing relationship between the patient and health care professionals, necessitating a safe health care system with well-trained staff and adequate resources. Services should be transparent and flexible, anticipating patient needs and fostering cooperative care, particularly in contrast to competitive private health care. Identifying best practices in care design and sharing knowledge with local communities can enhance engagement and reduce stigma. Quality measures should reflect local needs.

Quality of care can be compromised due to technological complexities and increasing longevity, leading to multiple comorbidities requiring effective self-management. The fragmentation of health care systems, lack of evidence-based care, and managerialism can worsen outcomes by possibly benefiting staff over patients.

As technology and AI become more advanced, there is every likelihood that these tools will be used effectively by individuals to manage their health and well-being and by clinicians to support decision-making, ascertain outcomes, collect data to measure these outcomes, and share the data. In theory, AI should enhance patient/clinician communication, but this will happen only if both sides are familiar with and comfortable using the technologies. In addition, issues related to confidentiality and privacy must be considered in the context of ethical interventions. In many countries, AI is being used to write case notes and histories, as well as for interpretation and report writing. Educating staff and patients about the role and impact of AI will be very helpful.

To deliver quality services in psychiatric care, safety must be a top priority, with patient and staff safety programs in place. Threats to the safety of patients and staff are the end result of complex individual and systemic causes. Cooperation among clinicians and other health care professionals, with proper and appropriate information-sharing, is crucial to ensuring safety. Any health care system must have in-built safety features so that patients and staff feel safe and are safe. System errors can cause untold damage. Errors are essentially failures of planned actions to be completed, or they occur when the wrong plans are used to achieve that aim. Effectiveness is defined as care that provides evidence that a specific intervention—whether it be diagnosis, medication, or prevention—works well and produces a desired outcome that is beneficial for the patient. These therapeutic decisions must be made based on the best research evidence but also on patient values (which indicate patient preferences and expectations, whenever and wherever possible) and individual clinical expertise. Quality assurance is about eliminating defects. Total quality management as defined by Kelly (2007) includes strategic objectives, customer focus, and continuous improvement in teamwork implemented through practice and supported by various techniques.

In service design and development as well as delivery, patient care must be based on continuing healing relationships with clear control by patients and services tailored according to patient needs, shared knowledge, and decision-making. Services must focus on the patient, and clinicians need to be compassionate, empathic, and responsive. It is good clinical practice that patients and those who care for them are given appropriate information in a language they can follow and understand. Patients and their carers and families must be able to rely on good quality, easy-to-understand information about the illness, its management, and potential outcomes. Pathways to formal and informal care should be well explained; here, "maps" can make information easily accessible. Whenever possible, patients and their families should be allowed to hold the information about their illness. A strong focus is needed on providing the right level and degree of information while encouraging and supporting self-management.

Organizations need to create and articulate their vision and goals. They must create the right environment for learning and invest in workforce training and support. Any therapeutic interventions must be evidence-based, integrating the best research with clinical expertise and patient values. The evidence can be synthesized in a variety of ways. Cultural values, both local and institutional, as well as differences must be taken into account. IT can be used in consumer health services, such as online assessments and prescribing. Clinical care and financial transactions can and do make use of IT, as can public health measures and professional development.

It is important that the response capacity of systems and services for people with mental illness, substance use disorders, and developmental disorders across the lifespan be evaluated regularly and that this capacity be adjusted appropriately where necessary. The rights of individuals, their carers, and their families must be monitored carefully and regularly, and relevant toolkits should be employed to record this information. Data on quality of care must be ascertained regularly to ensure that standards are met and improvements are maintained.

Workforce Planning and Training

Each nation must consider workforce planning and appropriate training for mental health services. Although often there are standard recommendations per capita of population, it is impossible to have clear-cut recommendations for the minimum number of mental health professionals needed to deliver services. Nevertheless, overall workforce numbers must be planned. The key to effective workforce planning is understanding the needs of the local population, followed by identifying those most capable of delivering services and providing them with adequate training. Therefore, regular mental health needs assessments may serve as the first essential step.

At the best of times, in many countries (including high-income countries), mental health service providers face challenges in recruiting and retaining adequately trained and qualified staff. The scenario is much worse in low-income countries: In sub-Saharan Africa, the average is about 0.1 psychiatrists per 100,000 people, with some countries having as few as one psychiatrist per million inhabitants (UNICEF, 2023) compared to 8–27 per 100,000 people in the European Union (Eurostat, 2018). Even if sufficient numbers are attracted to the specialty, clinician migration to richer countries ("brain drain") often depletes local workforces (Oladeji & Gureje 2016). Two steps are crucial and depend on local needs. First and foremost, key principles for the creation of a sufficiently skilled mental health workforce must be created and agreed on across stakeholders as well as the public. Second, in order to deliver these skills, required competencies must be identified (see appendix 2). The key competencies to deliver accessible and appropriate services are based on nondiscriminatory clinical practices irrespective of religion, gender, age, sexual orientation, culture, or disability.

The recommendation on the minimum number of workforce personnel needed must be tailored to cultural and national needs. Cultural models need to be remembered and considered while developing services. Existing recommendations and numbers put forward in one culture may not be entirely applicable in other settings. The needs of the local population must be carefully studied and understood and be made an integral part of workforce planning. In some settings or at certain times, a scaling up of the mental health skills of health professionals may be sufficient.

It is important that policymakers carry out workforce planning in a proactive manner. Levels of recruitment and retention of staff must be monitored regularly, and the morale of staff must also be evaluated. A range of health care professionals will be needed, from specialists to trainees to psychologists, occupational therapists, nurses, and social workers. Patient, carer, and family engagement at all levels of health care delivery needs to be monitored regularly as well. As mentioned earlier, patients, their carers, and their families should be encouraged to be part of the evaluation team of the health services and involved in advising on service development, planning, and delivery, as well as evaluation and research questions. They must be offered a range of occupational activities to ensure maximum social involvement and participation, which could lead to greater self-esteem, better engagement, and better outcomes.

Delivery of mental health services depends on partnerships across specialties and disciplines. Specific individual disciplines require specific training. Only sustained national action can produce a clear change that will deliver services that are accessible and appropriate. Depending on the basic needs of the population and relying on good epidemiological data, clear workforce planning should be encouraged. National planning will determine the number of health professionals, and training in mental health for all health professionals must be mandatory, especially in countries where the number of health professionals is insufficient. More workers, whether they are community support staff or volunteers (as in many low- and middle-income countries), may require specialized training. Training is discussed in detail below.

Standards of Service

No matter where in the world an individual who develops mental illness is, minimum standards of service must include early and rapid detection and diagnosis, easy access to affordable treatments, and subsequent habilitation and rehabilitation if needed. Care provided must be aimed at optimizing engagement and functioning, then preventing relapse. Every individual who requires hospital admission should be able to access it, and the admission should be the least restrictive possible for the individual and as close to home as possible.

Every country must attempt to collect adequate epidemiological data on levels of psychiatric disorders, frequency of various psychiatric disorders, and health care needs of individuals who have these disorders. Data collected in other countries may not be easily applied across countries for several reasons, including category fallacy. Cultures are relative and not entirely similar. Services should develop a set of standards following the assessment of local needs. These standards must be established in discussion with local mental health professionals, patients, and their representatives and carers, as well as families and other stakeholders.

Community Services

The essential components of community-based services are listed in box 2.3. Such services can be within either specific community mental health care settings or primary care collaborative settings. These services must be local, with intersectoral collaboration in the planning and delivery of services. Services must be culturally appropriate, equitable, and free from discrimination based on gender, religion, race, sexual orientation, social class, or psychiatric conditions.

Long-stay hospitals (or asylums) should be closed, but gradually and carefully, with a planned discharge of patients into the community after providing for training, support, and suitable accommodation and networks of care. A basic model for setting up community services is shown in box 2.4.

Primary Care Services

A majority of people who experience mental illnesses will be looked after in primary care, no matter where they live in the world. This has both advantages and disadvantages. The advantage is often that the services being used are local, far less stigmatizing, and—in countries where patients or their families must pay—often cheaper.

Primary care in the UK, as in many countries, manages most patients with mental illnesses, with only a very small proportion being seen in

Box 2.3

Principles of Community-Based Services

1. Providing comprehensive services across the lifespan
2. Focusing on recovery
3. Combining biopsychosocial models
4. Committing to human rights and equity
5. Undergoing regular evaluation
6. Addressing the particular needs of vulnerable groups
7. Ensuring scalability of services in times of disasters
8. Maintaining adequate staffing levels with a proper skill mix
9. Promoting mental health, preventing mental illness, and supporting rehabilitation and social reintegration
10. Expanding and decentralizing mental health services

Box 2.4
Requirements for Setting Up Community Services

1. Clear definitions of mental ill-health
2. Community epidemiological data
3. Bottom-up information systems
4. Agreed components of the service and their function
5. Shared systems for priorities
6. Shared systems for resources
7. Patient and carer/family involvement
8. Clearly documented plans, policies, and strategies
9. Competent trained staff with ongoing training
10. Evaluation and understanding of outcomes

secondary care and even fewer in tertiary care. Some patients, depending on available resources, will continue to require regular and ongoing care from specialist services, although in many countries, this may not be possible or even feasible. Among the various needs of individuals with mental illness, psychological and social interventions may be required, such as supportive and interpretive psychotherapies, accommodation, and employment, whether that assistance is ongoing or stable or independent.

Depending on health care systems, in many countries, primary care physicians act as guides and control access to specialist care. Primary care staff must therefore be trained to identify various psychiatric illnesses so that suitable referrals are made.

Various models of integration between physical and mental health need to be explored in any individual country. In some settings, mental health professionals can provide advice, whereas in some psychiatric settings, physicians or specialist nurses can offer face-to-face consultations as part of primary care. In some primary care services in the UK, for example, primary care psychiatrists or community psychiatric nurses are readily accessible online or by phone, whereas in others, they are physically present in primary care facilities. Regular evaluation of services by both those who work in them and external bodies, with the active involvement of patients, their carers, and their families, may raise early questions about pressures on services and help identify the resources needed. Increasingly, countries around the globe are developing regulatory bodies to inspect the services and structures through which they are being delivered.

Bearing in mind that many countries may not even have a well-organized primary care system, it is important for policymakers to assign it the level of importance it deserves. Furthermore, since community health workers such as community midwives and health visitors are present in most countries, it is important to build these links as they may make secondary psychiatric services more acceptable and less stigmatizing. Any individual who is distressed because of a psychiatric or substance use disorder should have timely access to services.

It is critical that individuals in need of care can access primary care without delay. To achieve this, health services must be adequately funded, ensuring sufficient capacity and capability in primary care settings. In low- and middle-income countries, even when resources are limited in primary care, community health visitors, traditional midwives, and nongovernmental organizations can be trained to help identify common mental disorders within the community and, if necessary, refer individuals to primary care physicians or specialists. There have been excellent examples of implementing intervention protocols; for instance, depression treatment algorithms have been utilized in primary care in the UK. Several protocols have received local approval and need to be widely publicized and made accessible according to local health care systems. Secondary care services, including nursing staff and other health professionals, may act as liaisons and provide advice to primary care staff.

Research has indicated that after educating school students about schizophrenia, those experiencing the illness find it easier to discuss their symptoms and seek assistance (Yamasaki et al., 2016). It appears likely that teaching the basics of serious mental illness can encourage openness, ultimately leading to improved access to services. Patients, their caregivers, and families often receive better support in primary care and home environments through educational initiatives and emotional assistance. In low- and middle-income countries, due to a shortage of human resources, caregivers may have to forgo their employment to care for someone with a mental illness. This imposes an additional financial burden that national governments must consider when developing services.

Services for People with Serious Mental Illnesses

Traditionally, serious mental illnesses have included psychoses, schizophrenia, personality disorders, and bipolar disorders, among others. People with serious mental illness are likely to be the most significant out-group. Often, they are also the most vulnerable. They may lack the capacity to seek help and might not be able to defend themselves, feeling powerless as they are often socially and economically dependent on others.

Everyone who experiences severe mental illness must be assessed thoroughly and promptly to determine their treatment needs and suitable therapeutic interventions. Individuals with severe mental illness exhibit higher rates of physical morbidity and mortality. Furthermore, in various countries and contexts, they are at substantial risk of social isolation and alienation, as well as discrimination related to employment, participation in social activities, and other acts that we all take for granted. Those with severe mental illness may present risks to themselves or others, requiring comprehensive assessment and appropriate management. Because of the nature of their condition, they may well have complex needs that must be addressed. A range of step-up and step-down services may be necessary, from inpatient facilities to day hospitals, day centers, or drop-in services with a range of accommodation options and possible short-stay homes.

Traditional Medicine and Traditional Healers

The World Health Organization (WHO, 2019) defines traditional medicine (TM) as "the sum total of knowledge, skills and practices based on the theories, beliefs and experiences indigenous to different cultures, whether explicable or not, that are used to maintain health, as well as to prevent, diagnose, improve or treat physical and mental illnesses." Traditional healers (i.e., those who practice TM) are often more approachable and accessible to patients and their families than formal health care services, especially if their explanatory models are culturally sensitive. They include faith healers, religious leaders, spiritual healers, and practitioners of Indigenous or complementary and alternative medicine. They form part of the unrecognized health care system in many countries, but often perform a valuable service, especially when dealing with common mental disorders such as anxiety. There are many reasons for their approachability. First, they align with the explanatory models of illness that patients and their families may have.

Second, they are more likely to take a holistic approach, and third, they are easily accessible. In addition, they are more likely to spend more time with patients, thereby providing better engagement. Thara et al. (2004) reported that often this group of healers has very high acceptability and accessibility and can work well with conventional mental health professionals. A project from Gujarat in Western India reflects one way of engaging with faith-based healers, observing that when they work well together, they are very effective, but it takes a lot of time and preparation to overcome distrust (Shields et al., 2016; appendix 10).

Mental Health Research

Every country and nation-state must align research and development funding for physical health with that for mental health. Research can take various forms, from basic sciences to translational research, as well as health services and population studies. While not all countries may possess the infrastructure to conduct basic science research, every nation should strive to enhance its capacity for conducting population and health services research. It is crucial that health services are evaluated appropriately and regularly, although this will depend on the specific health care systems in place. When private providers deliver health care, the assessment of quality often becomes increasingly relevant and patient led. In this case, the following areas are worthy of examination:

- Evaluating service delivery through quality assessment and patient satisfaction
- Investigating variations in service delivery in different parts of the country
- Investigating variations in diagnosis and management of comorbidities between physical and mental ill-health, between mental ill-health and addiction, between primary and secondary care, and between secondary mental health care services and tertiary mental health services

Research should evaluate clinical interventions, developing practice guidelines without viewing them as the only approach. Both efficacy and effectiveness of psychological, psychosocial, and psychiatric interventions must be assessed. Outcome comparisons for conditions like suicide and self-harm are straightforward, while prescription rates of drugs such as antidepressants and antipsychotics can vary even within the same culture because of geographical and other factors. Cost-effectiveness and user satisfaction can serve as additional indicators. In many cultures, alternative and complementary therapies are preferred and could be included in therapy assessments. Additionally, genetic factors influencing pharmacodynamics and pharmacokinetics, and cultural factors influencing diet, smoking, alcohol and drug use, religious practices, and taboos must be considered in service evaluations. In many countries, most drugs are available over the counter, and the prescriber may not know what is being sold (including quality of the medication) and what is being taken. Sometimes, patients may afford to buy medication only one day at a time. This must be explored by clinicians, bearing in mind that clinicians and patients, although from the same broad culture, may have very different worldviews.

Hyman et al. (2006) note that randomized control trials mainly involve highly selected populations in specialized settings in industrial countries, raising concerns about the generalizability of findings, particularly across cultures. The timely diagnosis and application of research-based treatments lag in both high- and low-income countries, compounded by a lack of funding for translational research. Researchers interested in randomized trials often struggle to see their findings applied in real-life situations and may overlook potential pitfalls.

Training in clinical research should emphasize translational research, acknowledging that not all mental health workers will pursue research, yet they should understand how to apply research findings to their practice based on their roles and responsibilities.

The Information and Support Infrastructure

Clinical Decision-Support Systems

A wide range of guidelines for clinical decision-making have been developed by various professional bodies and organizations and are widely and easily available. However, for a variety of reasons, clinical guidelines should be taken as guidelines only. These reasons include the quality of the trials and research, publication bias in favor of positive results, recruitment of more homogeneous samples included in trials, variations in cultural and clinical settings, and a mixture of comorbidities that may affect treatment choice, treatment adherence, and therapeutic responses.

Audit

Clinical audits in varying settings must be encouraged so that clinical services can be improved. In many countries, including the UK, clinicians are encouraged to carry out clinical audits for specific purposes of service improvement and annual appraisal and revalidation. It is important to ascertain patient, carer, and family satisfaction with services, but these perspectives must be seen in the context of clinical settings and cultural values. In many cultures, patients and their families will hesitate to give negative or less than positive responses lest they upset their professional caregivers. Both the structure and the processes within the health care delivery system must be regularly evaluated and suitable improvements and amendments made to the services. Service development and its evaluation must be seen in the context of national plans, policies, and priorities, but their application must be local.

Information Systems

Information systems are essential for adequate, appropriate, and proper delivery of services. Information systems must provide easy access to the knowledge base for service delivery and support individual service user care to inform clinical and management decision-making. Outcome scales can be used within information systems. However, access to these systems depends on the IT infrastructure in different countries. Patients in the private sector must have access to the same level of information systems as those in the public sector. In many countries and cultures, patients hold their own records, whereas in others, they have limited or no access to their notes. Some innovative simple solutions, such as giving patients all their data and information on a USB stick or in a notebook, make it easier for patients to carry their data across services. Copies of the information can still be stored centrally so that easy access is possible. Data-sharing across services or between departments such as health, education, employment, and justice must be encouraged within the existing framework of confidentiality.

Finance

Although clinicians are not typically trained to understand financial issues, it is important and helpful to know how and where financial resources are being spent. It is important for clinicians to understand financial costs of services, especially in times of economic downturn, when mental health services are most needed and yet are most likely to face severe financial cuts. Often, mental health services are the first to take a hit when resources are tight. We also know that economic downturns can lead to mental ill-health, thus creating a double jeopardy (Reibling et al., 2017).

The Role of Medicine and Psychiatry

Psychiatry's Social Contract

For centuries, a "social contract" has existed between medicine and society, with specific implications for psychiatry. As one specialty capable of depriving individuals of liberty and enforcing medication against the patient's will, psychiatry exemplifies this contract. Originally, the term referred to the relationship between monarchs and their subjects, where taxes were paid in exchange for public protection. Under the divine right of kings, subjects surrendered some natural rights for the assurance that their remaining rights would be safeguarded (Gough, 1936; Figgis, 1914). This relationship between the state and populace is central to the social contract. Gough (1936) identifies two types of contracts: the social contract, in which individuals agree to relinquish some rights for protection and care, and the contract of submission, where subjects define their governance. This latter form is particularly relevant in democratic societies.

The delivery of medical services (including psychiatric and mental health services) is dictated directly or indirectly (through its representatives) by society and the relationship between medical practitioners and society (as represented by its policymakers or rulers). It is evident that as societies change and develop, the ethical and moral imperatives embedded in medical practice must also evolve. Policymakers, guided by health care professionals, determine the levels of funding for services, training, and structures. The practice of psychiatry is heavily influenced by social norms and attitudes, which must be recognized in developing and delivering services and the legal and regulatory frameworks supporting them. Medicine's initial contract with society was rooted in the formation of guilds, which in Great Britain transitioned to Royal Colleges and other similar institutions that assumed responsibility for professionalism by setting standards and evaluating the functioning of these organizations. With technological advances and innovations, this implicit contract requires revival and renewal on a regular basis. It is important to recognize this contract for a variety of reasons: it concerns patients and health care professionals working together to ensure that sufficient funding is available along with reasonable expectations of each other from both sides.

Governments often bring together key stakeholders to develop health care strategies and objectives as part of medicine's social contract between society and the medical field, particularly psychiatry (Bhugra, 2014, 2024). This contract involves patients, doctors, and health care workers, on the one hand, and the government on the other, setting mutual expectations and responsibilities. A strategy imposed by the government is unlikely to succeed; instead, collaboration among patients, carers, health professionals, and policymakers can lead to shared ideas, strategies, and agreed outcomes for decision-makers. This collaborative approach fosters ownership and ensures adequate resource allocation while clarifying needs and expectations. Historically, it has influenced ethical codes in medicine, evolving in response to societal changes and advances in clinical practice. The tripartite contract with private health care providers holds significant importance, especially as telehealth and AI become more prevalent.

Society rightly expects the highest ethical standards from the medical profession. Medical professionals are anticipated to fulfill the role of a healer—someone who is moral, competent, transparent, and accountable (Cruess, 2006). Furthermore, these individuals are expected to exhibit altruism and offer unbiased, objective advice to society. The rights and duties of individuals and the state are reciprocal, accompanied by shared expectations and obligations. As long as this mutual understanding persists, both parties remain reasonably content. However, when this understanding begins to shift and diminish—particularly as medicine becomes increasingly alienated and complex, leading to perceptions of its inability to self-regulate—the focus on issues such as lay control of the profession in certain countries starts to surface. Consequently, regular assessments of the competencies of medical professionals through revalidation structures begin to emerge.

Clinicians have a dual role: they are both members of society and professionals advising it. In return, medical professionals expect a degree of autonomy, self-regulation, fair remuneration, and respect from the society they serve, recognizing their expertise and professionalism. Additionally, external factors such as the media and regulatory bodies significantly influence this unwritten contract. Cruess (2006) points out that the notion of medicine's social contract reflects the monopoly granted to the profession due to its knowledge base. With the rapid expansion of the internet, this knowledge is readily accessible to all. Therefore, the development and delivery of services must consider these social changes and how they, including social media, can be used to enhance service delivery. Similarly, psychiatry's contract with society requires careful attention.

The British Medical Association (BMA, 2019) highlights a chronic lack of investment in the UK health care workforce, which has led to a breakdown in the contract between the government and medical professionals. Strikes by nurses, ambulance staff, and even doctors reflect this issue. Party political ideology and differing expectations within the compact confirm the role of political factors in health care. The new government formed after the July 2024 elections managed to resolve these issues. Doctors face time constraints with patients, risking their contract and struggling to balance high-quality care with limited resources. Consequently, doctors and medical students are increasingly at risk of stress, psychiatric disorders, and burnout (Bhugra et al., 2019) as the practice of medicine grows more complex.

Psychiatry's Contract with Society

The Mental Health Foundation (MHF) examined the UK's social contract in psychiatry and found that mutual expectations play an important role. Their report highlighted significant challenges for psychiatry in fulfilling this contract, such as a lack of resources and psychiatrists' reluctance to take on leadership roles. Society, in turn, has high expectations, including a clear separation between the social and health sectors and better communication of these expectations. Based on two surveys, qualitative interviews, and focus groups, the report revealed that most respondents felt the contract between psychiatry and society was not meaningful. To fulfill its social contract, psychiatry must become credible by acknowledging its issues, increase its visibility, and ensure it is useful by providing appropriate support where needed.

As mentioned earlier, challenges to psychiatry include ongoing stigma against the subject (its patients and practitioners) in many countries, continuing negative attitudes, and perceived low status in the medical profession, all of which affect patients and families as well as funding, recruitment, and retention. It is not only clinical services that need adequate funding but also research funding, which must be on an equitable basis with research into physical illness. In the UK, after dozens of members of Parliament stood up in the House of Commons in 2013 to speak of their own personal experiences of mental illness, the nature and the focus of the debate on mental health changed dramatically and led to major changes in policy.

In the past few decades, the progress of psychiatry has been impressive, with newer investigations and interventions such as transcranial magnetic stimulation, the development and use of newer antidepressants like psychostimulants, and the use of avatar therapy and AI. A better understanding of the impact of epigenetics, childhood attachment patterns, brain development, and genetic influences on pharmacodynamics is influencing therapeutic interventions.

Changes in the practice of psychiatry related to biological discoveries, social changes resulting from globalization and rapid urbanization, and the advent and rapid spread of social media mean that this contract needs an urgent review. This contract is at the heart of the design, development, and delivery of psychiatric services. These developments occur in both the investigation and the management of psychiatric conditions; inevitably, they will contribute to increasing costs that will need to be considered in any social compact. This has led to Robertson and Walter (2011) highlighting the need for a clearer understanding of the values of psychiatrists as a professional group. Developments in clinical psychiatric practice over the last half century and ongoing show that psychiatry's imperative has changed, and this needs to be understood by the profession. These authors highlight that psychiatry's contract has failed when the "dual role dilemma" kicks in, which concerns the role of the psychiatrist as both a professional and a member of society. In the same way, the person with a mental disorder has the role of both a patient and a member of society. There is a tension in moral imperatives on both sides. This tension can be resolved in a pragmatic, open way.

A report by the British Medical Association (BMA, 2019) highlighted that the social contract approach can certainly be helpful in negotiating a variety of factors that affect the health care system. As mentioned above, this is an implicit "contract" with three interlocking societal components (see figure 2.1):

1. The government, employers, health care managers
2. Patients, patients' groups, and the public
3. The medical profession and its professional bodies (e.g., regulators, Royal Colleges)

It is important to acknowledge that social expectations are molded by how psychiatry behaves as a profession (Bhugra, 2011). Society's attitudes and expectations of the profession, alongside broader social attitudes, are likely to be influenced by several factors, including the individual's social, economic, and educational status, various geopolitical conditions, and prior experiences with health care system. Attitudes and expectations are also likely to be affected by funding available for services, which affects availability and accessibility of services. Psychiatry as a medical specialty deals with both the mind and the brain, as well as the relationship between the medical discipline and individuals with mental illness and their carers and families. This may well create a tension between the real role and the social expectations of that role, especially as psychiatrists often have the power of taking away patient's liberty and treating them against their will by force. Bhugra and Malik (2011b) point out that it is society that not

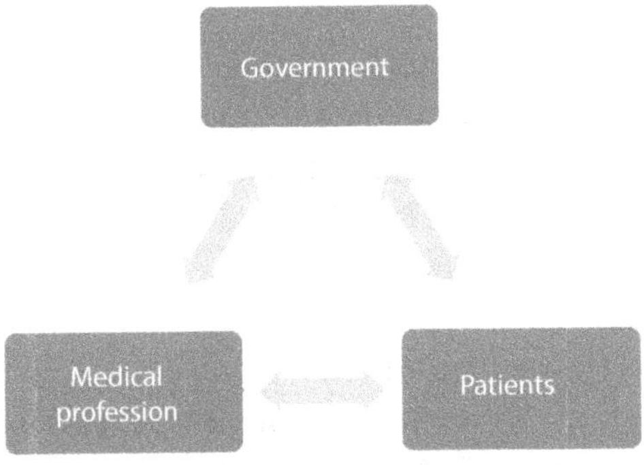

Figure 2.1
Three interlocking components of psychiatry's social contract.

only defines abnormal and deviant behaviors but also sickness roles and pathways into health care. Hence, there needs to be an ongoing dialogue so that simple deviant behavior is not turned into a sickness and medicalized.

Mental health clinical services may be separate from physical health facilities, but they are also an important part of society. Thus, the dialogue between society and psychiatrists (both as professionals and as citizens) takes on a different level of meaning. Patient expectations for health care and health professionals have changed. In many countries, doctors are not only seen as paternalistic but are expected to take charge, whereas in other countries, patients expect an equal say in their own treatment planning. In addition, the younger generation of patients are likely to be savvier with social media and may bring in information on their mobile apps that health care professionals may not be aware of. Challenges and changes in psychiatry continue to affect social and societal attitudes, which may well contribute to certain behaviors and changing expectations. Social structures need to be clearly understood by policymakers when building policy, but equally important is an understanding that these social mores are dynamic and fluid.

Primacy of patient welfare and advocacy for patients, as well as for caregivers, and eliminating social discrimination are the cornerstones of better services through better contracting and enhanced professionalism. As professionals, doctors need to possess up-to-date technical knowledge and competence

Education and Training

Training and education can be viewed from different levels: the first is the general population (i.e., public education, as discussed previously) and, for example, mental health and psychological first aid (see chapter 6); the second is the medical and health care professions; and the third is those working in the field of mental illness.

The Medical and Health Care Professions

The second level involves training all health professionals regarding the causation, identification, and fundamental understanding of mental illnesses. This may eliminate the artificial distinction between physical and mental health and encourage all health care workers to consider mental health and its disorders, regardless of their specialty and the settings in which they operate.

Every health care professional should receive basic training and opportunities for professional development, including those who do not act as gatekeepers to secondary or specialist services. While guidelines for diagnosing and treating common mental health issues are beneficial, the distribution of these guidelines should not be viewed as a replacement for ongoing developmental training for primary care doctors and staff. In many countries, it will be community health workers who are on the front line. Minimum competency criteria for mental health practitioners are proposed in appendix 2. World Psychiatric Association (WPA) guidance for training is outlined in appendix 3, along with roles and responsibilities for psychiatrists. WPA guidelines detailing the role of psychiatrists are also illustrated in appendix 3.

In many low- to middle-income countries, especially in South Asia, medical students receive only two weeks of psychiatry training in their fourth year, while the duration of postgraduate training varies from two to five months in Mongolia (Byambasuren & Tsetsegdary 2005) to seven years in the UK. Undergraduate students in Mongolia receive 80 hours of training in psychiatry and an additional 25 hours in child psychiatry, amounting to exactly 15 days. These disparities indicate that the profession has a moral responsibility to establish agreed-on standards for training and methods of delivery. Psychiatry and mental health education must commence at the beginning of the undergraduate course, enabling students to consider mental health aspects of illness, regardless of the specific illness or the settings and specialties in which they work. By incorporating medical humanities, particularly principles of anthropology and sociology, at an early stage, students will be better equipped to understand the societal role in relation to disease and illness. It is imperative that we examine and revise curricula and training accordingly.

In a similar vein, all nursing students should be taught the basic principles of psychopathology and the definitions of mental illness. Skill mix of nursing staff, whether they work in medical settings or psychiatric settings, must be judged at the levels of the local population's needs. Perhaps integrating medical, social work, psychology, and nursing training in the early stages of training, before going into specialist training, may help. Multidisciplinary training and learning should be encouraged.

Mental Health Professionals

The third level pertains to individual professions in health care. Core competencies for mental health workers, detailed in appendix 2, encompass four key areas: subject knowledge (and staying updated), attitudes and attributes, and skills for managing themselves and others. These competencies involve providing practical daily living skills to patients while being sensitive to cultural, religious, social, racial, and lifestyle variations, as well as recognizing individuals' physical, mental, spiritual, emotional, and psychological health needs. Interventions must be evidence-based, but individual patient needs take precedence. Mental health professionals should be aware of community resources and strive to demonstrate clinical competence, empathy, and flexibility while supporting individuals with mental illness and their families, particularly in uncertain situations.

Although there is a lot of common ground between psychology and psychiatry, in many countries, tensions between the two disciplines need to be resolved as a matter of urgency. The challenges to psychiatry from within itself also add to these tensions. There is no doubt that psychiatry as a profession has an imperative, but it is also a profession in transition. Embattled and bitter divisions within psychiatry, especially between social and biological psychiatry and increasingly bitter debates between anti-psychiatry psychiatry and psychiatrists, need to be resolved urgently. The profession must take this responsibility on so that appropriate training can be offered to the next generation.

Globally, training standards in many mental health disciplines vary dramatically. In many countries, postgraduate specialist training in psychiatry lasts two or three years, whereas in many other countries it is four years, and some require six years or longer after qualifying from medical school. This global variation in training brings with it major challenges in development and delivery of services, for a variety of reasons. First, as a result of globalization, psychiatrists may choose to move to better developed and more advanced countries for educational or financial advancement or may choose to migrate for political reasons. Psychiatry as a medical specialty is perhaps more strongly influenced by society's attitudes and the prevailing culture, in comparison with other medical specialties. Similarly, migration of nursing staff from one country to another will affect not only the service development of the new settings, but also that of other countries left behind. A commission jointly established by the WPA and the Asian

Journal of Psychiatry that examined psychiatric education has made recommendations, including a period of joint training across disciplines (Bhugra et al., 2023)

Conclusion

Doctors and often other mental health care professionals are interested in managing *diseases* as pathology (often following a mechanistic model), whereas patients are interested in managing *illness*, which is the impact of disease on their social relationships and functioning. For severe mental illness, these impacts may also include housing and occupation (which may encompass education as well as employment). Whether individuals have physical illnesses or mental illnesses or a mixture of the two, more often than not, they can manage to cope with their symptoms as long as they can function in social and personal spheres. They need reasonable accommodations, some kind of occupation whether it is employment or sheltered work, and some economic gains that can help them form, maintain, and deal with relationships. Therefore, in many cases, it is important for clinicians to move their focus away from symptom reduction. Hence, the outcomes need to be carefully identified and monitored during implementation of mental health services.

Policymakers have a moral and ethical duty to ensure that mentally ill people are looked after in an appropriate way, that services are accessible, and that the workforce is well trained. A significant number of countries do not have stand-alone policies on mental health. Furthermore, the resources allocated to psychiatric services are often inadequate, even in high-income countries. The increased mortality and suffering associated with mental illness makes it important and urgent to ensure that wherever possible, physical and mental health are looked after together. Closer working relationships between health and social care and between primary and secondary care can make patients' pathways into care easier.

3 Geopolitical and Social Determinants of Mental Health

Introduction

Social environments in which human beings are born, live, work, and play have a tremendous impact on the genesis and perpetuation of mental ill-health. Equally important, these factors play a vital role in physical and mental well-being. Furthermore, these social and cultural factors are intertwined with the way individuals experience illness, how they identify these experiences and respond, and where they seek help from. There is no doubt that individuals are part of a social fabric, and this two-way interaction affects their individual responses.

Several social factors can be identified that play an influential role in the causation of various mental illnesses. Although the etiology and treatment of psychiatric disorders looks at biopsychosocial models, some biological and psychological vulnerabilities can themselves be caused by social factors. Across the age span, social factors can determine health and well-being. From early adverse childhood experiences (ACEs), education, employment, poverty, inadequate or poor housing, the built environment, and food insecurity can contribute to poor physical and mental health and recovery. In addition, negative life experiences and chronic negative stressors such as discrimination can add to the development and sustenance of poor physical and mental health (Krieger, 2014). Social determinants can push people out of the main groups of society, and when they look in, they may feel hurt and inferior, contributing to low self-esteem and a sense of entrapment. This in turn may lead to alienation and the development of psychiatric disorders.

In this chapter, some of the research evidence on the role these factors play is discussed with explanations of geopolitical determinants. It is argued that there needs to be an international development of certain policies to ensure that political, commercial, geographical, and other determinants are recognized along with their impact on social determinants and that all of these matters are considered when developing mental health care policies and services.

Geopolitical determinants include political, geographical, commercial, economic, and cultural determinants in addition to factors that may be man-made, such as climate change, wars, and conflict, as well as natural disasters such as earthquakes, hurricanes, tsunamis, and so on. These may all lead to internal or external migration. Geopsychiatry is the emerging branch of psychiatry that aims to study determinants that influence social determinants, which in turn affect physical and mental health of individuals as well as total populations. Geopsychiatry aims to bring together geography, sociology, anthropology, political sciences, psychiatry, medicine, and other stakeholders to understand the impact of geopolitical determinants on health including mental health. Of these, geographical, political, and commercial determinants are being studied increasingly (Bhugra & Ventriglio, 2023a, 2023b, 2023c; McGeachan & Philo, 2024; Persaud & Ventriglio, 2023). In understanding the impact of social determinants, it is crucial to make sense of geographical factors as these influence various social factors.

Geographical Determinants

Geographical determinants focus, unsurprisingly, on geographic location. They include terrains, differences between rural and urban areas, and other factors such as levels of pollution.

Geography as a discipline looks at not only terrain but also environment and climate, which are influenced by geography. The discipline of health geography has been identified as being similar to medical geography as both subjects look at social models of health and wellness. These disciplines focus on health rather than disease or illness. As health geography also goes beyond traditional biomedical models looking at environment, it strengthens the psychiatric biopsychosocial model of etiology and interventions. Whereas medical or psychiatric models may look at bodily or brain dysfunction, medical or health geography focuses on health-related behaviors such as diet, drinking, smoking, and exercise with provisions of health care outside traditional settings (Moon, 2009).

Climate change is an emerging determinant of mental ill-health, with effects ranging from eco-anxiety to the psychological distress experienced by climate refugees. Forced migration due to environmental disasters increases the risk of post-traumatic stress disorder (PTSD), depression, and anxiety (Cunsolo & Ellis, 2018). Moreover, the concept of ecological grief, or mourning the loss of biodiversity and stable environments, has been identified as a growing mental health concern among affected populations (Albrecht, 2011).

Determinants of health go beyond genetics and include diet, education, employment, work environment, living conditions, clean water, sanitation, housing, and health care services, which to a degree influence individual and community health but are in turn influenced by geographical factors (see WHO, 2022 b). These geographical factors not surprisingly focus on cultures and thus also affect cultural values as well as socioeconomic and environment factors. Health geography highlights inequality and political ideologies, and certain psychiatric conditions are strongly influenced by environment (Moon, 2009). Although we are discussing geographic, political and commercial determinants separately they are strongly interlinked. Geographical determinants have a clear place awareness, that is, the physical place and space where people live, work, play and age, all of which are strongly influenced by cultures. Neighborhood factors affect pollution and the rates of smoking and drinking (Moon, 2009). Economic geography, too, has a role to play in mental health and well-being of individuals and communities. Living in iodine-deficient areas can cause high rates of myxedema, which can cause psychiatric problems.

Where we live affects our health and well-being (Elliott, 2014). Urban rural variations in rates of various psychiatric disorders have been identified for a considerable period. Faris and Dunham (1939), in one of the earliest studies, noted that rates of schizophrenia were higher in urban areas. They postulated that this may be a result of social drift. They considered the possibility that as people became more ill, they moved to cities perhaps for easier access to health care or to distance themselves from families because of stigma or other factors. Krabbendam and van Os (2005) noted that rural areas had lower rates of schizophrenia, which were attributable to better cognitive ability. This may also reflect social cohesion. Reid (2019) noted that rural health is strongly influenced by geography and topography. Lu et al. (2018) pointed out that air pollution is linked with criminal behavior, which is likely to be higher in urban areas. Zhang et al. (2018) found that sustained exposure to polluted air damages cognitive ability across the population, with the aging brain particularly vulnerable. In a large survey from India, Patnaik et al. (2023) reported that there were substantial variations in rates of ill-health that were associated with age, income, and also rurality. It is worth noting that these may be associations rather than direct causality. In a study of COVID-19 in four rural counties in Minnesota in the US, Wheeler et al. (2022) observed that there were community hot spots that had much higher rates of infections and appeared to be related to ethnicity and socioeconomic disparities, thereby suggesting that targeted interventions may be needed. Furthermore, medical care facilities are often largely congregated in urban areas, thus leading to delays in help-seeking for rural people, which may produce adverse outcomes.

Chen et al.'s (2020) overview suggests that geographical psychology examines the spatial distribution of psychological phenomena across various levels of geographical analysis. It is noted that characteristics of neighborhoods, cities, states, and countries are linked to diverse political, economic, social, public health, and other consequences, thus services and interventions must consider these factors. Rentfrow (2010) observed differences in rates of personality traits and clusters across different regions in the US. In a subsequent study, Rentfrow et al. (2013) examined a large US population sample and found that individuals with similar psychological profiles tended to cluster together geographically. It remains unclear whether people with similar traits gravitate toward each other or whether they develop these traits once together. Rentfrow et al. (2008) proposed a model to conceptualize how individual characteristics contribute to the clustering of people, with distinct personality profiles emerging in specific geographical areas. In a subsequent study, these authors (Rentfrow et al., 2015) replicated their findings in Great Britain, examining personality variations through the five-factor model: extraversion, agreeableness, conscientiousness, neuroticism, and openness. They found geographic patterns, with higher agreeableness in parts of Scotland and the north, southwest, and east of England. Extraversion was prominent in London, South and Southeast England, Yorkshire, Manchester, and some areas of Scotland, while conscientiousness was high in the south of England, the Midlands, and the Highlands of Scotland. Neuroticism clustered in Wales and parts of the Midlands. Similarly, Rentfrow et al. (2009) found that in the US, states with higher well-being levels correlated with wealth, education, tolerance, and emotional stability. The influence of geographical determinants on health (both physical and mental) merits further detailed investigation.

Cultural Determinants

As mentioned above, geographical variations may also be associated with cultural differences and cultural determinants, as well as political determinants. Emphasizing that cultures are not homogeneous, Vandello and Cohen (1999) found that within the US, individualism and collectivism varied and that state-level collectivism is related to low levels of alcohol abuse.

When cultures are divided into egocentric (individualistic) and sociocentric (collectivist) cultures, it is possible that behaviors change in response to cultural expectations. In collectivist settings, the focus is on the community, group, or tribe rather than the person. Interesting differences have been reported. For example, in sociocentric/collectivist cultures, rates of bribes are said to be higher (Mazar & Aggarwal, 2011). On the other hand, higher rates of happiness in individualistic cultures have been reported by Diener et al. (2003) but also higher rates of divorce, suicide, and crime. Interlinked factors such as loneliness and social isolation (discussed later in this chapter) and lack of social cohesion may affect rates of anxiety and mood disorders, which have been shown to be higher in egocentric cultures (see Maercker, 2001; Chiao & Blizinsky, 2010). Bleidorn et al. (2016) had observed that the self-esteem of individuals living in a city correlates with self-esteem of the city population, but again, cause and effect need teasing out here. Cultural perspectives on individualism and collectivism play a crucial role in shaping mental health care approaches. In collectivist cultures, communal support and family involvement are central to healing, while stigma toward mental illness remains prevalent, discouraging individuals from seeking professional help (Ahad et al., 2023; Kim et al., 2021). In contrast, individualistic societies prioritize self-reliance and personal agency, often with more positive attitudes toward seeking mental health care but potentially resulting in weaker communal support systems (Smith et al., 2018; Hofstede, 2001). These cultural orientations significantly influence treatment adherence and the effectiveness of mental health interventions, necessitating culturally tailored approaches to care (Triandis & Gelfand, 2012; Kirmayer & Ryder, 2018). It is important to note that these classifications emerged from the West, and knowledge of cultures in many parts of the world, including Africa, is not very clear.

Gelfand et al. (2011) differentiated cultures into tight and loose categories. Tight cultures are more likely to be autocratic and have stricter laws, and cultural tightness has been shown to be negatively correlated with happiness (Harrington & Gelfand, 2014). Similar findings have been reported from China (Chua et al., 2019). Moriarty et al. (2009) studied frequent mental distress (FMD) using data from the Centers for Disease Control (CDC) with a sample of 2.4 million people in the US. They found that the prevalence of FMD among adults overall was 9.4 percent. However, it ranged from a low of 6.4 percent in Hawaii to over twice that at 14.4 percent in Kentucky. There were intrastate variations, too. These authors noted that rates had increased by 1–4 percent in some states over the study period. They pointed out that these variations were related to a number of factors, including educational status, disability, employment, veteran status, marital status, chronic physical and mental illness, and levels of well-being. interpersonal abuse, smoking, and alcohol intake. They recommend that it is better to study the statewide picture rather than local levels because it is likely to give a better idea understanding that can then be incorporated into policies. Rates of FMD are said to be higher in excluded and vulnerable groups (see chapter 5) that may fare worse in collectivist cultures rather than individualistic ones. Understanding these geographical and cultural variations can help develop appropriate strategies for public mental health campaigns and service development.

Studies such as the International Pilot Study of Schizophrenia (Sartorius et al., 1974) and DOSMED (Jablensky et al., 1992) have shown clear countrywide variations in rates of schizophrenia and psychoses. However, as cultural and community-based variations were not explored either for etiology or outcomes, geographical and cultural variations could not be studied. From a policy perspective, it is crucial that geographical and cultural determinants are recognized so that appropriate services can be designed, developed and delivered. As geographical determinants are likely to be associated with cultures, it is important that the two are studied in association to understand the impact of these determinants on etiology, engagement, and outcomes.

Political Determinants

Political determinants of mental health have an impact on social factors such as poverty, poor housing, unemployment, lack of green spaces, poor public transport, and limited access to healthy food or good education. These are strongly influenced by government ideology, policies, and politics. These policies are also molded by the type of political system. If the general population is invested and engaged in the political processes, it may be easier to influence policy, whereas in autocratic societies, it may be more difficult, if not impossible. Depending on the electoral system, people vote for policies that are being put forward by a political party or individual. The elected representatives then deliver these promises and policies that may affect public mental health and population-level health.

In an interesting overview with a US perspective, Dawes (2020) highlights lessons that may be applicable to other societies. As mentioned earlier, the key principle in any policy must be equity between physical and mental health. Inevitably, in many societies, political systems do not value each group equally. Another point worth emphasizing is that politicians often do not have long-term vision because they concentrate on the next election and electoral cycle. This is particularly important for mental health as policymakers do not consider the impact of their policies on health at all, much less on mental health. Dawes (2020, pp. 41–42) reminds us that like many other high-income countries, the US has high rates of obesity, diabetes, high maternal and infant mortality, depression, opioid addiction, substance use disorders, and (especially the US) gun violence, which he attributes to a lack of political action. Similar lack of response to high rates of infections with HIV/AIDS was observed in many countries in Africa. Eisenberg-Guyot and Prins (2022) observe that in the US, between 2000 and 2017, rates of drug poisoning went up by 44 percent, alcohol poisoning by 40 percent, and suicide by 35 percent. They cite Marx (1990), who described capitalism as a socioeconomic system where the focus is on the means of production, and because the system is in private hands, the emphasis is on resulting profits. Thus, this emphasis on work, life, and play often tends to ignore individual welfare, working conditions, and the environment (further discussed in the chapter 9 on mental health in the workplace). Political determinants of health involve systematic processes of structuring relationships, distribution of resources, and how and where power is held and administered. These then shape opportunities that may advance health equity or exacerbate health inequities (Dawes, 2020). These opportunities are used by large corporations to lobby governments and parties in power to maximize their profits, often at the expense of health and well-being of workers and populations.

As described in chapter 2, a social contract, social compact, or social covenant carries with it certain mutual expectations. Through political alliances, a power nexus may develop that then goes on to influence people's lives and their working conditions directly and indirectly. Political determinants will influence social determinants in various ways. Political ideologies shape funding for education, employment, health, and social care. Health disparities and health inequity are direct outcomes of political ideologies and their associated determinants. It is recognized that sociopolitical factors affect both population and individual health and well-being, with Yang and Mak (2020) arguing that the longitudinal impact of sociopolitical values and political ideologies deserves further detailed study. In a follow-up study, X. Yang et al. (2020) observed that social political factors can negatively affect people's mental health. Following political unrest in Hong Kong, these authors conducted a telephone survey and observed that nearly three-quarters of their sample (71 percent) were pessimistic, and 11.3 percent could be classified as having possible depression. Thus, it appears that wider sociopolitical factors will influence current mental state but also have an impact on long-term well-being.

Related to discrimination, factors such as a recent rise in populism and political polarization in many countries have significant mental health implications, particularly by exacerbating social stress and anxiety. Political instability leads to uncertainty and chronic stress, affecting mental resilience (Levitsky & Ziblatt, 2018). Additionally, misinformation on health issues, including COVID-19, has led to widespread health anxiety and distrust in mental health services (Freeman et al., 2022) as well as governments. In the US, following the presidential election of 2016, a national survey conducted by the American Psychological Association reported that 69 percent of Blacks, 57 percent of Asians, 56 percent of Latinx, and 42 percent of non-Hispanic whites reported that the outcome of the 2016 presidential election was a "very significant" or "somewhat significant" source of stress (American Psychological Association, 2017). After that same election, the number of preterm births among Latinas increased between 3.2–3.6 percent (Gemmill et al., 2019), and there was a notable reported increase in hate crimes and harassment (BBC, 2016).

In a review of reviews, McCartney et al. (2019) emphasize that politics, economics, and public policy are important determinants of public health. They point out that countries with social democracy welfare, countries that focus on public health, and those with lower-income inequalities have better self-rated health in their population. It is thus possible that happiness levels and life satisfaction are higher in these countries. They remind policymakers that interrelationship between governance, politics, power, macroeconomic policy, public policy, and population health are important and should be considered while developing policy.

In the context of mental health, political ideology influences detention of patients and compulsory treatment. The Basaglia reforms in Italy in the latter half of last century at the behest of policymakers led to closure of psychiatric asylums with patients moving into community (Badano, 2024). Thus, political ideologies dictate the structures and funding of health care systems and clinicians, and researchers must be aware of these influences.

Commercial Determinants

Political determinants are often intertwined with commercial determinants by the lobbying and tax revenue power of big businesses. In many countries, multinational corporations (MNCs) not only tend to have a bigger say, in overt and covert ways, in the politics of a country but often their turnover can exceed gross domestic product of many countries. MNCs are in the business of making money for their owners and shareholders and delivering profits. However, by virtue of their size and geographical spread, they can influence the policies of governments in many ways using direct and indirect means.

Kickbusch et al. (2016) defined commercial determinants of health (CDoH) as the strategies and approaches used by the private sector to promote products and choices that are detrimental to health. WHO (2022b) defines CDoH as various private-sector activities that have an impact on public health. These can be either positive or negative influences, which in turn can work on political or economic systems and norms. These influences are obtained through various market strategies, working conditions and production. In order to maximize their profits, these MNCs are likely to indulge in direct and indirect political activities. In addition to lobbying and making donations to parties in power, these corporations may withhold information or share partial selective information that makes them look better. In some settings, these companies may develop and use instrumental, structural, and discursive power to undermine public health policies that threaten their profits. This was seen in Scotland a few years ago, in response to government policy on alcohol pricing, distilleries got together and took the government to court. Multinational corporations influence policies that may further contribute to inequalities within and across countries. WHO (2022b) has observed that MNCs indulge in "profit shifting," and the aggressive use of trade agreements by the unhealthy commodity industries are particularly detrimental to the Global South. Anaf et al. (2023) recommend that a corporate health impact assessment framework (which includes global economic, political, and regulatory contexts in which MNCs work) should be used to explore and understand the structures, products, and operating policies of MNCs, which then go on to affect daily living conditions.

MNCs significantly influence regulatory frameworks and trade agreements, impacting governmental decision-making. Their role in society's physical health is well documented, while their effect on mental health, both direct and indirect, warrants attention. For instance, the gambling and alcohol industries directly affect mental health, while unhealthy food products contribute to obesity and related physical conditions that can lead to depression. The King's Fund (Holmes, 2021) and UK Department of Health and Social Care (DHSC, 2020) report that over a quarter of Great Britain's population is obese, with the National Health Service (NHS) spending on diabetes projected to rise from £9.8 billion to £16.9 billion by 2035 (Hex at al., 2012). Nestle, the world's largest food company, was noted by Share Action for having 40 percent of its UK food sales high in salt, sugar, or fat (BBC, 2023).

The tobacco industry has often resisted regulation, and with increased pressures in the West, the industry started targeting countries like China and India that are relatively economically poor but aspire to Western standards (also see WHO, 2021d). The link between smoking and cancer was established in the 1950s, yet it took decades to regulate sales. Knai and

Savona (2023) highlight that to address public health concerns that could threaten profits, these companies invest heavily in strategies to promote their interests, defining the commercial determinants of health.

Physical and mental well-being are influenced by CDoH in both subtle and direct ways. Advertising by the food, drink, and gambling industries affects our health significantly. Fast-food marketing presents unhealthy options as smart and convenient choices. In a personal observation in India over two different days and different times, the author noted that a youth music channel had 14-minute advertising breaks featuring almost 40 ads each time. Over 95 percent showcased young, attractive characters, often Bollywood stars or well-known cricketers. Almost half of the ads promoted fizzy drinks, energy drinks, or fast food. Although alcohol advertising is banned on Indian TV, a beer brand promoted nonalcoholic beer, while others employed soft drink strategies to connect with alcohol, indicating that MNCs can bypass certain rules. In addition, MNCs often donate large amounts of money to policymakers both directly and indirectly through lobbying.

Digital Platforms

The commercialization of digital platforms has been a mixed blessing. While access to information at low cost has improved, information quality is highly variable. Not everyone has access to smartphones or the internet, and low-income countries have poorer internet coverage than richer countries. Such digital divides disproportionately affect lower-income students, leading to further educational disparities (Pierce & Cleary, 2024). Conversely, excessive social media use has been linked to negative mental health outcomes, including increased risks of depression, anxiety, and feelings of loneliness and isolation. Adolescents spending more than three hours daily on digital platforms are particularly vulnerable (Keles et al., 2020; Twenge & Campbell, 2018). Psychological effects include the fear of missing out (FOMO), which fuels anxiety and compulsive behaviors (Baker et al., 2016), cyberbullying that elevates depression and anxiety among victims (Kowalski et al., 2014), and body image issues stemming from exposure to idealized images, often leading to low self-esteem and potentially to disordered eating (Fardouly & Vartanian, 2016). Additionally, excessive screen time has been associated with poor sleep hygiene and lower academic performance (Hale & Guan, 2015).

Additionally, disrupted sleep patterns caused by late-night social media engagement particularly in younger users may exacerbate these mental health struggles, highlighting the complex and often detrimental impact of social media on overall well-being (Levenson et al., 2017). Social media "addiction," while not yet a recognized psychiatric disorder, further compounds these challenges, as users become reliant on validation from likes and comments on their postings, triggering anxiety when it is absent (Pallesen et al., 2012).

Similarly, online gambling, facilitated by the ease of digital access, has heightened risks for compulsive gambling disorders in vulnerable users, particularly younger populations (Gainsbury et al., 2015). Tompson et al. (2022) have emphasized how rates of online gambling are on the rise while the impact of commercial determinants on mental health often goes unrecognized. In the UK, increasing number of charities are resorting to running their own lotteries in order to raise funds, thus increasing the potential of addiction.

Other Global Forces

In addition to the impact on consumers, the effects on workers and their working conditions must also be considered. A factory that manufactures products or consumables can create pollution and other hazardous environmental and working conditions that contribute to the ill-health of workers and possibly their families, too. In an ever-shrinking globalized world, many factories are set up in low-income countries with poor working conditions and weak pollution regulations, so the health of workers is often also a low priority.

The transport of raw materials and finished products from one part of the world to another further contributes to pollution and climate change. The transport and storage of goods may well require police and political protection, thereby adding a further layer of corruption. Macro, meso, and micro factors contribute to pressures faced by workers as well as neighborhoods.

At a macro level, de Lacy-Vawdon and Livingstone (2020) suggest that the dynamics of CDoH are linked to globalization, with corporate structures, neoliberal trade policies, capitalism, and marketing contributing to global health issues. Globalization also increases job insecurity and financial instability, leading to stress and anxiety (Colantone et al., 2019).

Lacy-Nichols et al. (2023b) identify market, political, scientific, employment, and financial factors as influential in commercial determinants of health. At the meso level, production conditions affect worker health, while at the micro level, these determinants shape consumer purchasing power. The concept of unhealthy commodity industries, defined by Knai and Savona (2023), emphasizes the production and marketing of unhealthy goods and their political strategies. The influence of MNCs on public health policy is evident through lobbying and political donations and the complex impact on policymaking. Chronic physical conditions are often linked to psychiatric illnesses, necessitating integrated treatment approaches.

From a public mental health perspective, it is crucial that clinicians, researchers, and policymakers understand both the direct and indirect impact of the commercial activities of MNCs on mental health of individuals and their families. The systems-thinking framework of Meadows (2008) provides public health professionals with tools to identify patterns, understand dynamic relationships, and implement interventions that produce sustainable improvements in population health. Meadows focuses on leverage points where lasting impact can be achieved, such as offering clear overviews in addition to detailed, small-print labels to describe the contents of food packets. It is critical that people are given the right information early on and that examples of good practice are shared widely so that they can make their own informed choices. In Chile, for example, ultra-processed foods are marked with a symbol so they are easy to spot.

Lacy-Nichols et al. (2023a) argue that CDoH must include the complexity and complicity of commercial actors contributing to health outcomes by looking at the overall prevalence and development of health inequalities. Casswell (2023) proposes a policy agenda that includes understanding and acknowledging the impact of commercial determinants on each policy affecting health, including mental health.

Clinicians and researchers should become aware of which unhealthy MNC products their patients are exposed to in order to advocate for them, particularly at public health levels. The interaction of commercial and social determinants is intricate. By collaborating across disciplines with colleagues from diverse backgrounds, mental health professionals need to explore, understand, and respond to the impact of these determinants. Managing tobacco control serves as an excellent example of a public health approach in numerous countries. Similarly, alcohol pricing represents another potential solution, as does increasing taxes on gambling organizations.

Social Determinants of General Health

It is widely acknowledged that the social determinants of health are the circumstances in which people are born, grow, work, age, and die (Marmot, 2010; WHO 2008a). These factors and conditions can significantly affect families, relationships, and communities, which can ultimately lead to inadequate support, further isolating individuals. Poverty, unemployment, substandard living conditions, low educational attainment, and various social and physical environments affect mental health and well-being. Although health care professionals may not have control over social determinants and their assessment, they can effect change by advocating for policies that consider how they impact health, particularly mental health. Collaborating with and educating policymakers is a vital strategy for health care professionals acting as advocates. The artificial dichotomy between physical and mental health—perhaps stemming from Descartes and the Cartesian mind-body dualism—has inflicted substantial unintentional harm on the well-being of populations in numerous countries. As mentioned earlier, individuals with mental illnesses are likely to have shorter lifespans, while those with chronic physical illnesses are more susceptible to developing psychiatric disorders. Managing complex comorbidities poses significant challenges. In this context, prevention is indeed the best cure.

Social determinants are regarded as complex circumstances that include intangible factors such as political, socioeconomic, and cultural constructs, alongside various place-based and individual-based conditions (NEJM Catalyst 2017). These circumstances are inevitably shaped by the distribution of money, power, and resources at global, national, and local levels (WHO, 2008a). Such conditions can lead to stratification or the creation of a "caste" system, resulting in health inequities among different populations, which may arise from factors such as gender, wealth, ethnicity, and sexual orientation. In certain contexts, belonging to a specific religious affiliation or group can also contribute to health inequality. Examples of social determinants are illustrated in box 3.1.

Box 3.1
Some of the Social Determinants of Health

- Age
- Gender
- Ethnicity
- Migrant status
- Religious affiliations
- Sexual orientation
- Early childhood adverse experiences
- Education
- Insecure employment
- Unemployment
- Poverty
- Lack of or inadequate/poor housing
- Lack of access to affordable transport
- Lack of access to green spaces
- Access to clean water/clean air
- Recreational activities limited
- Food insecurity

Social determinants must form a crucial part of assessment and management of ill-health. The COVID-19 pandemic has shown, if indeed any evidence was required, that ethnic and racial minorities in high-income countries have been disproportionately affected, while in low- and middle-income countries, often poor urban migrants have suffered (Abrams & Szefler, 2020). These determinants also influence access to health care and quality of care if equitable services are not available. Within the social, community, and cultural context, these determinants also affect access to education and quality of education. Biological and genetic factors, healthy behaviors, and physical environment are all important aspects of social determinants. From Japan, comparing county-level data from across the country, Kataoka et al. (2021) found that life expectancy and healthy life expectancy were lower as the deprivation index worsened. Braveman and Gottlieb (2014) emphasize that, in addition, health-related features of neighborhoods—for instance, safe spaces, green spaces, ease of accessibility for walking, a nutritious and affordable diet, and recreational areas—can be influential in health-related behavior. Medical care often focuses on curing diseases and illnesses after they have set in, whereas perhaps more emphasis needs to be paid to preventive and public health measures including mental health. Marmot (2015) has illustrated differences in longevity based on socioeconomic status. Social and environmental influences are said to contribute 45–60 percent of variations in health status (Donkin et al., 2018). Shim et al. (2015) point out that social determinants can often be dealt with at the population level whereas medicine focuses on individuals. Others note that mental illnesses are highly prevalent, affecting nearly half the US population (Kessler et al., 2005). Associated epidemics of drug dependence, gun violence, pollution, and road traffic accidents further contribute to changing circumstances and poor mental health.

Addressing inequalities in the social determinants of health is vital for public health strategy. Managing individual illnesses amid technological advancements necessitates multilevel policy development, as shown in figure 3.1. Access to health care is determined by social and cultural factors that shape health care systems and individual pathways to care, which are also influenced by urban and rural settings. Many of these factors can adapt to changes in policy. Funding and resources hinge on health care policy and its consideration of population health needs, creating a complex system. It is essential for all policies to include health impact assessments, but as mentioned earlier, it is particularly important for mental health. Doctors must collaborate as advocates and policymakers to address health inequalities. Health care professionals may need training to effectively contribute to policy. The effects of social inequalities are significant for the physical and mental health of individuals and communities.

The impact of these determinants at various levels can be extremely complex. Some individuals, with their early childhood adverse experiences, may cope with subsequent stressors whereas others may not manage it. Thus, it is important to explore the impact of various factors both cross-sectionally and longitudinally with specific hypotheses explored.

Social Determinants of Mental Health

Social determinants for mental health are not dissimilar from those of physical health. Mental illnesses are complex entities with multiple causative

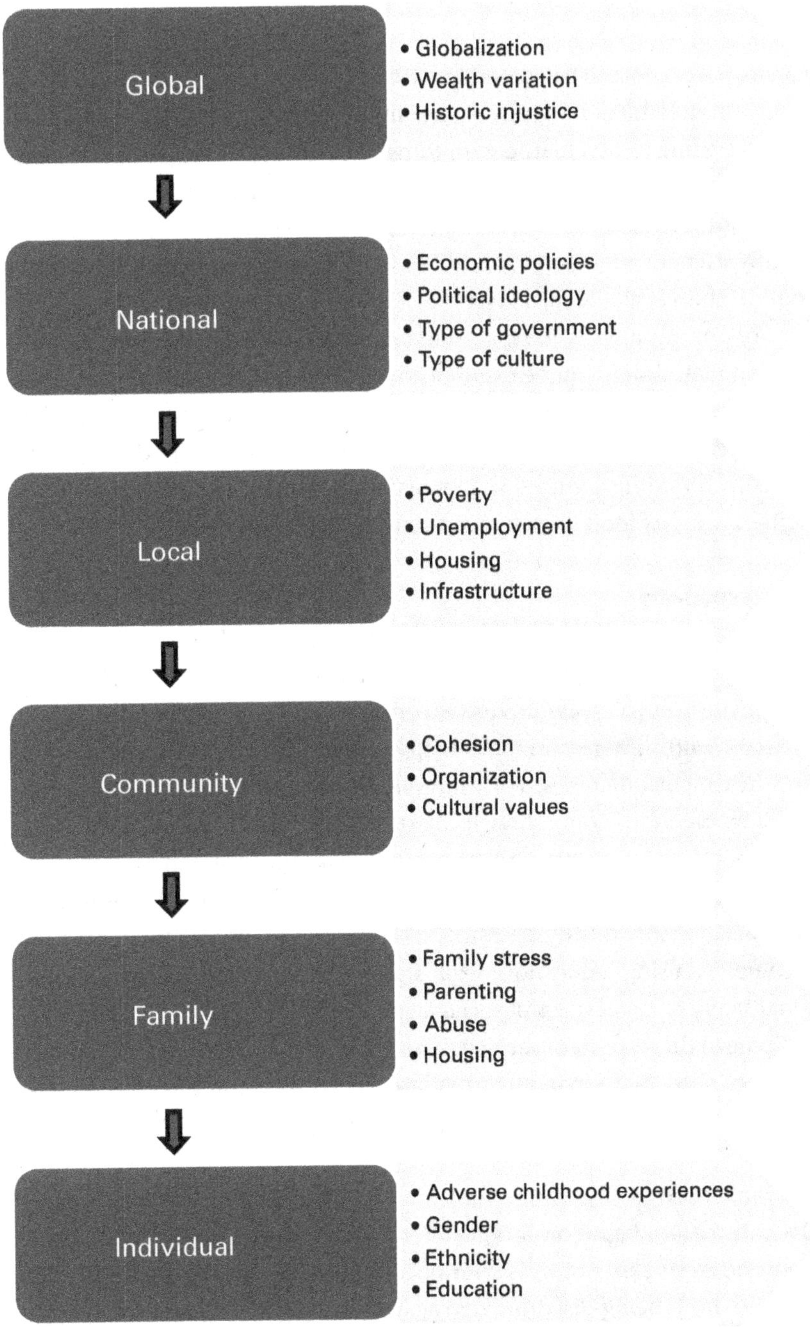

Figure 3.1
The social determinants of health, from the global to the individual level.

factors. They can also be comorbid with other mental or physical conditions, some through the same pathway (e.g., myxedema caused by local iodine deficiency leading to psychiatric symptoms). Physical illnesses can affect mental well-being and contribute to mental illnesses (e.g., diabetes and depression). Under these situations, both conditions need to be treated properly and thoroughly. Genetic vulnerability and the role of epigenetics must not be overlooked. Shim et al. (2015) add a note of caution, emphasizing that within the network of causative factors, personal choices and behaviors, such as smoking and diet, should not be overlooked. They also highlight that the notions of social determinants are not recent and have been recognized for a considerable period. Complex interactions between poverty, poor education, and difficulty affording a nutritious diet may push vulnerable individuals toward high-calorie fast food, thereby contributing to obesity.

Intersectionality

Intersectionality, a term coined by Crenshaw (1989), highlights how multiple social identities such as race, gender, disability, and socioeconomic status intersect to create unique experiences of oppression or privilege. In mental health, intersectionality helps explain disparities in access to care and treatment outcomes. For example, Bowleg (2012) demonstrated that Black women face compounded mental health risks because of the simultaneous effects of racism and sexism, necessitating tailored interventions. Kenyan et al. (2007) recommended the use of acronym I-HELP to ascertain social history during assessments—referring to income (including food income); housing, education, legal status (if indicated); literacy; and personal safety at domestic and social levels.

Some of the important social determinants are described below. Although they are described separately, they are interlinked and affect each other. Their cumulative effects may prove devastating.

Discrimination

Discrimination, based on race, gender, religious affiliation, sexual orientation and even skin color, is common around the world. As a result, the person who is being discriminated against is likely to feel inferior, may feel trapped, and could develop depression. Underlying reasons for discriminatory behaviors are related to identity and the creation of "otherness" (Bhugra et al., 2022; see also chapter 4).

Minority Ethnic Status and Discrimination

Studies from the UK (Pinto et al., 2008; Office for National Statistics [ONS], 2017) and elsewhere have shown that rates of schizophrenia among African Caribbean individuals and other ethnic minority groups are between 2 and 14 times higher than the local population; this has been a consistent finding in the past six decades or so. People of ethnic minorities living in communities with high levels of racial prejudice are at an elevated risk of mortality (Chae et al., 2015; Lee et al., 2015; Leitner et al., 2016). Prejudice, discrimination, and social exclusion do contribute to poor physical and mental health (Rafferty et al., 2015). These authors highlight that the psychological and physiological stress mechanisms are similar no matter the cause of the discrimination.

Discrimination is associated with high rates of various psychiatric illnesses and with poorer outcomes (also see chapter 4 on stigma, discrimination, and human rights). But what is even more intriguing is that the *perception* of discrimination is more problematic than discrimination itself (Berg et al., 2011; Pearce et al., 2019; Stickley et al., 2019), which can lead to delayed help-seeking, poor therapeutic alliance, and chronicity of symptoms. Rafferty et al. (2015) note that chronic stress can contribute to the lifetime prevalence of mood and depressive disorders across all racial and ethnic groups. One discrimination experience is sufficient, they note, in making individuals experience symptoms of anxiety. Among Black individuals, experiences of discrimination lead to higher reported rates of depression and mood and anxiety disorders. The impact of discrimination on mental health and well-being may not be explored or discussed in clinical settings. Heterogeneity of groups and experiences, as well as responses to discrimination, must be acknowledged. Minority individuals with mental illness may experience double jeopardy.

Similar discriminatory experience are reported by lesbian, gay, bisexual, transgender, queer (LGBTQ+) individuals who also show higher rates of anxiety, depression, suicidal ideation, and suicidal acts (Gilmour, 2019; Ross et al., 2018; Meyer et al., 2007; Russell & Fish, 2016; Figueiredo & Abreu, 2020). Prejudice and social stress play a major role in contributing to the rates of psychiatric disorders in LGBTQ+ populations (Meyer, 2003). Social isolation, lack of connectedness, and policy/environment influence the rates of depression in LGBTQ+ youth (Wilson & Cariola, 2020). McLaughlin et al. (2010) found that Black respondents in their group reported the highest levels of past discrimination followed by LGBTQ+individuals, thereby contributing to anxiety and depression. This may lead to double jeopardy for Black LGBTQ+individuals. However, once equality in law is established, these rates of psychiatric disorders start to drop (Hatzenbuehler et al., 2009, 2010, 2012, 2016). Thus, equity and equality in law can lead to better acceptance, possible lower prejudice, and certainly improved self-esteem and self-image, thereby making vulnerable individuals feel valued. There is a difference between equity and equality, and for funding, research, clinical services, and law, equity is of prime importance. Multilevel stigma needs to be understood, and research and appropriate policies at the national, state, or local levels may be necessary to tackle discrimination so that individuals' mental health and well-being, along with functioning, can be improved.

Adverse Childhood Experiences

Adverse childhood experiences (ACEs) include maltreatment; emotional, physical, or sexual abuse; labor; prejudice; bereavement; and adult responsibility such as being a carer for an adult. ACEs are defined as highly stressful, traumatic, and acute or ongoing traumatic events that affect the individual. Domestic circumstances such as violence, alcohol, substance misuse, poverty, unemployment, and chronic long-term conditions can all contribute to these adverse experiences. ACEs may occur at familial, social, community, and personal levels. About 16 percent of adults report having experienced two to three ACEs, and almost 10 percent experience four or more (Kelly-Irving et al., 2013). There is evidence that a cumulative effect may be seen and cause worse outcomes (Geoffroy et al., 2014; Bellis et al., 2014a, 2014b; 2015). These childhood adverse experiences—reported as adverse early life experiences (AELEs) in the US literature with similar pathologies—can have a significant impact on individuals during their lifespan, affecting both physical health and mental health (Bellis et al., 2014). However, it needs to be recognized that not everyone experiencing the same ACEs will report similar resulting symptoms.

ACEs have been strongly linked to an increased risk of psychiatric disorders in adulthood. Longitudinal studies show that individuals with multiple ACEs are at significantly higher risk for depression, post-traumatic stress disorder (PTSD), and substance use disorders (Felitti et al., 1998). Neuroscience research indicates that early trauma alters brain development, particularly in regions responsible for emotional regulation (Teicher & Samson, 2016). Anda et al. (1999, 2006) reported an association between ACEs and smoking and neurobiological changes affecting patterns of smoking, whether associated with physical abuse or emotional abuse. Bellis et al. (2014a; 2014b) found that four or more ACEs predicted elevated odds of health-harming behaviors including smoking, perpetrating violence, and unintended teenage pregnancy. Koplan and Chard (2015) see AELEs as a mixture of circumstances such as hunger, poverty, inequality, and discrimination, but perhaps more importantly, interactions with adults who are supposed to be their caretakers whether at home, school, or communities. They see these experiences as inconsistent, stressful, threatening, traumatic, or neglectful experiences in utero, infancy, childhood, or young adults. The CDC (CDC, 2024a) indicates that ACEs cause social, emotional, and cognitive impairment, contributing to maladaptive health behaviors and leading to physical and mental ill-health, with premature death a potential consequence. Those experiencing six or more ACEs have a shorter lifespan (Brown et al., 2009). The impact of COVID-19 pandemic on children and young people leading to poor socialization, isolation, and quarantine can be seen as an adverse experience, and it will be interesting to do long-term follow-up studies to ascertain how it affects their development.

Traumatic experiences act as chronic stressors and can increase levels of depression, alcohol use, and substance use (Anda et al., 2002). In a meta-analysis, Norman et al. (2012) reported that physical and emotional abuse and neglect are all significantly associated with a range of poor mental health outcomes. They also reported that there is a close response relationship between adverse experiences and mental health outcomes.

Maternal stress and maternal behaviors such as drinking or substance use during pregnancy, along with other factors, can lead to alterations in a fetus's stress response system (Huizink et al., 2004) and cause preterm birth, low birth weight, and smaller head size at birth (Lou et al., 1994; Cooper et al., 1996), which may lead to cognitive impairment (Gale et al., 2006). As mentioned above, political factors can lead to early birth with potential accompanying stressors and potential long-term consequences, which are likely to influence structural development of brain and eventual functioning.

Adverse early life experiences can also occur in schools; bullying and discrimination are prime examples. Bullying can lead to self-harming behaviors (Arseneault et al., 2006), generalized anxiety disorders (Sourander et al., 2007), and suicide (Brunstein Klomek et al., 2010). As the body-brain stress response develops due to adverse experiences, epigenomes can lead to structural and functional changes. Koplan and Chard (2015, p. 63) point out that some of these changes are reversible, and positive relationships can reduce toxic stress caused by adverse experiences and thereby lowering the risk of long-term poor mental health and mental disorders.

Thus, early recognition of ACEs, interventions through education, suitably trained caregivers, and support for families to reduce violence and drug and alcohol use are all essential. To realize those objectives, policy changes in support of prevention, assessment, early intervention, and the provision of safe, stable, and nurturing environments are required.

Education

Education at all levels of one's life is crucial. Education not only improves one's life chances but also makes it easier to make friends and access peer support. It improves the chances of finding gainful employment as well as better job prospects. Beginning with pre-nursery education, which can start at home, all the way to grade school, high school, university, and continuing education, individuals gain skills to cope, manage life stresses, and in turn nurture others. Learning alongside others can help a person feel like they belong, and these social interactions can help them grow. These feelings of belonging can be reinforced in school settings (Powers, 2015). In addition, to academic achievements and qualifications, the individual can learn certain psychological, social, and communication skills, forming supportive relationships, regulating emotions, and learning about social rules, norms, and values.

Educational attainment influences physical and mental health and wellbeing. As Powers (2015) emphasizes, literacy can help emotional literacy. Rates of smoking, obesity, cardiovascular disease, asthma, cervical cancer, depression, and mortality are all higher in those of the lowest levels of education and income (Freudenberg & Ruglis, 2007; Adler & Rehkopf, 2008). Galea et al. (2011) reported that six factors contributed to mortality rates: low education, low social support, poverty, income inequality, racial segregation, and area-level poverty. It can be argued that all these factors are interrelated, but further work is needed to explore the directionality of causes. Lower levels of education are certainly affected by poverty and poor housing as well as the home environment. School environments in poor areas often have very high teacher/student ratios, affecting teachers' capacity to give sufficient attention to those who need it. Poor grades can then add to a poor sense of self-achievement or self-esteem. High-quality preschool programs for young children living in poverty can promote cognitive and social development in childhood. Consequently, this can unsurprisingly improve economic attainment in adulthood with a reduction in criminal activities (Powers, 2015; Schweinhart et al., 2005).

Education is a key social determinant and one where policy and adequate resources can make a tremendous difference. Clinical staff must be explore this connection and be encouraged to work with schools, teachers, and educational bodies to emphasize the importance of education and to reduce bullying. This also highlights the need to view health not in isolation but as interconnected with well-being. School mental health is covered in detail in chapter 8.

Employment

Unemployment or insecure employment can add stress to a person as these possibilities may not allow enough financial renumeration. Precarious employment, including reliance on short-term contracts, is a growing source of mental health stress. Job insecurity is strongly linked to heightened anxiety and depression rates (De Witte et al., 2016). The rapidly growing "gig economy," while providing flexibility, often lacks stability and employee rights, leading to financial and psychological stress (Muntaner, 2018). Poor educational attainment may lead to insecure employment, daily wages, zero-hour contracts, and uncertainty. Furthermore, long-standing unemployment can contribute to low self-esteem. The work environment contributes to a sense of purpose, belonging, and peer support. However, in high-pressure environments, individuals may feel increased stress, experience burnout (see chapter 9 on mental health in the workplace), or turn to alcohol and substances.

The longer someone is unemployed, the more likely they are to think about suicide (Classen & Dunn, 2012). Unemployment and job insecurity affect society; the social and cultural factors and micro-level internal stressors lead to poor self-esteem, hopelessness, psychosocial problems, and personal insecurities (McGregor & Holden, 2015). Clinicians will often inquire about job status, but they need to explore the quality of employment and job satisfaction. In some cases, social prescribing (see chapter 12) and social scaffolding may provide additional support and training to help people into employment.

Employment is one of the fundamental human rights, and this is where policies can make a huge difference. Job creation schemes and support for retraining, learning, and secure employment can be set at various policy levels. Work needs molding to people's skills and needs. As McGregor and Holden (2015) note, it behooves mental health providers to engage patients in discussions about employment-related issues. As advocates for their patients, they can attempt to influence policymakers so that suitable policies are framed. It is worth recognizing that unemployed people have high rates of mental illnesses, but those with mental illnesses are also likely to become unemployed.

Poverty

Poverty can be absolute or relative, and within the same community, there can be different levels of deprivation and poverty. Measurement of absolute and relative poverty can be problematic in some settings. Communities and geographical areas living in poverty are probably relatively easy to measure. Poverty also functions as a proxy measure for deprivation of material goods. It is observed that the world's 2,153 billionaires have more wealth than 4.6 billion people who make up 60 percent of the planet's population (Lawson et al., 2020). In this report for Oxfam, the authors observe that the 22 richest men in the world have more wealth than all the women in Africa. Thus, gender-based poverty needs further attention.

Economic inequality has been consistently linked to poorer mental health outcomes, with studies showing that countries with higher income inequality experience greater rates of depression and anxiety (Wilkinson & Pickett, 2006, 2009). Case studies from the UK and the US demonstrate how financial precarity is associated with increased psychological distress and reduced access to mental health services (Richardson et al., 2013; Ryu & Fan, 2023).

Like other social determinants, rates of various psychiatric disorders can be higher in individuals living in poverty, and those with mental illnesses may drift into poverty, thus creating a vicious cycle. Rural and urban poverty may differ. Rural poverty can be associated with increased substance use and limited opportunities for employment (Simmons et al., 2008, Smokowski et al., 2013). Manseau (2015) goes on to draw a distinction between social causation and social selection. Like all other social determinants, economic factors also work at different levels. Economic inequality can influence wealth in the same way education does. Poverty and neighborhood deprivation can contribute to family stress, domestic violence, and increased substance misuse (Evans & Kim, 2013). Lower household incomes show high rates of suicidal behaviors (Kingston 2013; Sareen et al., 2011). Poverty increases rates of anxiety, depression, psychological distress, and cognitive depletion (Sareen et al., 2011; Mani et al., 2013).

Manseau (2015) identifies that factors influencing the link between poverty and mental health exist at both the individual and family levels. Variables such as marital stress, parental traits, emotional deprivation, and neighborhood poverty further affect this relationship. Social security benefits can hinder social interactions and cognitive development, particularly in children and youth. Areas with concentrated poverty, like favelas and slums, are especially harmful to children's mental health. Wahlbeck et al. (2017) note that evidence on the mental health effects of policy interventions is limited and advocate for a cross-sectoral approach. Clinicians should recognize how poverty can affect nutrition, leading to malnutrition and stunted growth. Addressing poverty challenges often extends beyond clinical settings and requires policy-level action. Lawson et al. (2020) argue that requiring the wealthiest 1 percent to pay an additional 0.5 percent tax over the next decade could fund 117 million jobs in education, childcare, elderly care, and health care, benefiting women and girls. However, do governments and international organizations have the courage to act?

Food Insecurity

Nutrition is a complex, multilayered construct that must take quality, quantity, and access to food into account. Apart from the issue of affordability, poverty, access, and availability all play a role. Poor education may lead to unemployment, which contributes to poverty and results in food insecurity. In England alone, 1.3 million children reportedly rely on free school meals, and in the middle of the COVID-19 pandemic, the UK government stopped these meals because schools were closed—although the government subsequently relented as a result of a campaign led by a soccer player. The Food Foundation (2020) estimated that another 900,000 children in the UK registered in the new term. Over a quarter (29 percent) of children between the ages of 8 and 17 are registered for free school meals.

Even when families can afford meals, the increasing cost of fresh vegetables and fruit can begin to make it unaffordable. Hence, individuals from certain groups and families tend to rely on calorie-dense fast (ultra-processed) food, which can then lead to obesity and, consequently, physical conditions such as diabetes. Uncertainty about where their food comes from and when is defined as food insecurity (Compton, 2015). Food insecurity is likely to lead to malnutrition, especially for young children and adolescents whose brains are still developing. Food insecurity in early childhood is associated with long-term cognitive and emotional challenges. Malnutrition affects brain development, leading to increased risks of ADHD, depression, and generalized anxiety disorder (Whitaker et al., 2006; Liu et al., 2020). Case studies from low-income communities highlight the impact of chronic food scarcity on children's emotional regulation and academic performance (Weaver & Hadley, 2009). Mental health consequences of food insecurity include anxiety and a sense of powerlessness, hopelessness, and depression (Alaimo et al., 2002; Huddleston-Casas et al., 2009). Thus, parental and familial stress can change the domestic environment and affect children's attachment patterns and growth, both in terms of their physical and mental health. Furthermore, a reliance on inexpensive fast food can lead to obesity with its associated problems.

Those with mental illnesses may also face food insecurity due to inadequate finances and support. Here, once again, social prescribing may help. In most psychiatric institutions, patients were given vegetable patches and flowerbeds to look after as part of their occupational therapy, and vegetables thus acquired were used in the hospital kitchens. With closure of asylums, this changed. Many patients with chronic severe mental illnesses may not be able to shop for their food or cook, and thus they may go hungry, thereby worsening their mental state.

Once again, clinicians need to be on the lookout for signs of malnourishment and assess the situation as part of their physical and mental state examinations. Screening tools may be used to help the clinician obtain a broader picture. As advocates, clinicians can influence policies and, at local levels, work with food banks, schools, and nongovernmental organizations and charities to help improve access to food and reduce food insecurity.

Housing

Human beings' basic needs include food and housing. Inadequate, poor quality, or insecure housing can all influence the mental health and well-being of families, communities, and individuals. Housing insecurity is a significant determinant of mental health, with studies indicating that individuals experiencing homelessness have a much higher prevalence of psychiatric disorders such as depression (Gutwinski et al., 2021). In addition, the built environment, lack of green spaces, and poor access to affordable transport affect mental health. Urban areas have consistently shown high rates of psychiatric disorders, but that is not to say that the rural idyll is somehow always protective (see Bhugra et al., 2019). Built environments in urban areas also contribute to difficulties. Housing influences health, including mental health, in a variety of ways through psychological, physical (or structural), and social facets. Inadequate cramped space with dampness or mold, lack of privacy in some cultures, and pest infestation will adversely affect physical and mental health, while secure housing tenure will contribute to psychological solace. The built environment and neighborhood also foster a sense of social connectedness (Shaw, 2004; Suglia et al., 2015). As Shaw (2004) highlights, housing affects health both directly and indirectly. Deterioration in the quality of housing, insecurity, and lack of homeownership can all negatively influence one's housing status. Repeated moves, insecure tenancy, and housing conditions affect the quality of housing. Homelessness itself has illustrated high rates of psychiatric disorders, and without safety nets, individuals with severe serious mental illnesses are likely to fall into homelessness, thus creating a vicious cycle.

Quality of housing, if poor, affects both physical and mental health and well-being. Structural problems in housing will influence physical health (e.g., mold or pest infestation can cause allergic disorders or asthma). Insecure housing can lead to anxiety, hopelessness, helplessness, a sense of feeling trapped, and then depression. Housing instability and insecurity may further contribute to domestic violence, alcohol abuse, and inadequate schooling for children. Children and young people may go on to develop emotional and behavioral problems (Miller & Rasmussen, 2010). Homelessness affects individuals and may contribute to anxiety, depression, substance misuse, and suicidal ideation, among other disorders (Magdol, 2002). Insecure housing has been associated with attention and behavioral problems in children (Ziol-Guest & McKenna, 2014). Evans (2006) has demonstrated that specific features of one's housing influence the mental health of individuals, especially children. Indeed, poor and inadequate housing will affect the whole family. Furthermore, Todman and Holliday (2015) highlight some of the components of built environments that are essential for mental health and well-being; these include transportation, communication, waste management, and green spaces.

Using culture broker or community link worker models, individuals with long-term conditions can be referred for suitable secure housing. Policy changes are a crucial contributing factor. As a result of the mass sell-off of social housing since the 1980s in the UK, the number of homeless individuals has gone up and created a homeless population who are either living in hostels or in insecure and overcrowded settings. Stable housing initiatives, such as "Housing First" programs, have been successful in improving long-term mental health outcomes (Padgett et al., 2016). In addition, clinicians and policymakers must work together to link clinical needs with housing assistance as and when required.

Loneliness and Social Isolation

Humans evolved as social beings, hence social relationships and connections are vital to our well-being. Research has linked chronic loneliness to adverse health outcomes including anxiety, depression, dementia, increased cancer risk, and early mortality (Hawkley & Capitanio, 2015; Park et al., 2020; Wang et al., 2023). Loneliness has also been linked to depression and anxiety among children and adolescents with existing mental health distress, suggesting a bidirectional relationship (Hards et al., 2022). Persistent loneliness is associated with higher rates of depression and anxiety due to the lack of emotional support and reduced opportunities for social interaction (Cacioppo et al., 2015). Social isolation also alters brain function, increasing activity in the amygdala and hypothalamic-pituitary-adrenal (HPA) axis, leading to chronic stress, elevated cortisol levels, and heightened vulnerability to psychiatric disorders (Matthews et al., 2016). Loneliness and isolation have been linked to accelerated cognitive decline and a higher risk of dementia, possibly due to reduced mental stimulation and increased stress-related neuroinflammation (Holwerda et al., 2014).

Loneliness is a significant predictor of suicidal thoughts and behaviors, particularly among adolescents, older adults, and individuals with preexisting mental health conditions (Calati et al., 2019). Mental illness itself can also lead to increased loneliness and isolation, suggesting a bidirectional relationship; people with psychiatric disorders may withdraw from social interactions because of stigma, lack of motivation, or cognitive impairments (Santini et al., 2020). Loneliness is moderately positively correlated with internet addiction according to a large meta-analysis (Wang & Zeng, 2024).

Positive and authentic relationships are a key component of mental well-being and assist individuals in coping with ill-health, as well as reducing loneliness. Evidence-based interventions tackling loneliness across the course of one's life (Victor et al., 2018) include social prescribing (see chapter 12); structured peer-support programs (see chapter 7); school- and work-based social connection programs (see chapters 8 and 9, respectively); cognitive behavioral therapy for individuals with mental barriers to connecting with others (Cattan et al., 2005) through social prescribing; digital connections (online peer-support groups and therapies—see chapter 10); and public health loneliness campaigns (Gardiner et al., 2018).

Role of the Clinician as Advocate

In chapter 2, the role of the clinician as an advocate was described at some length. In this section, we shall relate it to community activities. Younan et al. (2020) suggest that social prescribing may be one way of tackling social determinants (see chapter 12 on social prescribing). Mental health professionals thus have a moral imperative to advocate for their patients, carers, and families. To advocate, clear scientific messages in a straightforward language have to be created. If the individual clinicians feel that they are not interested or do not wish to be involved, they should work with local community organizations and local parliamentary representatives to help tackle health inequalities and social determinants that contribute to these inequalities. Fundamental causes of health inequalities, as we have seen in this chapter, include social determinants but are also affected by broader global economic forces, geopolitical factors, national political ideologies, and societal attitudes to equity and fairness. Within countries, the effects of discrimination, institutional racism, inequality (of opportunities and access to health care), and the legacies of traumatizing societal injustices need to be addressed in order to give every person a fair chance at a healthy life. Social determinants as described herein are related to wider environmental influences that mold an individual's experiences. Thus, public health and public mental health are crucial to improving individual physical and mental health.

To tackle these inequalities, there must be employment opportunities that provide secure, reasonably well-paid jobs. Those who have psychiatric disorders need to be supported in their gradual return to work at the pace of their choosing. Dealing with workplace discrimination in an appropriate manner is important. Employment should be adjusted according to individual needs. Organizational policies must reflect and accommodate these needs. Policies must provide a fair and universal social security system. The economy must change through a fair tax system that is progressive and leads to redistribution of income from the more affluent to the less affluent. Consequently, this will improve the life chances and circumstances for families and individuals across all age ranges, allowing their living, learning, working, and relaxing environments to change.

The mental health of children and young people should be an urgent priority, and sufficient resources need to be made available at home and in schools and communities according to age-based needs. Public services must involve local communities in the design and development of services according to their needs and not their ability to pay. Equal access to services must be enshrined in law. Furthermore, policymakers must change discriminatory policies and encourage public health measures such as regulating the sale of alcohol and food products. As mentioned earlier, they must ensure that all policies undertake an impact assessment on health, including mental health, as a matter of routine. Adequate, affordable social housing must be available to those who need it with sufficient green spaces and ease of access to public and affordable transportation. New housing must incorporate energy-efficient approaches.

Inequalities in well-being, the improvement of healthy life expectancy, and the reduction of morbidity and mortality can be achieved by addressing political determinants, provided there is political will. Often, laws and policies may exist, but their implementation is poor or limited because of a lack of public health and different priorities. Policymakers need to develop integrated policies across public health (including mental health), education, employment, housing, access to affordable food, relaxation, sports, and physical activities throughout the lifespan. It is crucial for community organizations to be involved in developing these policies and providing advice to the communities. Furthermore, examples of good practice must be shared so that other groups and communities can learn from them rather than reinventing the wheel.

Conclusion

Social determinants are essential to mental health and well-being. However, the impact of geopolitical factors on social determinants must not be overlooked. Social determinants encompass housing, education, employment, and other elements that may contribute to both material and emotional poverty. The research evidence confirming the significance of these factors in maintaining both individual and community health is robust. To ensure that health (including mental health) is integrated with other elements such as education, employment, judiciary, and housing, policymakers must avoid working in silos. Every policy should include an impact assessment on health and mental health. Policymakers need to comprehend scientific evidence and collaborate with researchers, clinicians, communities, patients, and their carers and families to develop and implement appropriate policies. Affordable education, housing, and health care, particularly in the context of reasonably well-paid employment during the COVID-19 pandemic, have taken on significant importance. Addressing adverse childhood experiences through education, early recognition, and early interventions are crucial steps that can support the next generation of adults. A better and clearer understanding of various social determinants can assist in reducing health inequalities. The influence of local cultural values and expectations needs to be considered when formulating and delivering policies on equity and equality. Society and its environment impact policies, along with policymakers, should also address the long-term effects of their decisions. Learning from and collaborating with other organizations to achieve sustained change is vital. Clinicians, managers, and community organizations must work alongside policymakers to foster integrated thinking in improving the population's mental health.

4 Stigma, Discrimination, and Human Rights

Introduction

Stigma and discrimination are not new phenomena. Stigma against people with mental illnesses and their exclusion from the communities in many settings is exemplified by constructions of asylums often outside towns and cities to keep these patients hidden. The stigma often relates to the creation of the "other" to validate one's own identity and behavior.

Individual identity is what makes us who we are. In this context social, ethnic, and religious identity emerge, as well as the sexual components of identity. Although it is an essential aspect of human experience, identity is difficult to define neatly (Strauss, 2017). Philosophers have been exploring the idea of identity for millennia (Sollberger, 2013). Identity is about the self and self-identification influenced and defined by cultural factors. Identity is not only about how I see myself, but also how others see me, and in turn how I see them seeing me. In psychiatric settings, the notion of identity is similar to that of personality and is included in DSM-5 criteria for personality disorders (Schmeck et al., 2013). For a variety of reasons, identity is crucial in understanding stigma and discrimination (Bhugra et al., 2023).

The sense of self has been seen as fixed with intrinsic qualities (Zevallos, 2011), but all of us have multiple micro-identities related to our gender, sexual orientation, religion, qualifications, place of training, and so on (Wachter, Ventriglio, & Bhugra, 2015). This combination of micro-identities can be seen as a mosaic on which, when light shines, one specific micro-identity or multiple identities may be reflected. Certain identities can be hidden at times whereas others cannot, so, depending on the context, we may choose to show or hide aspects of our identities. These multiple social identities can augment psychological well-being and offer a sense of belonging and contribute to self-esteem. It has been shown that these may motivate individuals in helping them recover from some psychiatric morbidities, like substance use disorders (Chen et al., 2021; Dingle et al., 2015).

The Other, Othering, and Discrimination

As a result of these multiple micro-identities, individuals create the other who is opposite to them, and through this role, they validate their identity. Regrettably, these trends become binary and rigid and are pervasive across various ontological, cultural, and scientific spheres, including biological sex (male/female), species (animal/human), profession (layperson/expert), mental health (insanity/reason), and legal (criminal/noncriminal) (Bauman, 1991). Othering thus necessarily leads to the distillation of social identities into distinct classifications, and the otherness-related negative attitudes lead to misogyny, homophobia, Islamophobia, anti-Semitism, biphobia, transphobia, and other discriminatory behaviors. It has been argued that circumstantial factors can play a role in identifying the other as friend or foe (Kapuściński, 2009).

The process of othering is not new, either. According to Miller (2023), there are historical accounts where once people had stopped being on the move and settled down, those without permanent residences looked down on those who were nomads. In the Mesopotamian period (8000–2000 BC), the Marriage of Martu (Black et al., 1998–2025) illustrated this othering when describing Martu. Adjar-kidug's girlfriend speaks to her:

> Now listen, their hands are destructive and their features are those of monkeys; he is one who eats what Nanna forbids and does not show reverence. They never stop roaming about . . . , they are an abomination to the gods' dwellings. Their ideas are confused; they cause only disturbance. He is clothed in sack-leather . . . , lives in a tent. . . .and cannot properly recite prayers. . . . ignores the places of gods, digs up truffles in the foothills, does not know how to bend the knee, and eats raw flesh. He has no house during his life, and when he dies, he will not be carried to a burial-place. My girlfriend, why would you marry Martu?

This illustrates multiple characteristics which were not acceptable. Even in those ancient times, there was a hierarchy of status and strong prejudice against those who had not settled (Porter, 2012).

It is entirely possible that othering can contribute to stereotyping and prejudice based on divergences (either real or perceived) between social entities (Staszak, 2009). The resulting negative behavior leads to discrimination that can be based on race, ethnicity, or nationality and thus might be a by-product of the construction of the Other (Said, 1978). As Bhugra et al. (2023) point out, the perpetuation of Othering can culminate in discrimination predicated on different social identities. Othering of psychiatric patients and the resulting discrimination can have deleterious implications for resource allocation, training, professional relationships across medical disciplines, failures in help-seeking, therapeutic engagement, and consequent outcomes and patient well-being.

In addition to stigma and discrimination against people with mental illnesses, there are additional otherings and discrimination related to ethnicity, sexual orientation, and so on, thus creating "double" or even "triple jeopardy" for patients who may have other minority statuses. During COVID-19 pandemic, Thomeer and colleagues examined how minority ethnic groups in the US had higher levels of unmet psychiatric needs than white Americans (Thomeer et al., 2023). In Switzerland, minorities with substance use disorders had greater risks for comorbidities (Liebrenz et al., 2014). Although lesbian, gay, and bisexual individuals have elevated susceptibility for depression, anxiety, alcohol use disorder, and suicidality compared to heterosexuals (Wittgens et al., 2022), access to care is problematic, thus confirming their double jeopardy status. This can lead to negative cognitive effects, such as executive functioning impairments (Ozier et al., 2019).

Depending on the circumstances and the confidence the individual has in their micro-identity, people may show a side they feel comfortable with. They may also use strategies like "covering" (i.e., downplaying a stigmatized identity) or "passing" (i.e., hiding a stigmatized identity) (Goffman, 1963). Thus, using these perspectives from sociology (Zevallos, 2011) and public health (Akbulut & Razum, 2022), the concepts of othering, along with the resulting stigma and discrimination, need closer examination in psychiatry, especially as psychiatric patients can be severely stigmatized. Stigma-reducing interventions and techniques can be more focused on relevant micro-identities.

Stigma and Discrimination

Stigma and misconceptions associated with mental disorders contribute to the resulting discrimination and human rights violations experienced by those who develop mental illnesses and formal and informal carers who look after them, creating a sense of alienation and isolation. Discrimination related to mental disorders has been described as having worse consequences than the conditions themselves; therefore, raising awareness of mental health is fundamental to providing a better life to those with mental illness. However, it is crucial that any anti-stigma campaigns are culturally appropriate, humble, and sensitive. When these campaigns are launched, it is important to ensure that services are set up to cope with a potential increase in demand, otherwise people may feel even more stigmatized and abandoned by the services.

Not surprisingly and as noted before, the stigma related to mental health disorders and the discrimination against those suffering from them act as barriers to accessing mental health service. This is likely to delay people seeking care, preventing timely diagnosis, treatment, and recovery. This type of discrimination can affect an individual's education, employment, and access to care, and it reduces their status and capacity to contribute to society. In a series of surveys reported in 2017 on behalf of the World Psychiatric Association (WPA), Bhugra et al. (2016a, 2016b) and Nardodkar et al. (2016) looked at the laws in 193 countries and the rights of people with mental illness. They looked at four rights: the right to vote, the right to marry, the right to inherit property and make a will, and the right to employment. These social and economic rights are basic and crucial. These findings are described in some detail later in this chapter. Although all 193 countries were signatories to the United Nations Convention on the Rights of Persons with Disabilities, only around 40 percent of the countries allowed all these laws. The same group looked at the laws of countries that are members of the British Commonwealth and reported that of 52 countries, fewer than half (48 percent) had a mental health policy (as mentioned in chapter 2). This survey showed that a majority of the countries still believed in using asylum-based approaches rather than community-based approaches (Bhugra et al., 2017).

While a reduction in the stigma around mental illness can result from—and indeed bring about—improved knowledge and understanding, it does not necessarily lead to a change in long-term attitudes or behaviors toward mental illness, people with mental illness, and those who care for those with mental illness. As a result, the ability to form any meaningful social pressure to bring about government action often can be limited.

Governments must take a lead in mental health awareness, legislating to improve service provision and reducing discrimination. Most importantly, they need to ensure that there is a mental health impact assessment of all the policies; that is the only way things will change for the better.

Responses related to stigma against mental illnesses, those who have these illnesses, and those who care for these individuals can be attributed to othering as well as a lack of knowledge. Discrimination, by contrast, is often embedded in the law and may be legally sanctioned, creating further socially sanctioned stigma. Stigma and discrimination need to be differentiated from prejudice, which carries negative views about situations and people because of negative cognitions and behaviors. These experiences of prejudice against people with mental illnesses and their carers, whether informal or formal, affect their engagement with services and therapeutic alliances as well as their involvement in the processes of design, development, and delivery of services.

Discrimination and Mental Illness

There is no doubt that there are key advantages in focusing on eliminating discrimination to achieve social inclusion for individuals with mental illness. Historically, almost all movements for empowerment of vulnerable groups, such as sexual minorities, children, racial minorities, and gender groups, have focused on eliminating discrimination using legal tools rather than simply relying on increasing knowledge and hoping that it will result in changes in attitudes and behaviors, thereby reducing stigma. This strategy has had a reasonable degree of success around the globe. The need to eliminate discrimination is well understood by the general public as well as policymakers, whereas stigma itself may be seen as a stigmatizing concept. The policies developed by the state and legislative levers are themselves affected by different and interacting resources, historical context, and economic status.

Nondiscrimination in practice, whether it is psychiatric or social, forms the bedrock of international human rights law and is emphasized in all international human rights conventions. Thus, eliminating discrimination against individuals with mental illness is a matter for immediate action. A lack of financial or other resources is no longer a sufficient or indeed an acceptable reason for countries to fail to take action to eliminate discrimination against vulnerable groups. Human rights are embedded in the concepts of social justice. Social justice allows the development of institutions that can take over and further develop the equity principle. Furthermore, it is evident that it is possible to reduce discrimination through legal means if policy initiatives and legislative actions are in place. Governments (and individuals in some countries) can therefore go on to use laws to punish those indulging in discriminatory practices and obtain equity. Unfortunately, in many countries, laws themselves foster discrimination. Such institutionalized legal discrimination gives a message to the community that persons with mental illness are lesser human beings and contributes to increased societal stigma.

Equity and Mental Health

Equity for those with mental illness demands that all national, regional, and local bodies are charged with changing both the law and resources to ensure equity in access to mental illness prevention and treatment. Notably, countries that show the least inequity across incomes appear to have higher happiness indexes (Oishi et al., 2022) (also see WHO, 2022d). Interventions to promote mental health and prevent mental illness should seek to address the underlying determinants of poor mental health (see chapter 3). They should also have legal backing for antidiscrimination laws and regulations. Evidence-based interventions should be promoted in the appropriate social, cultural, and national context within which they are to be used.

Human Rights of People with Mental Illnesses

As noted earlier, there are several human rights covenants and conventions urging governments to ensure that individuals with mental illnesses experience equality. These include the United Nations Convention on the Rights of the Child, which sets out the civil, political, economic, social, health, and cultural rights of children throughout the world. It is thus important to note that laws in low- and lower-middle-income countries may be less likely to protect against inequality, discrimination, and human rights violations—although it is equally important to note that they may find innovative ways of delivering services and using their limited resources successfully. One of the major challenges for policymakers is to ensure that the laws keep up to date with changes in societies. Often, protection of human rights through legislative and policy measures requires government spending on mental health systems and parallel community and human resources.

Various international and national charters and conventions play an important role in raising awareness within the context of a rights-based approach. A treaty is defined as a written agreement between sovereign states and is governed by international law. Ratification of a treaty means that a signatory has accepted being legally bound by its provisions. On the other hand, accession means that a country accepts an offer to become a party to a treaty that has already been negotiated and signed by other states. It has the same legal effect as ratification. By "succession" of the treaty, a successor country consents to be legally bound by the obligations of the predecessor country to the international treaty, which has the same effect as ratification.

For the purposes of designing and developing services, it is crucial to use a standard definition of disability, and there must be a clear distinction between the concepts of medical and social disabilities. Inevitably, medical disability relates to individual bodily impairments that lead to or are associated with physical or mental dysfunction. Social disability is related to the concept of difficulties in social functioning. As far as mental dysfunction is concerned, social and medical disabilities are often strongly intertwined. Social disability limits participation in functioning and activities. The United Nations Convention on the Rights of Persons with Disabilities (CRPD) uses a social model to define disability, acknowledging that disability arises from the interactions between persons with impairments and the barriers society places in their way. This definition emphasizes the person's full participation in society on an equal basis with others, thus introducing the concept of equality (preamble p1).

International and Regional Human Rights Conventions

Legal systems are set up to protect vulnerable individuals, although sometimes they end up at one extreme, assuming that all individuals with mental illness have similar problems in severity as well as type. This can lead to the infringement of their rights, further adding to stigma directly or indirectly and inadvertently. Policymakers need to be cognizant of the fact that nondiscrimination is guaranteed under international law—for example, the International Covenant on Economic, Social and Cultural Rights—and that their countries have an obligation to ensure that laws do not discriminate against individuals with mental health problems within the national legal context. Policymakers, therefore, need to ensure and understand how persons with mental health problems may be enabled and indeed empowered to enter into valid contracts within the context of their testamentary capacity. The CRPD recommends that a supported decision-making paradigm be developed and provided in country legislation (Committee on the Rights of Persons with Disabilities, 2014).

Presently, in most member states of the United Nations, a person with mental illness is routinely judged as not competent to make decisions, and often a guardian may be appointed to make decisions on their behalf. The major problem with this substituted decision-making paradigm is that the guardian is assumed to have best interests of the individual with mental illness at heart, which ultimately excludes the individual from the decision-making process.

As mentioned earlier, in 2016, we decided to investigate laws of 193 countries to explore discrimination against people with mental illnesses. We explored four basic rights: the right to property, the right to marry, the right to employment, and the right to vote. The right to property includes not only the right to inherit property but also the right to make a will—hence the ability to enter into contracts.

Patient rights in inpatient psychiatric care require specific safeguards against coercion and involuntary treatment. International guidelines, such as the CRPD, emphasize the need for voluntary and informed consent-based treatment (United Nations, 2006). Alternatives to coercion, such as sensory rooms, open-door policies, advance directives, patient-controlled admissions, recovery colleges, peer-support services. crisis resolution teams, and open dialogue approaches, may all play a role in reducing involuntary hospitalizations and have other benefits (Torrents & Björkdahl, 2024).

The Rights

Right to Property

The ownership of property gives security but also economic benefits and social status. In the past, in many countries, only landowners had the right to vote; therefore, historically, these two rights—to property and to vote—should be seen as strongly interlinked. In Britain, for example, only landowners could vote or stand for parliament until relatively recently. In many countries, women were not allowed to own property, so they could not vote. The rights that we looked at in a series of studies all are connected. The right to own property means that people could vote and inherit property; this also gave them some employment. Therefore, the rights to consent and contract also become important. Furthermore, the right to own property also means the right to receive economic benefits from it. These rights are also linked very strongly with the potential to sell, gift, or dispose of the property through provisions made in a will. Thus, although rights are often seen in isolation, they are very strongly interconnected. Pathare et al. (2015) point out that there are additional problems in our understanding of differences based on acts of law, as a number of terms are used to express mental illnesses. This was illustrated by Nardodkar et al. (2016) and Bhugra et al. (2017), who observed that in law, the large number of terms that were used to describe psychiatric disorders included insanity, madman, mental derangement or imbecility, mental disorder, mental disturbance, lunatic, usual idiocy [*sic*], madness, mentally incompetent, and idiots, to name but a few. More importantly, in most cases, these terms are not defined in the law and were left open to interpretation by both lawyers and clinicians, which in itself further contributes to discrimination. In many countries, the use of these terms follows on from colonial times, and the laws and terms have not changed for centuries. The use of these pejorative terms in legislation contributes to and increases stigma against persons with mental health problems. This in turn contributes to misinterpretation of these terms, which may thus be detrimental to the interests of persons with mental ill-health, thereby setting up a vicious cycle. Laws dealing with contracts in many countries use the term "unsound mind" or "sound mind" to debar or allow, respectively, persons from entering into valid contracts. Again, it is difficult to describe and define these terms because a plain reading of the text does not necessarily mean that the term "unsound mind" equates with mental illness. Yet, often courts use the term unsound mind interchangeably with mental illness, thereby potentially denying legal capacity for persons with mental health problems. The Committee on the Rights of Persons with Disabilities (2014) has categorically stated that "the CRPD (Article 12) now makes it clear that 'unsoundness of mind' and other discriminatory labels are not legitimate reasons for the denial of legal capacity (legal standing and legal agency)." It further goes on to reiterate that "under article 12 of the Convention, perceived or actual deficits in mental capacity must not be used as justification for denying legal capacity" (Committee on the Rights of Persons with Disabilities, 2014).

For example, Article 17 of the Universal Declaration of Human Rights (UDHR) explicitly states that "everyone has the right to own property alone as well as in association with others" and that "no one shall be arbitrarily deprived of their property." However, the right to property is not specifically protected in either the International Covenant on Economic, Social and Cultural Rights (ICESCR) or the International Covenant on Civil and Political Rights (ICCPR). But other rights related to legal capacity that affect the right to ownership of property are protected by these conventions. The right to own property as well as to inherit property is protected under Article 5 of the International Convention on the Elimination of All Forms of Racial Discrimination. Article 15 of the Convention on the Elimination of All Forms of Discrimination against Women also recognizes women's right to enter into contracts. Article 16 of the same convention recognizes women's right to ownership, enjoyment, and disposal of property on an equal basis with others. Article 12 (5) of the CRPD specifically calls on countries to "take all appropriate and effective measures to ensure the equal right of persons with disabilities to own or inherit property, to control their own financial affairs and to have equal access to bank loans, mortgages and other forms of financial credit, and shall ensure that persons with disabilities are not arbitrarily deprived of their property." In a similar vein, regional human rights conventions also recognize the right to property. For example, Article 1 of the European Convention on Human Rights (1950) recognizes a person's "right to peaceful enjoyment of possessions." Also, Article 23 of the American Declaration on the Rights and Duties of Man (Organization of American States, 1948) states that "every Person has the right to own such private property as meets the essential needs of decent living and helps to maintain the dignity of the individual and of the home." Article 14 of the African Charter on Human and Peoples' Rights explicitly states, "The right to property shall be guaranteed."

Bhugra et al. (2016a, 2016b, 2016c) and Nardodkar et al. (2016), using various databases, studied legislation dealing with law of contract, law of succession/inheritance, and law relating to testamentary capacity (wills) of all UN member states (193 countries). In the case of federal countries, the laws of the most populous state as a representative state within that country were studied. Of the 193 countries, only 40 member states (21 percent) recognize or allow persons with mental health problems to enter into contracts. Of these, even fewer (only 16 countries, or 9 percent) recognize the right of persons with mental health problems to enter into a contract without any restrictions, while 24 countries (12 percent) allow a contract entered into by a person with mental health problems to be invalidated under certain conditions (Bhugra et al., 2016c). These countries also make the validity of the contract subject to the capacity to consent, based on the level of understanding of the person with mental health problems. They may allow individuals with mental health problems to enter into contracts only for transactions of an insignificant nature or involving personal rights. Furthermore, not surprisingly, there are significant variations between high-income and low-income countries. Policymakers need to consider that nondiscrimination is guaranteed under international law (e.g., ICESCR); therefore, their countries have an obligation to ensure that laws do not discriminate against vulnerable populations, including those with mental health problems. When examining the rights of people with mental ill-health to inherit property, over one-third of countries do not recognize their right to enter into contracts or write their own will and testament. The apparent nondiscrimination in the right to succeed or inherit property is of little benefit to persons with mental health problems as they are unable to enter into contracts (to sell or dispose of the property) or give it away in a will or testament. Hence, effectively, they are unable to enjoy the inheritance in many member states. In many settings, this may explain the rise in the number of homeless individuals who also have a psychiatric disorder or mental ill-health.

Right to Marry

Marriage is one of the oldest social institutions. It is culturally approved and supported, although types and contracts within marriage do vary across cultures. Cultures have been classified as sex-positive (where sexual activity is for pleasure) and sex-negative (where the sole purpose of sexual activity is for procreation) (Bullough, 1976). Resultantly, in some cultures, there will be an almost universal expectation that individuals will get married so that they can procreate and raise a family together as a unit. Furthermore, the attitudes toward marriage and settling down are changing in cultures in transition, so some of these observations need to be seen in the context of the period when data were collected. This is further complicated by other dimensions of culture (i.e., whether cultures themselves are egocentric or sociocentric). Sociocentric cultures are likely to be more traditional and also kinship-based, meaning that procreation is of great importance. Another dimension of cultures is whether they are masculine or feminine, which will influence male and female gender roles as well as how children are brought up (Hofstede, 2001).

Thus, the expectations of marriage and marriage partners are likely to be strongly influenced by culture. For example, in sociocentric or traditional cultures, marriages are often arranged, so individuals may have very little say in whom they marry. As in olden times, marriage is seen as being between families; individuals represent their families, and their expectations from marriage may differ. There is no doubt that the realization of the right to marry is not only an important part of one's life choices but also an exercise in personal liberty. It is clear, too, that every individual's right to marry or remain married is regulated by their country's family codes, civil codes, marriage laws, or divorce laws. However, social expectations also play a role. For example, anecdotally, it has been observed that in some countries, parents want to have their children (if they have mental illness) married off to ensure that they will be looked after when a parent dies.

Similar to the right to property, in the international legal scene, the right to marry, remain married, or dissolve a marriage has been enshrined in several human rights instruments. These include Article 16 of UDHR (1948) and Article 10 of ICESCR (United Nations, 1966). For persons with mental disabilities, provisions of Article 23.1(a) of the CRPD (United Nations, 2007) explicitly state that the state parties (countries) shall ensure "the right of all persons with disabilities who are of marriageable age to marry and to found a family on the basis of free and full consent of the intending spouses is recognized." State parties (countries) are also required to take "effective and appropriate measures to eliminate discrimination against persons with disabilities" in relation to the protection of the right to marry and found a family. In the context of Article 4 (b) of CRPD, these effective and appropriate measures include legislative measures "including legislation, to modify or abolish existing laws, regulations, customs and practices that constitute discrimination against persons with disabilities." Taken together, these obligations require member states to bring their marriage-regulating laws in line with the principles of CRPD so that persons with mental health problems or disabilities can marry on the basis of free and full consent of the intending spouses. Once again, the role of capacity to consent is incredibly important and relevant here.

Pathare et al. (2015) highlight that the laws of many countries have described conditions of unsound mind or insanity as lawful grounds for either not permitting marriage or annulling or dissolving nuptial ties. Such an approach is likely to be based on stereotypes that persons with mental health problems are incapable of consent and therefore unable to enter into a marital contract of their own free will. Other possible reasons for prohibiting marriage for persons with mental health problems may include concerns about whether mental illness could be inherited by the offspring of such a marital union and questions about the ability of persons with mental health problems.

In our study of domestic laws in 193 countries looking at the rights of people with mental illness with respect to marriage, we found that 37 percent of countries explicitly prohibit marriage by persons with mental health problems (Bhugra et al., 2016b). In 21 countries (11 percent), the presence of mental health problems can render a marriage void or can be considered grounds for nullity of the marriage. In 11 countries (6 percent), persons with mental health problems are allowed to marry, but the marriage is subject to approval from others. Of these 11 countries, four countries allow marriage only with permission from an appropriate court or family Council; in four countries, persons with mental health conditions may marry subject to consent from a parent, guardian, or custodian; and in two countries, marriage is permitted subject to approval from an expert or an institution Thus, in many countries, basic human rights related to marriage are being flouted. Furthermore, there is often an increased likelihood of getting divorce on the grounds of mental illness, which has been used in domestic disputes to find an easy solution, thereby further isolating and discriminating against those individuals with mental illness. This discrimination creates a double jeopardy, as people with mental illness face divorce or are not allowed to marry. Being single or divorced further adds to the stigma against them, perhaps more so in the case of women, as has been shown by Thara et al. (2003a, 2003b) in India. They reported that women and family members experience extreme stigma and distress from divorce related to mental illness, more so than from mental illness alone. It is a particularly difficult scenario for women who are most likely to be caregivers, thus creating further erosion of their basic human rights.

Laws in some countries require an expert such as a trained psychiatrist to decide whether a person with mental health problems can perform and fulfill duties in a marriage, but the definition of "trained" also appears to vary across cultures. Thus, the international picture appears to be extremely complex. Although decision-making capacity is task-specific, ill-defined terms such as "unable to reason" or "unsound mind" often get equated with mental health conditions and misinterpreted and misrepresented in courts. The Committee on the Rights of Persons with Disabilities (2014) has expressly stated in General Comment No. 1 that "perceived or actual deficits in mental capacity must not be used as justification for denying legal capacity." Moreover, use of terms like "madman," "demented," or "deranged" continue to perpetuate stigma of mental illness.

Right to Vote

In any democratic country, the right to vote is an important basic right that allows individuals to participate actively in the democratic process and affirms equality. This right is based on universal and equal suffrage and is also enshrined in international human rights treaties. Although these international conventions have been ratified by a large majority of United Nations member states, their application across the globe is patchy and problematic. In a civil society, democratic principles are enshrined and form an individual's basic right to participate in the decision-making processes affecting all citizens. Each vote has the same weight and value irrespective of gender, religion, or sexual orientation.

The right to vote is an important right representing full citizenship and is protected by international human rights treaties. Article 21 of the UDHR (1948) recognizes the right of "everyone" to take part in the political process, and elections should be based on universal and equal suffrage. Article 25 of the ICCPR (1966) also protects the right to vote and participate in the political process. More recently, the CPRD (2007) in Article 29 reinforces the right of disabled persons (including those with mental health problems and disabilities) to participate in political and public life on an equal basis with others. Article 29 of the convention also specifically mentions that persons with disabilities be offered the opportunity and the right to vote and be elected. These international conventions too have been ratified by a large majority of United Nations member states. The ICCPR, adopted by the United Nations General Assembly in 1966, has been ratified by 167 countries; the CRPD was adopted by the United Nations General Assembly in 2006 and has been ratified by 157 countries to date. There is a responsibility on UN member states ratifying these conventions to ensure that citizens in their respective countries are able to enjoy these treaty-based rights by taking "all appropriate legislative, administrative and other measures for the implementation of the rights recognized in the present Convention," according to Article 4 (1) (a) of the CRPD. This emphasizes that rights protected in international human rights documents can only be realized if they are translated into domestic legislation by the member states ratifying these conventions and treaties.

Bhugra et al. (2016a) in the same series of studies found that only 21 countries (11 percent) place no restrictions on the right to vote by persons with mental health problems, while 69 member states (36 percent) deny all persons with any mental health problems a right to vote without any qualifier. Again, many terms are used in legislation to describe persons with mental health problems; they include (suffering from) insanity, weakness of mind, unsound mind, lunatic, mental disability, mentally ill, psychiatric patient, "certified insane," "medically proven total mental incapacity," "mental derangement," "notoriously insane," mental incapacity, mentally incompetent, "lost his mind," "demented," seriously weakened mental state, mentally deficient, "insane or imbecile," certified to be insane, and "mental ineptitude," thus contributing to stigma. Worryingly, as noted before, these terms are not defined in the law and are left open to interpretation, making it possible for unscrupulous doctors or lawyers to misuse them. Another 21 member states (11 percent) deny detained persons the right to vote; of these, nine member states specifically do so for persons who were detained under the mental health law, while others apply it to all those who were interdicted or judicially interdicted. In 56 countries (29 percent), the restriction requires an order (declaration) from a court or magistrate. The ICCPR has been ratified in 57 member states (34 percent), and 57 countries that have ratified the CRPD deny persons with mental health problems the right to vote and therefore are failing their obligation under these international conventions. It has been shown that in countries with a federal state system, not all states offer the same rights. Corrigan et al. (2005) looked at the laws of the 50 US states and reported that 19 states denied all persons with mental illness the right to vote on the basis of mental illness, while 12 states did so on the grounds of incompetence or lack of capacity. Often, the argument made in order to disallow persons with mental ill-health from voting is the perceived need to maintain integrity of the electoral process, reflecting a certain level of informed choice by individuals who have the capacity to make such choices. This argument that all individuals with mental illness lack capacity to make an informed choice and thus should not be allowed to participate in the electoral process needs careful unpicking. We know that capacity is task-specific (i.e., a person may not necessarily have the capacity to make decisions on their finances or treatment but may retain the capacity to make other decisions, including voting choices), and it varies over time.

Right to Employment

Work is an important aspect of human functioning and social relationships. In addition to financial rewards and security, work provides an occupation, self-esteem, and pride. Work has both personal and social meaning. Employment offers a degree of confidence that can contribute to recovery, which, after all, is about social functioning. For people with mental illness, work provides an outlet and support system for better social interaction and integration. In many low-income countries, especially in traditional societies, joint families in rural areas can provide a degree of protection for individuals with mental illness who are not the sole earners. Even basic tasks and economic participation can keep people occupied and offer some income, no matter how small. We know that the rates of psychiatric disorders are higher in unemployed individuals, and this two-way relationship between work and social functioning at a number of levels is important. Yet, with the likelihood of stigma and discrimination in the workplace and indirect structural discrimination, the right to employment often gets eroded. It is important to recognize that stigma and discrimination can be reduced when individual experiences are shared openly.

In common with other rights, international law has adopted a human-rights-based perspective for promoting the participation of persons with mental disabilities in the labor market. Particularly, Article 23 of the Universal Declaration of Human Rights (1948), Article 6 and Article 7 of the ICESCR (1976), and Article 27 of the CRPD (2006) protect the rights of persons with mental disabilities to work and employment. CRPD holds historical significance for bringing about a paradigm shift in the perception of persons with mental disabilities from objects of charity to people with equal human rights. Article 27 expressly proclaims that state parties recognize that persons with mental disabilities have equal rights to work in an open, inclusive, and accessible environment and to earn their livelihood by the work they do of their own free choice. It requires states/parties to ensure that persons with mental disabilities are protected from harassment and bullying in the labor market and to promote the right to work through "legislation and other appropriate measures" (Article 27, para. 1). Moreover, according to the CRPD (Article 12), equal access to employment opportunities for persons with mental disabilities also reinforces their equal recognition before the law and enjoyment of legal capacity.

Despite the goodwill promoted in these international conventions and instruments, the delivery depends on national policies, the will of policymakers, and their awareness of the workplace environment and structural barriers. Nardodkar et al. (2016) reported that discrimination in the workplace against people with mental illness is likely to occur at many different levels and in different contexts; it is likely to be both explicit and implicit, taking forms that range from exclusion during short-listing to stigmatization that occurs when individuals do not receive any emotional or legal support at their place of work. Again, in their survey of the laws of 193 countries, when examining the right to employment, these authors reported that 28 countries (14 percent) do not even have laws that explicitly prohibit discrimination based on mental disability at the time of recruitment. A further 26 member states (13 percent) have laws with conflicting provisions. In 58 countries (30 percent), there are no explicit or implied provisions in the law for making reasonable accommodations for persons with disabilities, including mental disabilities.

Negative discrimination in the law inevitably gives permission and leeway to employers not to do anything to support individuals with mental illnesses. Laws of 56 countries do not explicitly define disability or mention "mental impairment/disability/illness" in the definition of disability, leaving room for uncertain interpretation and thereby contributing to the likelihood of unequal access to rights and resources for persons with mental disabilities and mental illnesses. In addition to the one-third of countries that deny equality to persons afflicted with mental illness by not prohibiting discrimination on the grounds of mental disability during recruitment, the laws of another 61 percent of countries pose barriers to retaining employment. As noted earlier, it is well recognized that work reduces not only incapacity but also fosters recovery from mental illness. Therefore, provisions of laws that give access to reasonable accommodations in the workplace can play an important role in the rehabilitation process. Services required to deliver support for the management of illness in the workplace and networking of mental health care professionals with employers can be adopted as part of reasonable workplace adjustments.

It may be that in some circumstances, positive affirmative action may help in supporting individuals with mental illness in the workplace. Anti-stigma campaigns can help reduce negative feelings and increase positive and supportive actions. Again, it is important to recognize that often laws in low- and lower-middle-income countries are less likely to protect against inequality, discrimination, and human rights violations. In many countries where laws date back to colonial times, urgent review is needed.

The Role of Legislation

Often, the protection of human rights through legislative and policy measures requires government spending on mental health systems and parallel community and human resources. In response to this, the WPA developed a bill of rights for people with mental illness. The bill of rights reiterates that persons with mental illness, mental disabilities, or mental health problems should not be discriminated against based on their mental health status. These individuals also have the capacity to hold and exercise rights and should therefore be treated on an equal basis with other citizens (Bhugra, 2016b). Harrowingly, only about 10 percent of countries have laws that are nondiscriminatory against people with mental illness. The dialogue between policymakers and stakeholders is critical in this case and needed urgently. Policymakers often argue that ICESCR rights, such as right to work, are subject to progressive realization (see General Comment No. 18, para. 19). However, 50 years after the ICESCR was adopted, countries have failed to amend or replace legislation that does not halt discriminatory practices. Policymakers must be held responsible and regularly reminded that discrimination against people with mental illness is unlawful, and because their country has signed on to international treaties and laws, they must change their laws to ensure that those with mental illness can lead a full and fulfilling life. A majority of countries are failing in their obligations under international human rights law when they not provide legal protection against discrimination in employment, inheritance of property, the right to vote, and the right to marry. The jumble of definitions used in laws to describe mental illnesses must be sorted out by the profession as a matter of urgency.

Mental health legislation must take into account changes in the way society *perceives* people with mental health problems, available resources (whether these resources are financial or human), and evidence-based treatments. The codification of social justice for those with mental illness at the national and international level needs not only urgent consideration but also immediate application.

Using the civil rights movement as an exemplar and following it to bring about substantial and sustainable change means that mental health pressure groups (including professional organizations and patient and family organizations) can play a significant role in advocating for humane care and treatment for individuals with mental illness. Mental health legislation is a powerful tool for codifying and consolidating these fundamental values and principles. However, the focus of most mental health legislation around the world appears to be limited to the regulation of involuntary detention in hospitals or other institutions and on the forced and involuntary treatment of mental illness. The underlying principles must be aimed at providing the best evidence-based care for those who need it while considering the wishes of the individual as much as possible. Legislation to prevent discrimination of people with mental illness—for example, by upholding parity of employment, testamentary capacity, and housing—is given considerably less emphasis. That needs to change. In fact, in some countries, there would appear to be no legal provisions or agencies to support mentally ill people. The negative consequences of an episode of mental illness often last longer than the duration of the illness itself. Many people will remain actively and unfairly discriminated against following their recovery. Dedicated mental health legislation is present in 77 percent of high-income countries, compared with only 39 percent of low-income countries. In addition to national wealth and prosperity, this may be related to cultural perceptions and values.

The fundamental aim of mental health legislation must be to protect, promote, and improve the well-being of citizens while looking after the most vulnerable citizens who need treatment sometimes against their will. Legislation offers an important mechanism to ensure adequate and appropriate care and treatment, the protection of the human rights of individuals with mental disorders, and the promotion of the mental health of the general population. There is little doubt that sometimes these tensions can be very difficult to resolve.

State commitment to mental health through its policies and laws is a key indicator for recognizing the needs of people with mental illness and consequently using these opportunities to develop, improve, and evaluate standards of services and care. There is no doubt that political will leading to sufficient and adequate resources—financial and human—and appropriately functioning institutions is critical in this endeavor. Without the necessary political will, resources and institutional structures dealing with social justice, policies, and legislation will be of little significance. Indeed, mental health laws require regular revision and updating, too. Such laws do and should evolve over time in response to changing social and economic structures of the nation.

Conclusion

In many countries, patients with mental illnesses are seen as second-class citizens with limited rights. Policymakers and advocates need to ensure that their rights are preserved in law and that laws are based on equity. Creating otherness allows discrimination and stigmatization to develop, which in turn can stop people from seeking help and engaging in therapeutic interventions, which impedes their recovery.

It is critical that patient organizations, mental health professionals, and policymakers work together to change discriminatory laws to provide equity to people with mental illnesses. An awareness of social identities and othering will allow policymakers to recognize potential sources of discrimination; public education focusing on the role of othering in creating stigma and discrimination can be helpful. Inequities and health care disparities can at least be reduced significantly, if not avoided completely. It is essential for both policymakers and health care professionals to be aware of the problems associated with othering and stigma and recognize the need for a deeper understanding of these issues, identifying the need for empathy and increasing professional and institutional awareness toward the stigmatizing paradigms of otherness. In doing so, mental health professionals can provide effective and inclusive leadership and treatment for individual and targeted patient needs and work toward more equitable environments that celebrate inclusivity, accentuate clinical diversity, and promote social justice and environments in which patients can flourish.

5 Epidemiology of Mental Illnesses across Cultures

Introduction

When designing, developing, and delivering psychiatric or mental health services, it is vital that mental health needs of the local communities are considered even when private health care is being provided. Thus, it is critical to use accurate local data to understand and explore the details of prevalence and incidence rates of psychiatric disorders as these rates are likely to vary across cultures. Furthermore, data may change over time, so services need to be nimble and flexible in their responses to changing demographics. It is entirely possible that local or even national data may not be available and that some kind of transposition of data may be required. There are other challenges in collecting and interpreting data. For example, in many languages, words describing certain psychiatric conditions (e.g., depression) do not exist. Does that mean that the conditions do not exist in those cultures or that the conditions do exist but are seen as something else and given local colloquial metaphorical descriptions? Once again, it is important to recognize that one size does not fit all. There is thus a problem with certain concepts of global mental health that seem to argue that psychiatric disorders are the same everywhere and that the treatment is likely to be the same medication.

We also know that expectations of medications and pharmacodynamic and pharmacokinetic factors vary across cultures. This is complicated by the observations that despite globalization, research instruments and assessment tools developed in Western countries may not assess the same factors if used in another without conceptual validation, thereby creating a category fallacy. The concept of "category fallacy," as defined by Kleinman

(1987), refers to the misapplication of Western psychiatric classifications to non-Western cultural contexts. For example, the Western diagnosis of schizophrenia may not fully capture culturally specific syndromes in other countries. A mixture of quantitative and qualitative approaches can help in making sense of the data from various epidemiological studies across countries and cultures. Mental health assessment depends on the accuracy of the diagnosis and its subsequent application in determining disability and social functioning and in developing services that will be culturally appropriate and sensitive.

Culture and Mental Illness

In the author's experience, the notion that cultures are unique often gets forgotten, and the relativist nature of cultures is often ignored in psychiatry. Culture is a complex, multilayered concept that can be defined in various ways, depending on the discipline and the viewpoint of the individual using it. Cultures comprise learned behaviors and patterns that influence lifestyles and are supported by knowledge, customs, beliefs, and values. These elements, in turn, shape human behaviors. Cultures fluidly influence human actions and affect how we experience and express distress help-seeking (Bhugra et al., 2021). Given the vast number and broad diversity of human cultures, this book can make only general statements regarding culture and mental illness. As reviewed by Bhugra & Bhui (2020), certain cultural groups may be more vulnerable to mental ill-health because of factors such as discrimination, low socioeconomic status, and acculturation stress. Conversely, cultural practices and community support can serve as protective factors, enhancing resilience and coping mechanisms. Cultural contexts mold the presentation of mental health symptoms. For instance, in some cultures, psychological distress may be expressed predominantly through physical symptoms—a phenomenon known as somatization, which is sometimes denigrated in Western psychiatry. Cultural beliefs, attitudes, and values significantly influence the stigma associated with mental illness. As mentioned in chapter 4, this stigma can manifest differently across cultures, affecting individuals' willingness to seek help and adhere to treatment (Abdullah & Brown, 2011).

Hechanova & Waelde (2017) identify five key components of diverse cultures affecting mental health practitioners, framed within disaster response in Southeast Asia. The first component is emotional expression, where some cultures believe that unhealthy emotional imbalances can lead to health issues. This concern is reflected in the view that discussing painful topics may heighten negative feelings (p. 33). Similar hesitance toward talking therapies is noted in research on African and Southeast Asian refugees (p. 5). The second component is shame, which the authors state affects Asians' willingness to seek professional help due to strong familial ties (p. 5). The third component, power distance, highlights the differences in power between therapists and clients in Asian cultures, influencing autonomy in therapy. Fourth, collectivism is examined as a source of resilience and coping. Finally, spirituality and religion are considered for their roles in attribution and coping strategies ([14], p. 34).

Mental illness prevalence studies from around the world have often used diagnostic instruments developed in high-income countries to carry out prevalence studies in other countries. While using similar assessment tools can provide for an easier comparison, these instruments, even when translated, may not measure psychopathology accurately within local culture. As mentioned above, Kleinman's (1980) observation on category fallacy (the forcing of categories onto those from whom they were not derived) is an important one that often gets ignored. Culture is an intimidatingly large subject to cover in a single book. In addition to the references, the interested reader is referred to the following works for a more detailed examination of the subject: Gopalkrishnan (2019), Bhugra et al. (2021), and the Canadian Mental Health Association's (2014) resources on cross-cultural mental health.

Rates of Disorders Around the World

Mental illnesses are seen across all cultures and all societies, although inevitably there are variations in rates as well as in the ways people perceive these disorders and the way in which they explain them and present with such experiences. Despite the methodological limitations of prevalence studies (discussed below, numerous international studies have attempted to quantify prevalence rates of different mental illnesses. Globally, as of 2019, over one billion people worldwide were thought to be living with a mental or addictive disorder (Rehm & Shield, 2019), and this burden appears to be rising (Patel et al., 2018).

There are many explanations for the increasing rates of mental illness. Life-changing stresses induced by a global pandemic, increased awareness of mental health issues among the public and clinicians, falling global stigma (which may lead to more help-seeking from professionals), improved screening and diagnostic capacity, and changing social determinants of health are all implicated (Kirkbride et al., 2024). These authors argue that other "shocks"—such as food and energy crises, global conflicts, and racial injustice—against a backdrop of persistent climate change and globalization further exacerbate the unequal distribution of mental health issues and resources across populations. Additional structural factors implicated in the twenty-first century include societal fragmentation, a (Western) shift toward external validation, and the rise of social media use, especially among younger people (Tkacz & Brady, 2021)

Rising prevalence rates may also reflect increases in overdiagnosis and self-diagnosis associated with the availability of online symptom checkers, social media content about mental health, and public health awareness campaigns (Monteith et al., 2024). Frances (2013) critiqued the tendency to label normal emotional variations as psychiatric disorders and warned against the overdiagnosis of psychiatric conditions, cautioning that broadening diagnostic criteria may lead to unnecessary medical interventions, especially within the cultural context. Boysen and Doonan (2014) compared revisions in the DSM-5 to its predecessor and found that 36 percent of disorders shifted toward inclusivity rather than exclusivity (25 percent). Also, seven out of ten types of DSM revisions showed a net shift toward inclusivity. Several studies have demonstrated how broadening diagnostic criteria in the DSM has contributed to inflated prevalence rates of conditions like depression (Hasin et al., 2018) and ADHD (Matte et al., 2015), although reasons for changing prevalence figures are many, including methodological changes, culture shifts, and substantive changes (i.e., true increases due to higher environmental risk factors) (Hasin et al., 2018).

The Research Studies

In an early attempt at exploring and understanding cross-cultural variation of rates of schizophrenia was the WHO-led International Pilot Study of Schizophrenia (IPSS). In the pilot study, Sartorius and colleagues (WHO, 1973, 1979) for the very first time were able to collect standardized data from countries and centers around the world. Using a narrow definition of schizophrenia based on Present State Examination (PSE) revealed rates of 0.06/1000 in the Czech Republic, but nearly double that at 0.14/1000 in the UK; broader definition schizophrenia rates were low at 0.09/1000 in the Czech Republic, but 0.42 in India. The IPSS also suggested better outcomes for patients in low-income countries compared to high-income countries. However, subsequent analyses reported concerns about selection bias, lack of standardized diagnostic criteria, and differences in health care systems that may have influenced these findings (Hopper et al., 2007). As different cultures evolve and move from traditional types to less traditional ones, it will be interesting to see if such variations remain or disappear.

The WHO pilot study was followed by the Determinants of Outcome of Severe Mental Disorders (DOSMED) study (Jablensky et al., 1992). This study provided data from 16 centers in 12 countries with similar findings. Jablensky (2018) points out that, in some isolated populations around the world, high rates of schizophrenia have been reported, along with an increased likelihood of developing schizophrenia. Similarly, higher than expected rates of psychoses, including schizophrenia, have been found in individuals who migrate or seek refuge or asylum as well as in other minority groups who are vulnerable. For example, LGBTQ+ individuals face higher rates of anxiety, depression, and suicidality due to minority stress and discriminatory policies (see the section on other vulnerable groups in this chapter). Focusing on migrant groups, the countries from which these migrants originate do not have high rates of schizophrenia, but migrants exhibit higher rates in their receiving countries, highlighting potential social causative factors. Blocked upward social mobility along with perceived and real discrimination have been put forward as potential explanations for increased psychosis rates among certain migrant groups (Bhugra et al., 1999). A meta-analysis finds that rates of psychotic disorders are greater among refugees when compared with native populations, and factors such as separation from social networks, social exclusion, discrimination, and poverty may contribute to these high rates (Brandt et al., 2019). Perceived discrimination has been put forward as a cause (Veling et al 2008). Other vulnerable groups, such as people with intellectual disabilities, are also more likely to have higher rates of psychiatric disorders.

Jablensky (2018) identified a higher risk of developing psychosis among genetic siblings, which has implications for early diagnosis and early intervention for vulnerable individuals. As mentioned above, the WHO studies showed that outcomes of schizophrenia varied across different cultures, with patients in developing countries showing a much better outcome than developed counties. Even within the same country, there were differences in rates of broad schizophrenia, which the researchers acknowledged but did not comment on. These observations indicate that rates of narrow schizophrenia were considered roughly similar, although there was a twofold variation in these rates. Interestingly, the proportion of patients who have never been hospitalized is higher in developing countries. This may reflect problems in accessing help, a limited number of beds available for admission, and family support perhaps combined with nonmedical explanatory models seeking help from other sources. But that begs the question about biological interventions and how they affect symptoms. However, the rates and outcomes may well be very different from the original studies, which are now nearly 50 years old. A similar attempt was made to compare the diagnosis of schizophrenia between the US and the UK, as it was believed that due to the preponderance of psychoanalysts in the US, schizophrenia was diagnosed more frequently. This project (Cooper et al., 1972) examined rates of diagnosis for schizophrenia and affective disorders in New York and London and found that case note diagnoses varied, with schizophrenia being much more commonly diagnosed in New York whereas affective disorders were diagnosed less frequently. However, when standardized assessment was applied, these differences disappeared, suggesting that there is a difference between clinical assessment and research tools.

Although old, the WHO outcome study (Jablensky et al., 1992) remains a classic cross-nations comparison. It showed that a subtype of schizophrenia-catatonic schizophrenia was almost ten times more likely to be seen in developing countries than acute onset cases of schizophrenia In the IPSS study, the outcome figures may also have been influenced by selection bias because patients were selected from inpatient units; this issue was overcome in the second study when cases of first presentation were included in the series. However, it is also likely that unless the symptoms are severe, some individuals experiencing their first onset may not seek help for various reasons and thus may not have been counted. Those studies were nearly 5 decades ago and in recent times, a majority of studies have looked at first contact, which can be problematic. Early interventions, although of great interest, also have the problem of potentially overmedicating individuals. Better outcomes in developing countries may reflect genetic environmental interactions. The other potential explanation was the low expressed emotion (hostility, warmth, and critical comments in communication by significant people toward the patient) observed in developing countries (Wig et al., 1987). Thus, it is possible that stress and stressors in different countries may well vary according to cultures and act in different ways. The services need to be reaching out and responding in a culturally appropriate way. Culture bound syndromes were originally described by Yap (1951), who argued that some conditions are specifically bound to certain cultures. A large variety of these syndromes was identified at one point, but DSM-5 counts only nine syndromes. In an increasingly globalized world, the impact of cultures on presentations appears to have changed. Over the decades, other symptoms such as catatonia appear to have declined in Western and high-income countries (Ungvari et al., 2023).

Some striking findings on the rates of various psychiatric disorders come from the UK and the Mental Health Foundation. Its report "Surviving or Thriving" (2017) states that only 13 percent of the population said that they had good mental health. Surprisingly, those over age 55 reported having better mental health, and they were also more likely to work toward it. Those who were unemployed had higher rates of poor mental health, and 40 percent of individuals acknowledged that they had had depression. The Mental Health Foundation concluded that the rates of mental illness among adults exceeded 26 percent, thus arguing that one in four adults will experience a mental illness of one kind or another. This has led to an assumption that this is the case worldwide, which is patently not true because rates vary across countries and cultures. Often, these findings are bandied about in the media and by professionals; the challenge for policymakers is to ensure that local rates are checked and double-checked.

In countries where suicide is deemed an illegal act, for example, it is common for those who attempt suicide or self-harm to hide the act or try to pass it off as an accidental death. In a similar vein, in countries and communities that do not allow alcohol for religious or other reasons, the rates of alcohol misuse are more likely to be inaccurate since people may attempt to hide their behavior out of fear of legal punishment. As mentioned earlier, there is clear research evidence that nearly half of all psychiatric disorders in adulthood start before the age of 15 and three-quarters before the age of

24 (Kessler et al., 2005), although Scott et al. (2018) point out that some disorders such as post-traumatic stress disorder (PTSD), major depressive disorder, and generalized anxiety disorders are likely to start later, in the third decade. Different psychiatric disorders inevitably will have a variable impact on overall individual functioning. Inevitably, some disorders, typically the severe mental illnesses, are much more likely to have a greater impact on functioning than others.

Rates of Specific Disorders: The Findings of the World Mental Health Surveys

Details of the survey method and findings are available in Kessler & Üstün (2008). A selected summary is provided here. Only a few psychiatric disorders will be discussed. Rates of various psychiatric experiences and disorders in the community vary, too. Psychotic experiences—defined as psychotic-like experiences or psychosis-like symptoms—become particularly important because they are seen in a variety of conditions such as schizophrenia/psychosis but also anxiety, mood disorders, and substance use disorders (see McGrath et al., 2018). It has been shown that those with psychotic experiences at baseline are much more likely to be hospitalized in the subsequent two decades (Kaymaz et al., 2012). It has also been shown that individuals who report psychotic experiences are also much more likely to have a significantly higher risk of suicidal ideation, attempts, and intent (Nishida et al., 2010; Saha et al., 2011a, 2011b, 2011c). In their report on the World Mental Health survey, McGrath et al. (2018) report a lifetime prevalence of any psychotic experience as 5.8 percent, any hallucinatory experience as 5.2 percent, and delusional experiences as around 1.3 percent. Psychotic experiences are significantly more common among men than women, as are hallucinatory experiences. Interestingly, these authors note that of the psychotic experiences, the commonest are visual hallucinations followed by auditory hallucinations. The 12-month prevalence among lifetime cases is reported to be highest in low-income countries; as income increases, the prevalence, too, increases.

McGrath et al. (2018) note that 5 percent of all cases would have had a psychotic experience by the age of 8; 25 percent by age 17; 50 percent by age 26; 75 percent by age 41; and 99 percent by age 62. Overall, 5.8 percent of respondents reported having one or more psychotic experiences at least once in their lifetime and 2 percent in the previous year. For the development and delivery of services, the question that needs to be addressed is the proportion of these individuals who may go on to develop and be diagnosed with a psychotic disorder.

Scott et al. (2017) point out the World Mental Health surveys clearly indicate that "there is a great deal of variation in disorder prevalence across countries as well as within each of the three country income groups . . . [in] the average prevalence for any given disorder in each of the three country income groups . . . [with] prevalence being lower in the low/lower middle-income countries than in the higher income countries." This is an observation worth emphasizing because as cultures change and societies move into higher-income status, the rates of mental illness may well increase in some settings. Whether these lower rates in low-income countries genuinely reflect a low prevalence requires further exploration. Therefore, culturally sensitive approaches in assessment, as well as when obtaining epidemiological rates of various mental illnesses, are urgently indicated. Rural settings may have better social capital that could act as a protective factor. Living in sociocentric cultures with a high reliance on community, religion, and spiritual elements may provide some degree of support. Pressures to achieve individual successful may also contribute to heightening stress and the risk of mental illness. Resultantly, with gradual shifts toward egocentrism in many countries, the rates may well increase. Maercker (2001), in a secondary analysis of the WHO data on the prevalence of common mental disorders in primary care, was able to show that rates of many psychiatric conditions are higher in more egocentric countries, as are the rates of crime and divorce.

Suicidal Ideation and Behavior

Suicidal behavior is seen around the globe, even in cultures where the act of suicide may be illegal owing to the influence of British colonial rule, dating back to the Victorian era. In cultures where religion proscribes suicide, acts of suicide do occur but may not be reported as such. WHO (2024) estimated that over 720,000 people around the globe took their lives. Globally, suicides account for 50 percent of all violent deaths in men and 71 percent of all violent deaths in women. Suicide rates are highest in people over the age of 70, with the second highest occurrence in the 15–29 age group. For every suicide, there are many more individuals who attempt suicide every year, and one of the major risk factors for suicide is a previous attempt. The average suicide rate, according to the WHO (2014b), is marginally higher in high-income countries compared to low-income countries, even though there appears to be a variation across countries. Furthermore, even within the same country, there are variations between urban and rural areas and across groups. Three times as many men take their lives in high-income countries in comparison with women, whereas it drops to about 1.5 times in low-income and middle-income countries.

Another study reported that globally, 746,000 deaths from suicide occurred in 2021, including 519,000 deaths among males and 227,000 among females. The age-standardized mortality rate has declined over time, from 14.9 deaths (12.8–15.7) per 100,000 population in 1990 to 9.0 (8.3–9.6) per 100,000 in 2021. Regional differences are striking, with the highest rates in Eastern Europe—19.2 deaths (17.5–20.8) per 100,000. The mean age at which males died from suicide progressively increased during the study period from 43.0 years in 1990 to 47.0 years. Female age increased from 41.9 years to 46.9 years (Global Burden of Diseases Report [GBD], 2025)

Although Islam proscribes suicide, rates have been shown to be higher in women in countries like Bangladesh, Iran, Pakistan, and Turkey (Canetto, 2015). In China, the suicide rates used to be higher for females, but this seems to have changed over the past decade (Zhang et al., 2014). Hjelmeland (2018) notes that rates of suicide are lower among children (especially those under age 15) and highest among the elderly (especially in low-income and middle-income countries). She goes on to caution that the reported rates of suicide need to be explored carefully and treated with caution. Suicide statistics are often underreported because of legal and cultural barriers; where suicide remains criminalized, for instance, it leads to misclassification of deaths as "accidents" or drug disorder deaths (Bakst et al., 2016; Schmeckenbecher et al., 2024). Additionally, family stigma can further complicate reporting especially when religious beliefs play a strong role in shaping attitudes toward suicide (Stack & Kposowa, 2011).

The ingestion of pesticides, hanging, and firearms are the most common methods of suicide globally, but the choice of method will inevitably vary according to the availability of the method, country, age, and culture (WHO, 2014b). There are culturally influenced methods, such as hanging among Aboriginal peoples in Australia and self-burning in Kurdistan and India. As the GBD (2025) study showed, guns are a common means of suicide in the US, Uruguay, and Venezuela, especially among men. The nature of stressful life events and their impact on suicidal acts will also vary across cultures. Vijayakumar et al. (2005) highlight social change as an example of a high-risk factor.

Mental disorders and suicide are often related, although not all cases of suicide have an underlying psychiatric disorder. Between 23 percent and 48 percent of suicides in India and China, respectively, have been shown to involve a psychiatric disorder (Rao et al., 1989; Zhang et al., 2010). In rural China, 39 percent of women who committed suicide had a psychiatric disorder (Yang et al., 2005). Studies from Africa have also indicated a low proportion of psychiatric disorders in cases of suicide (Mars et al., 2014). Hjelmeland (2018) suggests that the high rates reported in studies from the West reflect methodological issues. It is entirely possible that informants in psychological autopsy studies may choose to attribute the event to mental illness rather than other factors. Gender roles and responsibilities are also essential in understanding the consequences of masculinity. Rates of self-harm vary across cultures and ethnic groups. Fortune and Hawton (2018) remind us in their review that rates of self-harm vary not only across countries but also over time.

Bipolar Disorders

Historically, bipolar disorders were identified, classified, and discussed as manic depression. In recent decades, the diagnostic categories have shifted to bipolar disorders. Bipolar disorders are separate from depressive disorders. DSM-5 (American Psychiatric Association [APA], 2013) includes bipolar I, bipolar II, cyclothymic disorders, substance/medication-induced bipolar and related disorders, bipolar disorders resulting from another medical condition, and unspecified disorders.

Bipolar disorders are of three varieties—bipolar I, bipolar II, or subthreshold. Bipolar I consist of either an elevated or depressed mood lasting for at least seven days. Bipolar II is diagnosed when an individual has had episodes of both hypomania and depression, each lasting at least four days. At least one episode of major depressive disorder and at least one episode of hypomania are necessary. Cyclothymic disorders are experienced for at least two years among adults and one year for children and include both hypomanic and depressive periods without ever fulfilling the criteria for an episode of mania, hypomania, or major depression. Using data from

World Mental Health surveys from 21 countries, Kessler et al. (2018) found that the estimated lifetime prevalence of bipolar spectrum disorder averages 1.9 percent across countries. Again, the rates are higher at 2.5 percent in high-income countries, 1.6 percent in upper/middle-income countries, and 1 percent in low/lower middle-income countries. The geographical regions with highest rates are the Americas at 2.8 percent and Europe at 2.3 percent. Median age of onset is in the mid-twenties (around age 24) across nations. Marginally more common in women, bipolar spectrum disorder is also associated with being unmarried. It has been shown that depressive episodes typically have their first onset earlier than hypomanic episodes. Bipolar disorders have also shown significant impairments in functioning.

Major Depressive Disorders

Major depressive disorder is often severe and recurrent with poor role functioning, medical morbidity, and high mortality (often related to suicide or comorbidity with medical conditions such as hypertension, diabetes, and various cancers). The World Health Organization conducted a five-nation survey of depression and found that certain core symptoms of depression, such as sadness, were universal and most frequent across all centers, although even within the same country there was a variation in symptoms (Sartorius et al., 1980; WHO Collaborative Study on Standardized Assessment of Depressive Disorders & Sartorius, 1983). Malhi and Byrow (2018) note that there is a discrepancy between reported prevalence rates of depression, with higher rates observed in Western rather than non-Western cultures. These variations may be the result of biological, psychological, social, and lifestyle factors (Malhi et al., 2015). Major depressive disorders are said to be a Western concept. Various culturally influenced terms are often used to describe listlessness and feeling sad, low, and unhappy. Malhi and Byrow (2018) have argued that there are biological differences between individualistic (egocentric) and collectivist (sociocentric) cultures. There are clear biological/genetic predispositions to major depressive disorders. Furthermore, symptom profiles of depression vary across cultures. In a multination study, Weissman et al. (1996) were able to demonstrate that poor appetite was more common in Lebanon, Taiwan, and Korea; feelings of guilt and worthlessness were more common in New Zealand, the US, Canada, and France, whereas slow thinking was more commonly reported in Canada, Lebanon, Korea, and Taiwan, thus indicating clearly that assessment and recognition of depression varies across cultures. Some countries report higher levels of somatic symptoms. Similarly, Bhugra et al. (1997) from their findings in India noted that symptoms of depression varied even within the same country.

The World Mental Health surveys reported that the average lifetime prevalence of major depressive disorder is 10.6 percent (highest in high-income countries at 12.6 percent, ranging from 21 percent in France to 6.1 percent in Japan). Intermediate rates are reported from upper/middle-income countries at 9.2 percent (Sao Paolo at 16.9 percent and Romania at 2.5 percent), with the lowest rates in low-income countries at 7.1 percent (with Ukraine at 14.6 percent and Nigeria at 3.1 percent). Women are twice as likely (and in high-income countries, three times as likely) to experience major depressive disorders, so special attention must be paid to gender differences in service planning and ensuring that services are appropriate and accessible. In addition, major depressive disorder starts at a younger age in high-income countries. Being outside the workforce also makes individuals more likely to develop major depressive disorders (Paul & Moser, 2009). Thus, a linked-up policy approach is needed to prevent development of major depressive disorders.

Common Mental Disorders

Although the term common mental disorders was widely used a few years ago, its usage has now become less common. However, we use this term to describe a group of disorders that include anxiety, phobias, panic disorders, and other conditions that are common and often treated in primary care settings. The term may also include dissociative disorders, dysthymia, obsessive compulsive disorders, and bodily distress disorders (Desai & Chaturvedi, 2018). These authors suggest that stress (whether ongoing or acute), reactions to such stress, and evidence of being prone to anxiety are important aspects to consider in reaching a diagnosis.

Generalized, free-floating anxiety that is excessive, unrealistic, and accompanied by symptoms of anxiety related to multiple life circumstances is not uncommon. World Mental Health surveys showed a lifetime prevalence of generalized anxiety disorder of 3.7 percent; it is more prevalent in high-income countries and least prevalent in low/lower middle-income countries (Ruscio et al., 2018). It also appears to be accompanied by higher levels of comorbidity and role impairment. Median age of onset is 39 years, although it can begin at age 24–25.

Panic disorders and panic attacks also shows higher levels of prevalence in high-income countries. From the World Mental Health survey data, de Jonge et al. (2018) observe that the lifetime prevalence of panic attacks for all countries combined is 13.2 percent, varying from 2.1 percent to 18.5 percent in low-income countries, 6–20 percent in middle-income countries, and 6.6–27.4 percent in high-income countries. Lifetime prevalence of panic disorder varies from 0.8 percent in low-income countries, 1.1 percent in middle-income countries, and 2.2 percent in high-income countries. Nearly half (46 percent) of those affected by panic disorder show impairment in their functioning. Interestingly, these authors report that lifetime comorbidity with other mental disorders is 80.4 percent. The comorbidity levels are high for other anxiety disorders at 63 percent and mood disorders at 53.7 percent, but lower for substance use disorders at 26 percent. Other vulnerability factors include being under age 60, being female, being unemployed or disabled, being widowed/separated/divorced, and having low levels of education and poor household income.

From the same survey, Roest et al. (2018) report that lifetime prevalence of agoraphobia is 1.2 percent with low prevalence (0.7 percent) in low/lower middle-income countries; higher prevalence at 1.5 percent in upper/middle-income countries; and 1.4 percent in high-income countries. Agoraphobia is a moderately persistent disorder, and 41.9 percent of respondents report severe impairment in any domain (e.g., managing home, job, relationships, or social life).

For agoraphobia, lifetime prevalence in low-income countries is 0.7 percent (with China at 0.2 percent but Colombia at 2.5 percent); in upper/middle-income countries, the average is 1.3 percent (with Lebanon at 0.5 percent and Brazil at 2.9 percent); in high-income countries, the average is 1.4 percent, with 0.3 percent in Japan but 2.4 percent in the US and in Australia. Similarly, the prevalence rates of social anxiety disorder in high-income countries are three times those seen in low-income countries. Rates for low-income countries are at 1.6 percent (a low of 0.2 percent in Nigeria, but 5.0 percent in Colombia); in upper/middle-income countries, the lifetime prevalence is at 2.9 percent (with 0.8 percent in Bulgaria and 5.6 percent in Brazil); and in high- income countries, the average is 5.5 percent (with Japan at 1.4 percent and New Zealand at 9.5 percent). Social anxiety disorder is more likely to be seen in women, the unemployed, the unmarried, and individuals with low income and low educational status (Stein et al., 2018).

Anxiety disorders have a low prevalence in low-income countries, but even among this group, there appears to be a large variation. For example, in Nigeria, the lifetime prevalence is 0.1 percent, but in Iraq it is 5 percent, which should not be a surprise because of external stressful and life events such as wars and conflicts. Among upper/middle-income countries, the lifetime prevalence in Romania is 1 percent, but five times that in Brazil. Among high-income countries, Germany has a prevalence rate of 1.5 percent while Poland is at 0.9 percent; way ahead are the US (7.8 percent), Australia (8 percent), and New Zealand (7.9 percent).

Lifetime panic disorder is at 6.4 percent in low-income countries (with Nigeria at 2.6 percent but Colombia at 18.5 percent). In upper-middle-income countries, the average lifetime prevalence of the disorder is 11.1 percent, with Bulgaria at 6 percent and Colombia at 20 percent.

Related to anxiety are specific phobias that are characterized by the presence of a significant level of anxiety related to a specific object, situation, or stimulus. This contributes to fear and avoidance and immediate anxiety response. Wardenaar et al. (2018), reporting on the World Mental Health survey findings, found that lifetime prevalence is 5.7 percent in low-income countries (with low rates of 2.6 percent in parts of China and 12.5 percent in Colombia). In upper/middle-income countries, lifetime prevalence goes up to 8 percent (with 3.8 percent in Romania and 12.5 percent in Brazil). The lifetime prevalence increases marginally to 8.1 percent in high-income countries—for instance, 3.4 percent in Japan and in Poland but 12.5 percent in the US. Specific phobias are more common in females, retirees, households with low incomes, and those with low educational status, and 18.7 percent of individuals with specific phobias show role impairment in one of the domains.

Substance Use Disorders

Homo sapiens has experimented with, consumed, and misused a large variety of psychoactive chemicals over the millennia. The earliest record of beer brewing is from 13,000 years ago (Liu et al., 2018). The use and misuse of various substances including alcohol is strongly influenced by culture and cultural values. For example, the use of some stimulants like *khat* may well be limited to certain communities, whereas alcohol use is likely to be universal, except for countries where alcohol is prohibited by religious rules or political decisions on prohibition. While substance misuse and addictions represent a considerable burden of illness globally, there are national and cultural differences in prevalence rates, reflecting availability, affordability, legality, and cultural and individual factors.

Psychoactive substances are used across the globe, though the prevalence rates of different substance abuse and use vary across countries. In addition, their legal statuses are in a state of flux in many countries. The *World Drug Report* (United Nations Office on Drugs and Crime [UNODC], 2024) indicated that over 292 million people used an illicit drug in 2022. An estimated 39.5 million people around the globe are drug dependent or have drug use disorders, a figure revised upwards from 27 million in 2013 (UNODC, 2023). Only 1 in 5 of these individuals receive treatment (UNODC, 2024). The annual death rate from drug abuse is estimated to exceed 200,000 per annum, reflecting the growing impact of synthetic opioids and other drugs.

Nicotine, in the form of tobacco or synthetic nicotine, is the second-most used psychoactive substance globally. It is also legal and normally regulated. Tobacco use is associated with nicotine dependence and many forms of cancer. Synthetic nicotine, typically in the form of "vapes," is also dependence-inducing, and other health effects are as yet unknown. Nearly a billion people around the world use tobacco, although the usage is beginning to fall in some parts of the world and increasing in others. According to the World Health Organization (WHO), tobacco use kills more than 8 million people each year, including an estimated 1.3 million nonsmokers who are exposed to secondhand smoke. Approximately 80 percent of the world's 1.3 billion tobacco users live in low-income and middle-income countries (WHO, 2021c,d). Paradoxically, alcohol and tobacco both contribute a significant amount of revenue to most governments around the world.

The continuum of substance use and misuse remains of great interest in epidemiological studies. Normal use versus dependence, on the one hand, and disorder, on the other, are important in our understanding of what is needed in service planning and delivery. Using data from the World Mental Health surveys, Degenhardt et al. (2018) reported on drug use disorder, drug abuse, and drug dependence and noted that lifetime prevalence rates of drug abuse are lower in low-income countries, almost five times higher in high-income countries, and somewhere in the middle in upper/middle-income countries. Rates of drug dependence are also low in low-income countries and nearly six times higher in high-income countries. Similar observations occur related to drug use disorder (Castaldelli-Maia & Bhugra, 2022).

In high-income countries, the median age of onset for alcohol use typically ranges from 16 to 19 years, whereas in low- and middle-income countries, the age of initiation has traditionally been later (Degenhardt et al., 2018). However, there is a trend toward younger age groups (Kassew et al., 2023), which may reflect changes in cultures. Substance use disorders can lead to complex comorbidities as well as social burdens, criminal activities, and behaviors that contribute to the burden on health care. Decriminalization of certain drugs may increase the likelihood that criminal behavior will decline, while improved control over the quality of available substances could lead to fewer medical complications (Rêgo et al., 2021). However, there is an urgent need for data on the long-term impact of decriminalization.

Substance use disorders have many similarities with alcohol use disorder. Illicit opiate use can lead to dependence, resulting in an increasing burden of disease and creating problems not only medically but also in other spheres of an individual's functioning (Degenhardt et al., 2019). In the US, the opioid epidemic, driven by the overprescription of opioid painkillers, increased the availability of synthetic opioids like fentanyl, and rising heroin use has led to a significant public health crisis marked by high rates of addiction, overdose deaths, and economic burden (CDC, 2024b). Harm reduction strategies aim to minimize the negative health and social consequences of substance use without necessarily requiring abstinence. Marlatt (1998) pioneered the harm reduction model, advocating for safe injection sites and opioid substitution therapies. Babor et al. (2010) provide evidence that medication-assisted treatment (e.g., methadone, buprenorphine) significantly reduces overdose deaths and promotes long-term recovery from opioid use disorder.

Many non-opioid, non-cannabis, non-alcohol substances can significantly impact mental health, including stimulants (e.g., cocaine, methamphetamine), hallucinogens (e.g., LSD, psilocybin), inhalants, and benzodiazepines. Chronic stimulant use is linked to psychosis, paranoia, depression, and cognitive impairment (SAMHSA, 2021). Hallucinogens can trigger transient psychotic episodes or hallucinogen-persisting perception disorder (HPPD) in some users (Martinotti et al., 2018). Inhalant abuse is associated with neurotoxicity, depression, and cognitive deficits (Radparvar, 2023). Benzodiazepine misuse can lead to dependence, emotional blunting, and increased risk of suicide (Votaw et al., 2019).

The rise of synthetic drugs, such as synthetic cannabinoids ("spice") and fentanyl analogues, has introduced new psychiatric risks, including psychosis, severe withdrawal symptoms, and increased overdose mortality (Stoicea et al., 2019; Schifano et al., 2021). Synthetic cannabinoids and their chemical analogues may induce acute psychotic episodes, particularly in individuals with preexisting psychiatric vulnerabilities (Every-Palmer, 2011; Fantegrossi et al., 2018).

A co-occurring disorder, also known as a dual diagnosis, refers to the simultaneous presence of a mental health disorder and a substance use disorder that interact in complex ways, often worsening outcomes and requiring integrated treatment approaches (National Institute on Drug Abuse [NIDA], 2024). The comorbidity of drug misuse disorders and other psychiatric disorders is considerable, and the interaction between substance use disorder and psychiatric disorder is important in the management of both disorders. Their specialist management is outside the scope of this book. Similarly, substance use and substance use disorders are a vast area of knowledge, and the interested reader is encouraged to read specialized works related to substance use and public mental health (Babor, 2010; WHO, 2021b) and clinical treatments (El-Guebaly et al., 2015; Ruiz & Strain, 2021) in addition to the references in this text.

Alcohol Misuse

The sale and use of alcohol is legal in most countries and plays a sociocultural role in many communities (Sudhinaraset et al., 2016). Alcohol is one of the most common legal addictive substances that is widely available in a variety of forms, strengths, and culturally sanctioned venues (e.g., pubs and restaurants). Patterns of drinking are influenced by personal and cultural factors. However, the Global Burden of Disease study (GBD, 2018) reported that, globally, alcohol use was the seventh leading risk factor for both deaths and DALYs, accounting for 2.2 percent to 6.8 percent of age-standardized female and male deaths, respectively. This study also demonstrated that the safest level of drinking is none, contrary to most national health guidelines that claim moderate drinking offers health benefits. The WHO (2023) declared that no level of alcohol consumption is safe for our health. Drinking alcohol and driving under the influence can lead to accidental injuries; chronic alcohol misuse can cause cardiovascular and hepatic diseases and nervous system damage.

Drinking has been described at different levels: hazardous, harmful, and dependent. WHO (1993) defined alcohol dependence as meeting at least three of the following criteria: strong desire or compulsion to take alcohol; impaired control and physiological withdrawal if intake is reduced or stopped; tolerance; preoccupation with use; and persistent use despite harmful consequences. The DSM-5 (APA, 2013) integrated the concepts of alcohol abuse and dependence into alcohol use disorder (AUD) with mild, moderate, and severe classifications.

It has been estimated that per capita, consumption of alcohol has increased in most regions of the world (WHO, 2014c), although there are clear geographical differences. Glantz et al. (2018) point out that annual per capita alcohol consumption in France and Australia is 12.2 liters of pure alcohol, but the lifetime prevalence of alcohol use disorder is only 7.1 percent in France and 22.7 percent in Australia, indicating that cultural attitudes about alcohol and patterns of binge drinking may play a role.

The average lifetime prevalence of AUD is around 6.2 percent, varying from 0.5 percent in Iraq to 18.7 percent in Australia (Glantz et al., 2018). These authors note that following the World Mental Health surveys, the average 12-month AUD prevalence is 1.3 percent, ranging from 0.1 percent in Iraq to 1.7 percent in Ukraine. The average lifetime prevalence rates of alcohol abuse, alcohol use disorder, and alcohol dependence are higher among high-income countries and the median age of onset is between 16–20 years. Men are almost five times more likely than women to develop a lifetime AUD. The earlier the age of first use, the more likelihood of developing alcohol disorder.

Alcohol use is also highly comorbid with other psychiatric disorders, so treating services need to be carefully crafted to address both issues. Preventive strategies include a reduction in advertising and increased taxation on alcohol (WHO, 2018; Babor et al., 2010), which are important legislative actions any government can take. However, governments are often reluctant to do so, mostly because of the tax revenues generated. Advice and education about alcohol and dependence work very well as interventions to reduce heavy drinking (Knox et al., 2019). Various harm reduction approaches, such as minimum pricing policies, controlled alcohol distribution centers, and early intervention programs, have demonstrated mixed success depending on socioeconomic and policy contexts (Kilian et al., 2023). For example, Scotland's minimum unit pricing (implemented in 2018) led to a measurable reduction in alcohol-related hospital admissions (Holmes, 2023). In addition gambling as an addiction needs detailed evaluation.

Learning and Developmental Disabilities

In many countries, people with an intellectual disability (ID) are known as having a "mental handicap," "mental retardation," or "learning disability," all terms with potential stigmatizing associations. It is important to use a uniform term such as "intellectual disability" because this is probably the least stigmatizing and most descriptive. Learning and developmental disabilities include functional limitations often manifesting in infancy or childhood due to disorders or injury to the developing nervous system (Institute of Medicine Committee on Nervous System Disorders in Developing Countries, 2001). Inevitably, some forms of these disabilities are very mild, whereas others can be severe. The known causes of these disabilities are many and include genetic, infectious, toxic exposures, nutritional factors, and perinatal factors (Durkin et al., 2006). Rates of learning and developmental disabilities in high-income countries are said to be between 10–20 percent of children (Benedict & Farel, 2003). With improving child survival in low- and middle-income countries, it is difficult to be certain whether rates are going up or remain static.

People with ID have a higher risk of comorbid neurological and psychiatric disorders, including mood, anxiety, psychotic, and impulse control disorders (Pinals et al, 2022a). There are specific factors for these disabilities that can add to the burden of disease. These conditions are lifelong and will also likely affect educational attainment and employment prospects. Many of these disabilities can be prevented, and governments need to take this task on by investing in better control of communicable diseases and better perinatal health services, providing appropriate information on diet during pregnancy, and reducing exposure to environmental pollutants and toxins. Durkin et al. (2006) provide a useful road map for ID prevention strategies; for example, the simple addition of folic acid to the diet can help reduce rates of neural tube defects by up to 50 percent, thus making this a useful primary prevention tool.

Zisman-Ilani (2022) reminds readers of the "years of neglect, structural discrimination, and maltreatment of individuals with ID disorders." Moreover, even within mental health services, people with ID frequently encounter professionals with limited ID literacy, coupled with minimal training concerning their needs and treatment modalities. Consequently, these individuals are often misdiagnosed and prescribed psychiatric medications, while nonpharmacologic supports—such as social prescribing, behavioral and educational interventions, or psychotherapy—are insufficiently utilized (Pinals et al, 2022a, b). In many countries around the world, specialist services are not available or easily accessible, and families often struggle to manage children as well as adults with intellectual disability. These groups may also have associated neurological disorders that complicate access to therapeutic interventions. Resources and training are needed to develop a comprehensive service delivery system for working with persons with ID with and without co-occurring mental illness (Pinals et al, 2022b).

Other Vulnerable Groups

Many vulnerable groups have shown higher than average rates of psychiatric disorders, and often these groups are underserved populations. Vulnerable individuals are those who may be socioeconomically disadvantaged, homeless, or medically ill individuals; people living with HIV/AIDS; women and children in general, but especially those who may have been victims of sexual abuse or interpersonal violence; lesbian, gay, bisexual, transgender, and queer (LGBTQ+) people; migrants, refugees, and asylum seekers; Indigenous people in many parts of the world; prisoners; and ethnic or other minority groups in the national context (also see WHO, 2022c, 2022e). Each country should clearly identify vulnerable groups in the context of their national characteristics and context and make suitable and appropriate allowances to ensure that they receive care according to their needs.

Children

Even though retrospective historical data confirm a correlation between childhood abuse (sexual, physical, and emotional) and psychiatric disorders in adulthood, data on abuse and neglect can be difficult to obtain and confirm. As noted earlier, adverse childhood experiences and adverse early life events can contribute to mental ill-health in adolescence and adulthood. As mentioned, half of psychiatric disorders in adulthood start before the age of 15, and three-quarters begin before the age of 24. Children and young adults are at an increased risk of certain psychiatric disorders and suicide (see the previous section on suicidal ideation and behavior). Risk factors for children's mental health problems can be divided into those associated with the children themselves, their families, schools, and communities.

Risk factors for children Genetic influences, intellectual disabilities, chronic medical illnesses, developmental delays, and autism spectrum disorders are all risk factors that contribute to poor academic performance and subsequently affect self-esteem. Secure attachment, a positive attitude, and achievement can serve as protective factors.

Risk factors for family Parental mental illness, family disharmony, inconsistent discipline or parenting, parental discord, sexual abuse, physical or emotional neglect, poor role models, insufficient social support, parental death or loss, caregiving responsibilities, and parental criminal behavior are significant vulnerability factors. While it is theoretically highly likely that these factors have a cumulative effect, further analysis is needed. Family support, stability, and harmony—along with strong values, consistent messaging, support for education, and recognition of achievement—may help to mitigate some of these issues.

Risk factors for school Bullying, discrimination, lack of friendships, peer pressure, poor teaching, and ambivalent relationships with teachers are all potential risk factors. In contrast, a positive atmosphere in school, fostering a sense of belonging, peer support, and friendships that encourage participation in physical activities—along with safe spaces where children and young people can voice their concerns and receive support—should be regarded as protective factors.

Risk factors in the community These include social inequalities such as family unemployment, homelessness, a lack of green spaces, overcrowding, and a significant deficiency in support. High levels of discrimination can be viewed as potential risk factors. Conversely, a strong sense of purpose and belonging, reasonable living standards, positive social roles and role models, and a variety of leisure activities can serve as protective factors. Increasingly, the role of social media is understood as a risk factor for poor mental health in children (see chapter 8).

Women

Women are at a higher risk of mental illnesses such as depression, anxiety, and PTSD because of the complex interplay of biological, social, and structural factors (also see WHO 2022c). Gender inequality plays a significant role, as women are more likely to experience poverty, domestic violence, unpaid caregiving burdens, and workplace discrimination, all of which contribute to psychological distress (Seedat et al., 2009). Socioeconomic disparities limit access to mental health resources, while cultural norms may discourage help-seeking behaviors among women in certain societies (WHO, 2022i). Additionally, gendered expectations and exposure to gender-based violence increase the prevalence of trauma-related disorders (Oram et al., 2017).

Women are also more likely than men to be carers of both children and elders in many countries, thus adding to their burden This may be further compounded in more patriarchal societies and cultures where women may not have equal rights and face further discrimination on the basis of gender, gender roles, and gender role expectations. Often, this discrimination gets compounded by other factors such as fertility, caste, religion, sexual orientation, age, and socioeconomic disadvantage. Addressing gender inequality is essential for improving women's mental health outcomes, highlighting the need for policies that promote gender equity, economic empowerment, and access to mental health care. The scope of gender and mental health is vast. Interested readers are encouraged to read the 2022 textbook by Hutner and colleagues.

LGBTQ+ Individuals

In a number of countries around the globe, same-sex behavior is deemed a criminal act that is even punishable by death in some countries. LGBTQ+ individuals are often discriminated against at several levels, even in more liberal societies. As mentioned previously, numerous epidemiological studies confirm that these groups have higher rates of psychiatric disorders when compared with majority populations (Bhugra et al., 2022). Recent meta-analyses indicate that LGBTQ+ individuals are twice as likely to experience mental health conditions such as depression and anxiety compared to heterosexual and cisgender individuals (Malik et al., 2023). For instance, rates of depression among LGBTQ+ individuals have been shown to range from 30 percent to 60 percent, compared to approximately 10 percent to 20 percent in the general population (Ross et al., 2018; Semlyen et al., 2016). Similarly, the risk of suicide attempts is estimated to be four times higher in LGBTQ+ youth than in their heterosexual peers (Haas et al., 2011).

The elevated prevalence of mental illness within this group is closely linked to experiences of inequality, social exclusion, and discrimination, collectively referred to as minority stress (Meyer, 2003). Chronic exposure to stigma and prejudice, alongside internalized homophobia and transphobia, has been shown to contribute to poorer mental health outcomes (Russell & Fish, 2016). Importantly, research has demonstrated that these rates of psychiatric disorders tend to decline following the implementation of legislative changes that promote equality and inclusion. For example, in the years following the legalization of same-sex marriage in the United States, studies observed a decline in depressive symptoms and psychological distress among LGBTQ+ populations (Hatzenbuehler et al., 2012). These findings suggest that structural and legal protections play a critical role in improving mental health outcomes for LGBTQ+ individuals.

Ethnic Minorities

Long-established ethnic minority groups in Western countries often experience systemic racism that affects their mental health. Williams and Mohammed (2009) found that racial discrimination contributes to increased rates of depression, anxiety, and stress-related disorders. Schwartz and Blankenship (2014) showed that white psychiatrists are more likely to overdiagnose psychosis in Black patients, which may in part explain the higher rates of involuntary commitment and incarceration among Black men (Shea et al., 2022). Implicit bias in clinical settings has been shown to result in misdiagnosis and inadequate treatment for racial minorities (Hall et al., 2015).

Additionally, structural racism limits access to culturally sensitive mental health care, exacerbating disparities in outcomes (Bailey et al., 2017). In the UK, people with Black and African Caribbean ethnicity are overrepresented in mental health services, experience worse outcomes, and are over four times more likely to be detained under the Mental Health Act than white individuals (McKenzie & Bhui, 2007). Research indicates that compared with people who are white, Black and Indigenous people of color (BIPOC) are less likely to seek out and have access to mental health services and more likely to receive poor quality care (Williams, 2018). In the US, which is a high-income country, BIPOC have been disproportionately affected by the nationwide post-COVID increases in drug overdose and suicide deaths, and disparities in mental health care by race and ethnicity persist (Kaiser Family Foundation [KFF], 2023). Barriers to mental health care for ethnic minorities in the US include cost, difficulties finding providers with shared background and experiences, lack of information, stigma, and embarrassment (KFF, 2023).

The underlying reasons for these stark racial inequities are complex and cut across racism, stigma, individual and cultural trauma, socioeconomic disadvantage, "othering," and the legacy of colonialism (all described in different sections of this book). In his 1952 seminal text *Black Skin, White Masks*, Frantz Fanon analyzed how colonial subjugation led to feelings of inferiority and identity crises among the colonized, using psychoanalytic theory to explore the internalization of racism and its detrimental effects on mental health. He argued that the colonized individual's adoption of the colonizer's culture resulted in a fractured self-perception and mental distress. This possibility, combined with other social stressors and factors, may contribute to higher rates of psychiatric disorders in these vulnerable populations.

Migrants

Migrants, refugees and asylum seekers have shown higher than average rates of psychiatric disorders (Bhugra & Gupta, 2010). Here, too, socioeconomic and social discrimination can contribute to these higher rates. Migrant populations have a disproportionately higher risk of schizophrenia, with studies suggesting social stressors, discrimination, and genetic predispositions as contributing factors (Cantor-Graae & Selten, 2005). Acculturation stress, particularly in second-generation migrants, has been linked to an increased incidence of psychotic disorders (Bardol et al., 2020). However, this seems to indicate that it is the individual's fault, which is not really the case as negative attitudes, prejudice, and nonacceptance toward migrants further exacerbates the situation affecting migrants. People from refugee and asylum-seeking backgrounds have compounding risks for poor mental and physical health. For a deeper look at migrant mental health, readers may consider Bhugra and Gupta's 2010 textbook or the *Oxford Textbook of Migrant Psychiatry* (Bhugra, 2021).

Individuals with Intellectual Disability

Individuals with an intellectual or learning disability, whether children or adults, show higher than expected rates of mental illnesses (Cooper et al., 2007). Often borderline intellectual disability is not diagnosed, compounding the problem. Specialized services combined with pediatric or adult neurologists, educationalists, physiotherapists, occupational therapists, and others must form the core of service delivery targeting this group.

Older Adults

Mental ill-health in later life includes various types of dementia. As the average lifespan is increasing, rates of dementia are going up, too. People older than age 60 form 11 percent of the population, and this figure is expected to double to 22 percent by 2050. Those age 80 and older form 1.6 percent of the population, which is likely to rise to 4.3 percent by 2050 (UNFPA, 2012). The Mental Health Foundation (MHF, 2015b) provides collated figures for various disorders and estimates that the number of people living with dementia worldwide is 44 million—and it is likely to double by 2030 (Prince et al., 2014). In addition to discrimination, other key factors affecting the mental health and well-being of older people were identified as participation in meaningful activities, relationships, physical health, and poverty (Lee, 2006). Obviously, these factors will vary across cultures and societies, but it is imperative that all nations plan according to their needs. Systems must be in place to identify, help, and support individuals in later life who may be living with multiple comorbidities. Again, in many countries, older adults may be living alone, whereas in other countries, families carry the burden, and filial piety plays a major role. In each case, specific pressures emerge and need to be identified. Older people are also more likely to suffer from physical ill-health. Social support, especially from family and friends, is an important factor assisting older adults to be physically active (Smith et al., 2017). The neighborhood environment and loneliness have been reported to be important factors in contributing to morbidities in this age group (MHF, 2015a). Minority older adults may thus face double or triple jeopardy in seeking help. Chandra et al. (2006) point out that current rates of Alzheimer's disease are lower in low- and middle-income countries, but this is likely to change. It may be that either there are some protective factors or people do not live long enough for symptoms to emerge, or dementias may be conflated with aging.

Carers

In the vast majority of cases, family members—often women and sometimes parents or children—take care of the individuals with mental illnesses and carry the burden of care. Some families look after elders with physical and psychiatric conditions even when it may be difficult and the care is full-time. Many cultures see it as a filial duty. Often, the contribution such individuals make does not receive due recognition. Looking after a family member with mental ill-health can have a significant impact on a carer's own mental health. Younger carers may have to give up school and education as well as employment opportunities. It is essential that enough resources are dedicated to looking after the carers.

Caregiving for individuals with mental illness is associated with high levels of emotional distress, financial strain, and social isolation. Schulz and Sherwood (2008) identified caregiver burden as a major public health issue, advocating for targeted interventions such as counseling and respite care. Pinquart and Sörensen (2003) demonstrate that structured support programs improve caregiver well-being and reduce burnout. Minimum standards for information for carers are outlined in appendix 10.

The Burden of Mental Illnesses

This figure of one in eight mentioned earlier includes not only severe mental illness but also common mental disorders, including psychosexual problems, substance use disorders, and personality disorders. Recent observations suggest that the number of people with mental illnesses is on the rise in many countries, with a notable increase during the COVID pandemic (Winkler et al., 2020; Wu et al., 2023). It is likely that the burden on health care will also rise proportionately in these countries. It has been suggested that in the UK, the burden caused by mental illnesses is higher than for cancer and heart disease (Ferrari et al., 2013). Prevalence rates of some mental illnesses around the globe have been further described earlier in this chapter.

Hessel (2008) defines the term "burden of disease" as the total cumulative consequences of a defined disease or a group of diseases, considering health, social aspects, and costs to society. The gap between an ideal situation where everyone lives free of disease and disability and the cumulated current health status is the burden of disease. In 1990, the first study on the Global Burden of Disease looked at the health effects of more than 100 diseases and injuries in eight regions of the world (World Bank, 1993; Murray & Lopez, 1996a, 1996b). Age, sex, and regions were studied, and consistent estimates were generated (Murray & Lopez, 1996c). The study also introduced the concept of disability adjusted life years (DALYs), defined as years of life lost from premature death and years of life lived in less than full health. Estimates suggest that the worldwide economic cost of mental illness stands at around US$5 trillion (Arias et al., 2022). The authors indicated that in 2019, mental disorders were responsible for approximately 418 million DALYs, representing 16 percent of global DALYs. This figure likely contributed to about 4 percent of the gross domestic product in eastern sub-Saharan Africa and up to 8 percent in high-income North America.

In an overview, Hyman et al. (2006) highlight both attributable and avoidable burden of psychiatric conditions globally. The psychiatric conditions discussed were both major severe mental illnesses such as schizophrenia, other non-affective psychoses, and mood disorders (bipolar affective disorder and major depressive disorder), as well as common mental disorders such as anxiety, phobias, and panic disorders. These authors confirm that public-level interventions can and indeed do reduce the burden of disease. They indicate that the most cost-effective strategy for reducing the burden of severe mental illnesses such as psychosis and severe affective disorder is the use of possibly the lowest-cost drugs available in conjunction with psychosocial rehabilitation. Thus, using cheap medications (typically generic brands) in comparison with no medication would benefit more patients in low-income countries. The authors remind us that developing mental health policy for the nation is the first step in looking after the mental health of the population.

Conclusion

This brief overview of epidemiological data suggests that psychiatric disorders occur in all countries and settings, and their presentations may differ somewhat. This indicates that cultures and societies may well play a role in presentation, identification and help-seeking. Policymakers must be made aware of the prevalence and incidence of psychiatric disorders to ensure that sufficient resources are available. This will also enable policymakers to work with clinicians and public mental health officials to develop public mental health messages for mental illness prevention and mental health promotion. Clear linking of public mental health initiatives and design and delivery of psychiatric services is important, as is input from primary care and social care. Cultural values must be taken into account, bearing in mind that cultures in many parts of the world are in transition.

6 Public Mental Health

Introduction

Public mental health deals with population-based approaches to deliver better well-being and functioning. Any comprehensive mental health approaches must aim at reducing the likelihood of developing future mental health problems, reducing stigma around mental illnesses, and supporting recovery from mental ill-health. The aim of public mental health strategies is to improve mental health and well-being of society at a broader level through identification and elimination of social determinants of poor mental health, bearing in mind that these are strongly influenced by supranational geopolitical factors.

As mentioned in earlier chapters, it is essential that all countries must do an impact assessment of all their policies on the mental health and well-being of their populations. This process also needs to be fully supported by integrating public health (including mental health) measurements across the lifespan.

As noted in the introductory chapter, mental health and well-being can often mean different things to different people. Public mental health, an often-neglected element of public health practice, spans mental health promotion, prevention of mental illness, effective (evidence-based) early treatments, proper care, and recovery. Mental health should be seen as a spectrum, from mental health problems, conditions, illnesses, and disorders (as well as mental ill-health) through to well-being or positive mental health (LFPH & MHF, 2016), although a dual continuum is used to explain that psychiatric disorders per se do not exclude mental well-being and that a lack of diagnosis does not guarantee mental well-being. For instance, individuals who have certain psychiatric diagnoses may be mentally well in between episodes of illness.

In many low-income countries, public health is an integral part of undergraduate teaching, but often the focus remains on communicable diseases and nutrition rather than on public mental health. Public mental health includes prevention of mental illnesses and mental health promotion. Mental health promotion aims to encourage development and maintenance of well-being within communities that are connected, caring, content, and confident. Communities must have these characteristics to survive and flourish. Primordial prevention focuses on risk reduction with a focus on social and environmental conditions that can be influenced through laws and policies. For example, broader pavements or sidewalks encourage walking, and cycle lanes allow people to cycle safely. These measures can also reduce the likelihood of people developing diabetes, hypertension, and other conditions. Primary prevention is related to the promotion of well-being and reducing the likelihood of developing mental illnesses by focusing on vulnerable individuals. The focus is on reducing risk exposure. Needle exchange is one example. Secondary prevention focuses on early detection, especially in vulnerable groups, and offers evidence-based interventions. Tertiary prevention involves managing people with mental illnesses and enabling their rehabilitation to minimize further illnesses. Quaternary prevention focuses on preventing overmedicalization. The well-being of the population and those who care for people with mental illness is of paramount importance.

Well-being is determined by genetics, early childhood factors such as parenting, attachment patterns, adverse childhood experiences, personality factors, age, gender, marital status along with maternal well-being, employment status, intentional activities such as regular exercise, emotional and social literacy, self-esteem, and autonomy (Gautam et al., 2024). Various steps in promoting well-being include identification of the groups who should be involved in formulating the solutions. Addressing the root causes, especially those which are social determinants (e.g., unemployment, poor housing, overcrowding) is crucial in developing well-being. Developing appropriate and suitable strategies at all levels is important. Well-being approaches should be developed, maintained, and delivered across the lifespan. This life course approach (table 6.1) needs to start at an early age. Promoting good parental health, reducing parental alcohol abuse, addressing interpersonal domestic violence, preventing bullying at school, mitigating adverse childhood experiences, increasing physical activity and exercise, and helping build self-awareness and resilience are all important steps. These social interventions can play a significant role in optimizing well-being. Mental health promotion is vital in improving population mental health (WHO 2008).

Mental health and mental ill-health are not two ends of the same spectrum; they are interrelated and not either/or exclusive. The model of mental well-being and mental health can be seen in multiple ways. This is a multidimensional model and may require modification across different cultures depending on sociocultural factors. The concept of mental well-being, too, is multidimensional. It includes attitudes and behaviors toward oneself, toward others, and toward the environment and community at several levels. This positive state can be identified and recognized at personal, community, local, regional, national, and international levels. Feeling positive toward oneself and others at kinship, community, and group levels is important for individuals to function effectively in achieving their own personal goals and meeting community norms. This sense of purpose can foster supportive relationships and a strong sense of belonging and feeling connected, content, and confident, while also creating communities where people feel cared for.

Well-being and (positive) mental health are influenced by biopsychosocial factors. Of these, social factors are perhaps the most important and may impact other factors. Biological factors are both genetic and environmentally influenced. Parenting and parenting skills influence brain structures and brain development. Gender also plays an important role. It is likely that psychological factors include personality, cognitive abilities, emotional frameworks, and relaxation activities. Social factors include stress, socioeconomic factors, spirituality, life events, social capital, and social networks. Again, it is entirely possible that these factors may act in isolation or have a cumulative effect, especially if individuals are vulnerable because of genetic and other biological factors. Table 6.1 illustrates some potential interventions for public mental health across the life span. Interaction of social determinants and other vulnerability factors can play a significant role in improving mental health of populations.

Positive mental health and well-being can improve physical health and relationships and functioning in areas such as education, achievement, employment, productivity, and crime reduction. Furthermore, these

Table 6.1
Potential intervention measures across the life course

Stage	Individual interventions	Structural intervention
Prenatal and early childhood	Maternal mental health screening and support, nutrition supplements (e.g., folic acid), early parenting programs (Fisher et al., 2020)	Maternity/paternity leave policies, universal health care access, poverty reduction programs (WHO, 2021a)
Childhood	Social and emotional learning programs in schools, cognitive behavioral interventions for at-risk youth, parental training (Patel et al., 2018)	Anti-bullying laws and programs, school mental health services, access to health care and social services (Durlak et al., 2011)
Young people	Same as indicated for childhood, plus interventions for alcohol and drug misuse, sex education, and vulnerable groups such as LGBTQ+ individuals, those with intellectual disabilities, BIPOC	Reducing adverse childhood experiences Reducing alcohol use, violence, unemployment, overcrowding, and other social determinants
Adults	Building resilience, workplace mental health initiatives, stress management programs, mindfulness-based interventions (Harvey et al., 2021) Interventions to reduce smoking, alcohol, and drug use Social connection Healthy relationships	Flexible working conditions, social welfare programs, antidiscrimination laws (Lund et al., 2010) Improved economic activity, employment/training/meaningful activity Social connection Optimal nutrition, physical exercise, physical health
Older adults	Cognitive training, physical activity programs, social engagement activities (Livingston et al., 2020) Early detection and intervention in dementias	Same as indicated for adults, plus age-friendly urban planning, pension security, policies supporting social inclusion (WHO, 2021a)

Note: BIPOC, Black and Indigenous people of color; LGBTQ+, lesbian, gay, bisexual, transgender, and queer plus.

activities will inevitably contribute to better resilience and adjustment to stressors, leading to a positive impact on society and improved social and community functioning. Improved well-being of the population contributes to several spheres (box 6.1). These spheres are interconnected and influence each other in a bidirectional and indeed a multidirectional way. Positive mental health and well-being influence and produce social functioning and reduce social disability and antisocial behavior.

Good mental health is the key to overall better health, social and economic functioning of the individual, and society as a whole (WHO, 2022i). Good mental health is not simply the absence of mental illness. Box 6.1 illustrates factors for population well-being. Campion et al. (2012) highlight various factors associated with good mental health (see box 6.2). For purposes of mental health promotion and the prevention of mental illness, various protective and risk factors need to be considered. These are illustrated in box 6.3 and table 6.2.

These protective factors may help reduce the rates of various psychiatric disorders but may also support prevention approaches and help reduce the burden of disease as well as the severity of illness if it cannot be eliminated altogether. Risk factors are listed in table 6.2, but this is not a complete and exhaustive list and should be seen as indicative.

It is worth noting that these risk factors may also have a cumulative effect, especially in the face of adversity and biological vulnerabilities,

Box 6.1
Population Well-Being and Its Impact

- Improved cognitive abilities
- Better educational achievements
- Better employment opportunities
- Improved socioeconomic status
- Better physical health
- Lower antisocial behavior
- Reduced levels of suicide
- Better quality of life
- Reduced burden of health care
- Reduced absenteeism and presentism

Box 6.2
Factors Associated with Good Mental Health

- Improved educational attainment
- Improved productivity
- Reduced rates of sickness
- Improved cognitive ability
- Better physical health
- Reduced mortality
- Increased social participation
- Reduced risk of suicide
- Reduced risk-taking (e.g., smoking, alcohol, substances, gambling)
- Improved resilience to adversity

Box 6.3
Protective Factors Against Mental Illness

- Genetic factors
- Maternal perinatal health
- Parenting sills
- Personality factors
- Age, gender, marital status
- Social determinants, especially equality
- Socioeconomic and educational factors
- Employment
- Social capital and belonging
- Self-esteem, autonomy
- Emotional intelligence
- Physical health and well-being

Table 6.2
Broad risk factors for developing mental illness

Life stage	Biological factors	Psychosocial factors	Environmental factors
Prenatal & early childhood	Genetic predisposition, maternal stress, poor prenatal nutrition, birth complications (Gottesman & Shields, 1967; Cannon et al., 2002; Talge, et al., 2007; Van Os & Kapur, 2009)	Parental mental illness, neglect, adverse childhood experiences, growing up in care (Felitti et al., 1998; Patel et al., 2018)	Exposure to toxins, inadequate prenatal care, maternal malnutrition, poverty (Buss et al., 2012; WHO, 2021a)
Childhood & adolescence	Neurodevelopmental disorders, early childhood trauma, malnutrition (Green et al., 2010; Kessler et al., 2010)	Poor parenting, bullying, academic stress, family dysfunction, peer rejection, substance misuse, minority stress (BIPOC, LGBTQ+) (Durlak et al., 2011; Arseneault, 2018)	Neighborhood violence, unsafe housing, poor education, inequality and discrimination (Leventhal & Brooks-Gunn, 2000; Reiss, 2013)
Adulthood	Chronic illness, hormonal changes, substance use (Lund et al., 2010; Kendler et al., 2003)	Workplace stress, financial instability, relationship breakdown (Harvey et al., 2021; Butterworth et al., 2009)	Job insecurity, discrimination, urban stressors (Lund et al., 2010; Marmot, 2015)
Older age	Noncommunicable diseases, neurodegenerative diseases, sensory impairments, chronic pain, physical inactivity (Livingston et al., 2020; Prince et al., 2007)	Social isolation, bereavement, elder abuse (Holt-Lunstad et al., 2015; WHO, 2021a)	Lack of community support, elder neglect, unsafe living conditions (Livingston et al., 2020; WHO, 2021a)

Note: BIPOC, Black and Indigenous people of color; LGBTQ+, lesbian, gay, bisexual, transgender, and queer plus.

creating further difficulties for the individual. Interventions at a public health level must focus on individuals and communities. Interventions for communities include efforts to improve social cohesion and reduce loneliness through group activities and empowerment. Peer support, working with the community on educational projects, adult learning classes, and accessing green and blue safe spaces are increasingly recognized as important for human well-being. Recently, social prescribing using the arts, gardening, and time banks has become popular and can be used successfully to improve mental health (see chapter 12).

Building resilience should start at an early stage and be seen as a lifelong process. By promoting well-being, motivation and resilience across the lifespan can contribute to social capital and improved functioning, longevity, and health population.

Mindfulness, cognitive therapies, and other talking therapies can help improve well-being and resilience. In many cultures, religion, religious rituals, and spirituality influence social capital and thereby promote well-being and life satisfaction. Both education and leisure activities throughout one's lifetime can play an important role in building resilience and well-being, thereby reducing the likelihood of mental ill-health. Participation and community activities can help create a sense of purpose and belonging by reducing loneliness. Mental health improvement interventions should start at the general population level to reduce health and socioeconomic inequalities but can also be applied at community and individual levels.

Factors Affecting Public Mental Health

Vulnerability to mental disorders or ill-health can occur due to individual, social, cultural, economic, and political factors. Risk factors can be of any variety and may also have a cumulative impact. Cultures and child-rearing patterns can influence brain development, which continue throughout a lifetime (Stewart-Brown, 2005). Public mental health thus has a broad scope and encompasses physical, natural, social, and ecological environments. It has been suggested that a major function of public mental health must be empowerment to combat inequalities that contribute to a sense of powerlessness (LFPH & MHF, 2016).

The contribution of social factors to mental ill-health and poor functioning is well recognized. Abusive parenting, domestic violence, and drug or alcohol misuse in the family are all well identified as contributing factors, but often they are difficult to measure, unlike social or educational status (LFPH & MHF, 2016). However, as discussed in chapter 5, rates of mental illness vary across cultures, and cultural values give varying emphasis to these factors. Furthermore, social inequalities also vary, creating further inequalities and setting up a vicious circle. Child-rearing patterns and children's access to education, sports, and other activities are critical and require careful attention in eliminating disparities. Understanding, exploring, and measuring inequalities in any given society must be taken into account so that inequalities, irrespective of their variety, can be eliminated. Appropriate investment is needed with a lifetime approach. As has been argued (LFPH & MHF 2016), the relationship between inequalities related to socioeconomic status and protected characteristics—which under law include age, gender, disability, marriage, civil partnership, sex, sexual orientation, race, religion, and pregnancy—and mental ill-health is a two-way process.

Developing communities must also focus on reducing stigma and discrimination so that individuals can seek help at an early stage. In addition, creating and maintaining social networks requires safe green spaces where people can meet and interact. Ease of access to affordable public transport and sustainable interventions can facilitate well-being while, in the process, obviating the impact on climate change. Promoting positive thoughts and participation in the arts and creative activities can also help. Connected individuals lead to connected families and kinships, which contribute to contented communities, which in turn not only influence the environment but are also affected by it. The human being is not an isolated entity; rather, a person's interactions across different domains need to be acknowledged. The well-being and mental health of an individual are intricately linked to their physical health and influenced by current and past experiences and circumstances. And, for a number of reasons, there are specific vulnerable periods in the life span and vulnerable groups.

Health Inequalities

Health inequalities can be defined as the unfair and avoidable differences in people's health across social groups and within different population groups (NHS Health Scotland 2015). Health inequalities do not occur by chance or randomly, and they can lead to premature morbidity and mortality. As these factors are often beyond an individual's control, they are perceived as unfair. However, these inequalities are avoidable because they can be addressed through political and social will and decisions. For example, in Scotland, people living in affluent areas enjoy nearly a quarter of a century more of good health. Growing up in such areas can significantly shape the physical, cognitive, social, and mental development of children (Beeston et al., 2013).

Causes of inequality include low income (which may or may not be associated with power, which is the ability to do and control something), poor housing, and poor access to transport. Power can arise from additional resources such as knowledge, prestige, beneficial connections, and other sources (WHO, 2008a; Link & Phelan, 2002). The concept that power and privilege are derived from historical oppression of certain groups has been recognized. For instance, the American Association of Medical Colleges (2016) defines oppression as "the combination of prejudice and institutional power which creates a system that discriminates against some groups . . . and benefits other groups." This definition acknowledges that systemic advantages for certain groups are rooted in historical injustices. Additionally, the concept of the "matrix of domination," introduced by sociologist Patricia Hill Collins (2000), describes how interlocking systems of oppression, such as race, gender, and class, have historically structured power and privilege in society. As discussed in the chapter 5, health inequalities are also linked to marginalization and discrimination related to gender, religion, sexual orientation, age, intellectual disabilities, and so on (WHO, 2022d; Hatzenbuehler et al., 2024).

There is considerable research evidence to suggest that less equal societies (in terms of income, power, and wealth) are associated with poorer outcomes across a range of health and social indicators, including violence, homicide, drug use, social mobility, and teenage pregnancy (Wilkinson & Pickett, 2006, 2009). Some of these will also vary depending on whether a culture is egocentric or sociocentric. Table 6.3 illustrates the actions required to reduce health inequalities.

Policymakers and decision-makers must be targeted to build their will based on a solid base of research and evidence, both local and international. Innovative practices should be encouraged and examples of good practice shared through improved public awareness and public inclusion at all levels.

Table 6.3
Actions required to reduce health inequalities

To undo	**Minimum income**
	Sufficient support for welfare
	Progressive taxation at corporate and individual levels
	Equity in participation
	Social justice
	Social support
	Drivers of wealth inequality including gender pay gap
To prevent	**Green, blue, and open spaces**
	Playgrounds
	Price control of tobacco/alcohol
	Improved work conditions
	Efforts to reduce adverse childhood experiences
	Efforts to reduce adverse work conditions
	Improved childhood and adult education
To mitigate	**Training workforce**
	Support vulnerable/at-risk individuals
	Specialist outreach
	Accessible and affordable services
	Collaboration across ministries

Sources: MacIntyre, 2007; NHS Health Scotland, 2015.

Income, Wealth, and Poverty

There is little doubt that income and wealth go hand in hand, and differences in income contribute to health inequalities. Furthermore, these differences affect living conditions, with overcrowding, poverty, and malnutrition leading to poor physical and mental health and well-being. To reduce income and wealth disparities and poverty, the most successful interventions have to be at the policy level so that they can be enforced. Economic, social, and taxation policies can bring about changes in wealth inequalities, thus changing health inequalities. Income can be seen as the most important social determinant of health (Office for National Statistics [ONS], 2015). Better income often means better health.

Stable and secure finances can certainly improve one's health and well-being. Income can be seen as the amount of money received by an individual or a group of individuals living together over a period—daily, weekly, monthly, annually, or over a lifetime. The source of income can be wages, income from properties, shares, savings, pensions, or sales of other goods. The individual or their group may then choose to spend this income in several ways. Sufficient income is essential for individuals and their units to buy the essentials and the services they need to participate in society and maintain health (Morris, 2010). As wealth encompasses both material and capital assets, it provides an element of future security, and associated with economic status, it also provides social status. Thus, socioeconomic status offers privileges and position that give the individual power to bring about or block change.

Poverty is defined both in absolute and relative terms and generally recognized as being below 60 percent of median income. Wealth inequalities inform health inequalities (Beckfield & Krieger, 2009), and increased use of alcohol, tobacco, and psychotropic drug use is affected by social and material deprivation (Baumann et al., 2007). Stuckler and Basu (2013) provide convincing evidence that the economics of a country affects the physical and mental health and well-being of its citizens; in their book, they illustrate how events such as a stock market crash can affect an individual's health and well-being. Thomas et al. (2010) and Krieger et al. (2008) have demonstrated that poverty levels in the UK and the US fell between 1920 and 1970 because of investments in infrastructure and planned institutions; however, this trend was reversed from 1970 onwards, leading to stagnation and in some cases a decline in longevity.

Public mental health policies are often shaped by broader socioeconomic conditions, with wealthier nations generally providing more comprehensive mental health care (Lund et al., 2010). However, within high-income countries, socioeconomic disparities still affect service accessibility, as seen in the US, where Medicaid expansion has improved but not fully resolved gaps in mental health care (Bailey et al., 2017).

Actions to reduce wealth inequalities include raising the minimum wage and increasing employment, which in most deprived areas can help reduce health inequalities substantially. Other possible policy actions are shown in box 6.4.

Housing

Inevitably, access to adequate housing is strongly influenced by wealth and income. Overcrowding can affect physical health by allowing the rapid

Box 6.4
Key Strategies for Reducing Wealth Inequalities

1. Implementing an economic strategy to bring about equality and equity in income, wealth, and prosperity, which feeds into industrial policy
2. Expanding access to capital ownership
3. Enacting equitable and fair taxation to reduce inequalities
4. Raising the minimum wage and ensuring job security
5. Protecting workers' rights
6. Providing a social security net for those who need it

spread of communicable diseases and their sequelae. Homelessness impacts health—both physical or mental—and may also contribute to substance and alcohol abuse. Individuals who are homeless are much more likely to develop infections and psychiatric disorders. Housing is not simply a physical shelter or building; it is also a psychological concept that provides a foundation for social, psychological, economic, and cultural interactions that give an individual a sense of belonging, which positively affects well-being. In an interesting qualitative study that involved interviews with over 70 tenants in three different housing organizations over one year, Garnham and Rolfe (2019) found that tenants' health and well-being generally improved during that first year. A good quality property—one in good condition on the day of the move—contributed to overall positive well-being. Tenants valued a sense of safety, friendliness and amenities, thus confirming that housing is more than simply a building.

Homelessness (Gutwinski et al., 2021; Munoz et al., 2005; O'Connell, 2005) poor physical housing quality (Braubach et al., 2011; Fisk et al., 2010; Marsh et al., 2000; Thomson et al., 2013) dampness, cold, and moldy housing are all associated with poor mental health (Branbach et al., 2011; Liddell & Guiney, 2015; Thomson et al., 2013). Insecurity of tenancy affects both physical and mental health (Jelleyman & Spencer, 2008; Downing, 2016). A sense of belonging, achieved by converting a house into a home, improves physical and mental health and overall well-being (Kearns et al., 2000; Hiscock et al., 2001). Garnham and Rolfe (2019) conclude in their study that having a choice in where one lives is important; furthermore, a sense of belonging and a sense of home are crucial in developing well-being. These authors outline various mechanisms that link housing to well-being (see Table 6.4). There are multiple parallel mechanisms that should be considered in both individual and community contexts. In this study, participants viewed home as a sense of belonging based on strong, stable, positive relationships; quality; affordability; and community networks. A safe, secure, and comfortable environment, along with affordability, are important aspects of belonging.

Policymakers have a moral obligation to provide affordable and accessible housing to citizens and to ensure safety and freedom to turn houses into homes.

Access to Green Spaces

Green spaces and contact with nature can help people relax and improve their ability to cope with stress, illness, and injury. In settings like Hong Kong, often thousands of people gather in public green spaces to practice tai chi. In addition, activities such as mindfulness, gardening, and working in allotments can help improve mental health and well-being. Such activities can be encouraged by involving partner groups including nongovernmental organizations.

Social prescribing (see chapter 12) may include access to green spaces with the added benefit of social connection. The Royal Edinburgh Hospital partnered with a charity to create a community garden with flower beds, lawns, and summer houses. Cabins provide space for meetings and office work. The garden's design, developed through consultations with patients and stakeholders, allows patients to visit alone or with staff. Managed by a garden coordinator, the space fosters rehabilitation for mental health and

Table 6.4
Possible mechanisms for links between health and housing

Mechanism	Context
For tenants, having positive contact and a relationship with the housing provider reduces stress	Security; support; managed expectations
Quality housing and home	Capacity and freedom to improve
Affordability reduces stress	Income and rent levels; social security
Suitable neighborhoods	Supportive networks; sense of community

forensic patients, helping them feel calmer and more purposeful. Public events in the green space promote community participation, and the garden offers a tranquil escape from the noise typical of psychiatric wards.

Physical Illness and Comorbidity

Comorbidity between physical illness and mental ill-health is well recognized. Physical illness increases the risk of mental illness, while mental ill-health can also contribute to physical illness, thereby creating complex comorbidities that require treatment both conjointly and independently. Many psychiatric conditions, such as depression, can influence physical health, making it more challenging to treat physical conditions. Individuals with mental ill-health are more likely to smoke heavily, consume alcohol, and experience obesity, all of which can further lead to poor physical health. As noted previously in this book, those with mental illnesses are also much more likely to die 10 to 15 years earlier. Smoking itself can increase the risk of depression and anxiety, as well as suicide rates and the likelihood of developing psychiatric disorders (see Campion et al., 2012, for a more detailed discussion). Additionally, it is recognized that tobacco use, alcohol intake, and unhealthy diets are linked to negative mental health outcomes, which can further lead to increased levels of the former.

In their meta-analysis, Chida and Steptoe (2008) systematically reviewed prospective observational studies to examine the relationship between positive psychological well-being and mortality. They found that higher levels of positive psychological well-being were associated with a reduced risk of mortality in both healthy and diseased populations. These authors further suggest that the autonomic nervous system is integral to emotional states. Additionally, various systems in the body are regulated by the autonomic nervous system and contribute to resilience and well-being. Both positive affective states (e.g., joy, happiness, vigor) and positive trait-like dispositions (e.g., life satisfaction, optimism) were linked to reduced mortality risk.

Mental health issues have a direct impact on physical health, and vice versa. There is significant overlap in the risk factors for both, and social determinants play a crucial role in influencing resilience. It is widely accepted that there are intricate comorbidities between mental and physical health, necessitating suitable therapeutic interventions for both fields.

The Promotion of Mental Health and the Prevention of Mental Ill-Health

Mental health promotion focuses on what is needed to improve as well as maintain an individual's mental health and well-being. The concept of positive mental health is "an individual's perception of his/her life" in the context of the cultural and value systems in which the individual lives and in relation to goals, expectations, standards, and concerns (WHO, 2004). A healthy individual can contribute to the functioning and well-being of society and also save health care resources. Mental health promotion, similar to the prevention of mental ill-health, can occur at the community level, the personal social-environmental level, and the personal internal psychological level. Such interventions can thus be at universal, selected, and indicated levels, with the latter targeted at high-risk individuals. Selected levels are for those subgroups who may be at significant risk (Arango et al., 2018).

Many psychiatric disorders can be prevented. Using the types of prevention mentioned at the beginning of this chapter is helpful. For example, primordial prevention focuses on reducing risk factors for an entire population by addressing social and environmental conditions through laws and national policy. Primary prevention consists of measures aimed at a susceptible population or individual in order to prevent a disease from ever occurring. Thus, its target population is healthy individuals, and its focus is on limiting risk exposure or increasing the immunity of individuals at risk to prevent a disease from progressing in a susceptible individual to subclinical disease (e.g., immunizations, needle exchange). Secondary prevention aims to stop the development of the sequelae of an illness through suitable therapeutics, early detection using screening tools, and intervention. The focus of tertiary prevention is on reducing the risk of relapse and promoting recovery wherever possible by targeting the clinical and outcome stages of a disease. Its aim is to reduce the severity of the disease and any associated sequelae through evidence-based therapeutic interventions. Quaternary prevention is about preventing overmedicalization, which can cause more harm than good.

Selective prevention aims to deal with vulnerable groups so that they do not go on to develop psychiatric disorders. As mentioned earlier—and it is worth repeating—mental illness and mental health can coexist or exist separately. However, the promotion of mental health and the prevention of mental ill-health or illness may be seen in a constructive, interactive manner.

Public health interventions are universal for the whole population, groups, or settings; selective for groups or communities that show higher rates or risks of distress, vulnerability, and exposure to adversity; and indicated for those individuals who exhibit early detectable signs of mental ill-health or distress. Interventions can use several approaches. They include using digital means, such as social media. Online communities, through social networks and various groups, can be used to deliver educational materials and interventions. Mindfulness and other individual interventions can be made available through phone apps and other social media channels.

Needs Assessment

Before mental health promotion and mental illness prevention programs are set up, it is crucial to ascertain the mental health needs of the population. This involves understanding both the epidemiological data and carefully teasing out the cultural variables in each country. Working with key stakeholders and improving and strengthening family and community ties can be extremely helpful in enabling the development of social capital. Reducing isolation and loneliness—for example, through the use of social networks, leisure and recreational activities, shared interest clubs, and connections made in the workplace—can contribute to better well-being (Morrish et al., 2023). Campaigns based on public education models can be beneficial, but it is not always clear how long these changes in knowledge and attitudes last. Education can also lead to empowerment, which may reduce the likelihood and the severity of psychiatric disorders. Effective public health and social interventions can improve mental health, especially when implemented by key stakeholders. It is also important to recognize that these programs must be sustained with proper evaluation and resourcing. Educating communities and individuals about risk factors can be helpful in delaying or preventing mental ill-health and resulting poor social functioning. Through education and empowerment, people can look after their own mental health; equally important, they can seek appropriate and early help if needed.

Principles of Public Mental Health

The UK Faculty of Public Health and Mental Health Foundation (2016) set some key principles of public mental health based on the work done by Brown et al. (2015) and Knifton and Quinn (2013). These principles are interventions focusing on the positive (added value over preventing the negative); addressing social, economic, cultural, and environmental determinants; a proportionate universalist approach; community and individual engagement; and a life course approach, which is multidisciplinary and intersectoral.

Public mental health should be seen in an interdisciplinary manner. Psychiatric disorders, at least in the West, are seen as being caused by biopsychosocial etiological factors supported by anthropological and spiritual models. Therefore, prevention and mental health promotion can be developed using one or more of these approaches. Although the model uses biological substrates, it is now well recognized that biological factors are affected by epigenetics, creating a close relationship between biology and social factors. Furthermore, the interaction between biology and psychological factors is not necessarily unidirectional. Social determinants also play a major role, so the multidirectional interaction can become extremely complex in the context of well-being and mental health.

The relationship between general well-being and good mental health remains a topic of great interest in planning and delivering mental health services. Well-being is defined as feeling and functioning well, as recognized and evaluated in a personal and cultural context. Well-being and mental health often have different parameters (Patalay & Fitzsimons, 2016). People living with mental ill-health can lead satisfying and meaningful lives, even within the context of the symptoms they may be experiencing (WHO, 2014c). Paradoxically, those who have good mental health may not experience good levels of well-being. The two concepts are interrelated and can affect each other. For example, poor well-being may lead to mental ill-health, and mental ill-health can lead to lower levels of well-being.

Public health interventions should be developed and delivered at the following levels:

a. *Whole population*: through initiatives of parenting skills, training, healthy schools, healthy workplaces, healthy lifestyles, and green neighborhoods.
b. *Vulnerable or at-risk individuals*: new parents, the unemployed, those living in poor and overcrowded housing, and families in distress.
c. *Vulnerable groups*: migrants, refugees, asylum seekers, women, elders, LGBTQ+ individuals, the intellectually disabled, and prisoners.
d. *Antidiscrimination*: combating discrimination against people with mental health problems and promoting positive images of mental ill-health.

Each national government should set performance indicators according to local epidemiological findings and needs. Short-, medium-, and long-term targets must be agreed on with key stakeholders and standards set accordingly. The minimum standards of service expected for people in psychiatric inpatient care, for people with schizophrenia, for people with dementia, and for children and adolescents with psychiatric disorders are listed in appendices 5–8. These minimum standards are for guidance, and similar standards must be developed for other conditions and groups.

Mental Health First Aid

Mental health first aid (MHFA, appendix 13) originated in Australia in 2001 to enhance public mental health literacy. MHFA trains laypeople to recognize signs of mental distress, suicidal ideation, and substance use disorders, including identifying those at risk or in the early stages of mental health issues. MHFA provides skills for responding to mental health crises, including panic attacks, psychosis, self-harm, and suicidal ideation, making it a key component of suicide prevention efforts in workplaces, schools, and communities.

Separately, psychological first aid (PFA, appendix 14) is an evidence-informed, early intervention approach designed to reduce initial distress and build resilience in individuals exposed to trauma, disasters, or crises. Both are typically delivered by non-mental health specialists in a task-shifting model, expanding access to support and playing a role in the prevention of future mental illness.

The Life Course Approach to Public Mental Health

Mental health is crucial for ensuring personal and social growth, learning, and developing well-being and resilience that protect the body from stressors and distress. Mental well-being enables the adoption of healthy lifestyles and, in the case of illness, helps manage symptoms and experiences while facilitating processes of recovery. It contributes to the overall functioning of the individuals, their families, and communities at large. Contributing to general physical well-being, mental well-being also enables and facilitates positive interpersonal relationship and assists individuals in realizing their ambitions, coping with adversity, and living productive work and lives (Foresight Mental Capital & Wellbeing Projects, 2008; Chida & Steptoe, 2008; Pressman & Cohen, 2005). Key areas for action are illustrated in table 6.5.

Table 6.5
Types of intervention at different stages of life course

Pre-childhood:	Parenting skills Education about diet
Childhood:	Parenting skills Helping vulnerable families Helping vulnerable children School mental health programs Reducing adverse childhood experiences, bullying, emotional abuse Reducing alcohol use, violence, unemployment, gambling overcrowding Better housing
Young people:	Same interventions as employed in childhood, plus education about mental health literacy; alcohol and drug use and harm reduction; sex and relationship education; and targeting vulnerable groups especially LGBTQ+ individuals, those with intellectual disabilities, BIPOC, and minority ethnic groups
Adulthood:	Family support Mental health awareness Improving social networks Improving workplace support Building resilience, better economic activity, lower unemployment, better physical exercise
Older adulthood:	Social prescribing Health promotions Physical activity, occupation activities, cognitive improvement, early intervention in dementia

Note: BIPOC, Black and Indigenous people of color; LGBTQ+, lesbian, gay, bisexual, transgender, and queer plus.

Stigma and discrimination must be addressed throughout the life course. There is no single approach that works to reduce stigma. A combination of education, social contact, protests, and changes in the law may work to reduce stigma. Targeted approaches may be beneficial. Through targeted and universal approaches, change can be achieved. One-off programs may not be sufficient, however. Collaboration with stakeholders such as the judicial system can facilitate legal changes aimed at tackling and reducing discrimination in a way that is sustainable.

To promote public mental health awareness, it has been argued that a psychologically informed environment is a promising approach that centers on the emotional and psychological needs of service users in relation to modifications to the physical environment of services (Dekker et al., 2023). A major aspect that needs urgent and regular attention is providing mental health literacy training to care and housing workers. In addition to informing them about mental health and various mental illnesses and signs of relapse, it is important to enable them to support individuals with mental illness in the context of accommodation, financial management, debt, and social security. The key is to develop and design community partnerships that best serve those in need. When patients settle in the community, housing, welfare, education, employment, and health care pathways need to work together. The Asset-Based Community Development (ABCD) approach can help cultivate thriving communities and enhance population well-being (McKnight & Russell, 2018). Its aim is to identify and build on the existing strengths of the communities. Such an approach can foster community development and assist communities in managing distress. There is also a place for improving mental health literacy of carers and families who may be looking after the patient. Some of these tasks can be easily shared with nongovernmental organizations and other community bodies. Teaching about relapse signs, medication, side effects, and appropriate therapeutic interventions can be very helpful.

Box 6.5 and table 6.6 illustrate areas for interventions at different stages of the life course.

Box 6.5
Key Areas for Action

1. Addressing social determinants of health by recognizing their impact
2. Conducting a mental health impact assessment for all policies
3. Making mental health promotion a part of physical health promotion
4. Implementing specific mental health promotion strategies at the national level
5. Using a life course approach in partnership with schools, colleges and universities, workplaces, religious institutions, community organizations, public libraries, and other relevant social institutions

Table 6.6
Focus of intervention at different stages of life course

Stage	*Focus*	*Needs*
Intrauterine	Parents No alcohol/smoking Diet and exercise	Maternal health
Infancy	Parents Nourishment	Attachment
Childhood	Parents Peers Avoiding bullying	Attachment/nourishment Emotional attachment
Adolescence/Teens	Peers Individuation Support Avoiding alcohol/violence	Attachment/friendship
Adulthood	Family Peers Social interactions	Emotional/financial support Friendship/kinships
Older adults	Family Friendships Social interaction	Emotional/financial support
Parenting skills		
Infants	Nurturing Physical contact Warmth Attachment patterns Avoid alcohol/violence	
Children	Clear boundaries Discipline Nurturing/nourishing Personal sensitivities Avoiding bullying/ACE/abuse	
Adolescents	Provision, support Encouraging individuation Avoiding adverse experiences/ abuse Education	

Note: ACE, adverse childhood experience.

Box 6.6
The Benefits of Public Mental Health

1. Improved educational attainment
2. Improved cognitive abilities and social functioning
3. Reduction in domestic interpersonal violence
4. Reduction in risk-taking behavior (e.g., smoking)
5. Improved productivity and presence
6. Reduction in burden of mental ill-health
7. Reduction in suicide rates
8. Reduced morbidity
9. Better quality of life
10. Improved life satisfaction

Throughout the life course, education and information about risk factors such as obesity, smoking, poor diet, lack of exercise, alcohol dependence, and addiction must be delivered in a way that is engaging, culturally appropriate, and not perceived as patronizing. Some or all of these risk factors are related to increased levels of stress and distress and are likely to affect both physical and mental health. It is important for countries to set national standards and policies along with adequately and appropriately funded local services.

Maternal Health

Maternal health and well-being are important to the prevention of mental illness and mental health promotion for mothers, babies, and families. Infant programs, parenting skills, and maternal mental health are all interlinked and need to be developed in a consistent way. In countries where traditional midwives deliver children and may follow them for a while, it is important that they receive basic training in identifying early signs of postnatal depression and puerperal psychosis. Targeted programs are aimed at individuals who are at risk of perinatal mental health problems (e.g., teenage mothers, single mothers, those who abuse alcohol or drugs). Intergenerational violence, alcohol dependence, and physical, emotional, or sexual abuse can all contribute to vulnerability. Early recognition and appropriate interventions are critical. Parenting skills programs must focus on strengths and skills of parents and should be offered at different levels by trained individuals.

Women's Mental Health

Women's mental health is incredibly important. Very often, women are carers, but they are also prone to higher rates of many psychiatric illnesses. In addition, women are more likely to face interpersonal domestic violence, which needs to be addressed at multiple levels (WHO, 2022e). These issues need to be addressed in any educational program to ensure that everyone is aware of the sequelae and is involved in prevention (Chandra & Stewart, 2017).

Child Mental Health

Children who are at high risk of developing mental disorders either while still young or later in life include those in care, those who have parents with mental ill-health, and those in families characterized by violence or alcohol misuse. Early intervention is critical for childhood psychiatric disorders if long-term mental health outcomes are to improve. School-based programs, such as social and emotional learning (SEL) curricula, have been effective in reducing anxiety and behavioral problems (Durlak et al., 2011). Family therapy approaches, including Parent-Child Interaction Therapy, have been successful in managing childhood conduct disorders (Eyberg et al., 2008). School mental health is considered in some detail in chapter 8. However, as explored in chapter 5, children with intellectual disabilities will have additional needs that must be addressed (Totsika et al., 2022). WHO (2021b) makes some clear recommendations on adolescent mental health. School mental health is important to help children develop well (Council of Europe 2023). Cowie (2022) recommends pastoral care, although this may not be easily accessible across cultures.

College Mental Health

As in school settings (see chapter 8), universities and colleges are well placed to deliver public mental health interventions. Lavis and Robson (2015) propose eight principles for promoting a whole school and college approach to emotional health and well-being:

1. Designing curriculum teaching and learning to promote resilience and support social and emotional learning
2. Facilitating and co-partnering with students to influence decisions

3. Helping staff to develop their own well-being and that of their students
4. Identifying needs and monitoring the impact of interventions
5. Working with parents and carers
6. Providing targeted support and making appropriate referrals
7. Creating an ethos and environment that demonstrates respect and values diversity
8. Providing leadership and management to support and promote emotional health and well-being across all the areas above

Adult Mental Health

Providing mental health literacy to all adults is beneficial, along with ensuring access to employment, housing, and financial support (if needed) and promoting physical exercise and appropriate and adequate activities (e.g., time-banking, volunteering). Targeted interventions, such as improving the capacity to use psychological treatments and mindfulness, can be extremely helpful. Those who have mental illnesses will need support in navigating the health care system and require physical health assessments on a regular basis. Dental and optical examinations, vaccinations as appropriate, and access to smoking cessation and alcohol control programs must be essential parts of any targeted intervention. Health care services must be accessible and available. Peer support and appropriate navigators must be accessible when needed. Physical and mental health care must be delivered in an integrated manner, and suitable training must be made available to all staff on a regular basis.

Workplace Mental Health

Post-pandemic, as more people are working from home, office work has paradoxically become more stressful. Workplace well-being is important for many reasons. A healthy workforce is likely to be more productive and contribute to the economy, community, and the building of social capital. By creating happier workplaces, improvements in physical, environmental, and psychosocial factors can enhance the mental health of society as a whole. Health care services in the workplace need to be linked with human resources departments, occupational health, and other stakeholders. WHO (2022h) recommends some basic features dealing with mental health in the workplace.

As discussed previously, any interventions must include universal, selective, and indicated preventive strategies. Workload, job control, clarity in responsibility, and effective antidiscrimination and anti-bullying policies, among others, need to be put in place. Universal interventions must include options for baby care (for young parents, if needed), access to physical activities, and access to affordable nutritious food, if required. Targeted interventions may require anti-stress programs, increased availability and access to talking therapies (online or in person), and support for those who are returning to work after a period of absence due to mental ill-health. For employees who may have alcohol or substance use problems, there must be easy access to specific available interventions. For those who have developed mental ill-health, it is important to provide necessary levels of support. Early interventions, support, and ease of access to services are certainly important, but equally vital is reintegration into the workplace. Mental health first aid (see appendix 13) may support such steps. Unemployment can increase problems related to common mental disorders, so at a policy level, it becomes crucial to manage it. Additionally, as soon as any employee shows signs of developing mental ill-health, steps should be taken to provide easy access to help along with ongoing support.

Mental health in the workplace is equally important for individuals who are recovering from mental illness, and a gradual introduction can be helpful. Again, it is worth emphasizing that jobs should be tailored to people rather than the other way around bearing in mind that while certain jobs may be difficult to mold, every attempt should be made.

Later-Life Interventions

At a universal level, addressing loneliness and reducing isolation through befriending programs and various social group activities has proven helpful and shown excellent results in improving mental well-being. Targeted interventions that focus on older carers, peer-support groups, and drop-in day centers can also make a difference.

Suicide Prevention Initiatives

Suicide can be prevented, and each country needs to examine the basic data on rates—overall rates, age-specific patterns, methods used, and outcomes. WHO (2024) maps key risk factors for suicide onto systems based on the strength of interventions, urging clinicians and policymakers to follow these interventions accordingly. A reduction in suicide rates in each country must be viewed as a priority. As discussed in an earlier chapter, rates of suicide are influenced by underlying mental illness, but social and cultural causes can also contribute heavily to these rates. In nearly one-third of countries, the act of suicide itself is punishable under the law (Mishara & Weisstub, 2016) or proscribed on religious grounds, so it is difficult to know with certainty the exact rates of suicide or attempted suicide, which makes intervention difficult. However, it is possible to set targets that are achievable.

Community-level causes of suicidal thinking and acts include discrimination; stresses of acculturation; disasters, wars, and conflicts; and trauma-related to abuse. Educating key players to ask the right questions and providing formal training can help to reduce rates. At the level of relationships, especially if these individuals are isolated and face a cultural conflict, training and education to point them in the right direction can be helpful. At an individual level, risk factors include previous attempts, mental illness, alcohol abuse, financial difficulties, hopelessness, family history, chronic pain, and genetic vulnerabilities. Rapid access to helplines and assessment and management of mental and substance use disorders will be essential first steps.

Health systems may act as barriers for an individual who is feeling suicidal, and thus changes in accessibility through better mental health policies to improve access to health care will be an important first step. At the societal level, access to means and inappropriate media reporting may be contributing factors that must be addressed. For example, impeding ready access to pesticides by locking these products up in central locations have been shown to lead to a decrease in suicide rates (Pearson et al., 2017) and restricting the sale of over-the-counter medications such as aspirin and paracetamol may have contributed to fewer admissions to liver units and liver transplants, decreased hospital visits for paracetamol poisoning, and lower paracetamol sales (Morgan & Majeed, 2005).

Policy changes may be needed to remove the stigma of suicide as an illegal act so that accurate data can be obtained and, accordingly, comprehensive services offered. Figures require careful public education, as well as restricting access to means and reducing harmful use of alcohol. Such changes will go a long way toward reducing rates of suicide. Raising awareness of mental health substance use disorders and suicide, responsible media reporting, and gatekeeper training have all been shown to reduce rates of suicide (WHO, 2014b).

Vulnerable groups—including Black and Indigenous people of color, those from minority ethnic groups, migrants and refugees, prisoners, and LGBTQ+ individuals (see chapter 5 on vulnerable groups)—have all shown higher rates of suicide compared with the general population. Thus, specifically targeted educational materials and interventions are needed. To engage teachers, pupils, and parents in fostering social responsibility, the WHO (2014b) has recommended early upstream strategies, including programs to educate young mothers, mentoring programs, community-wide prevention systems, and school-based violence prevention and skills-building programs.

According to the WHO (2014b) data, only 28 countries around the globe have a national strategy or action plan to deal with suicide, while another 13 countries are planning such a strategy, with nearly half of them in Europe. Thus, an important first step is to urge all countries around the globe to implement a policy to reduce rates of suicide. Typical components of national strategies are surveillance of rates, means reduction, media guidelines and training on reporting, ease of access to services, treatment, crisis intervention, post-attempt support, awareness, stigma reduction, and coordination among various agencies.

The Economic Case for Mental Health

It is well recognized that poor mental health in individuals can contribute major costs to families, societies, health care systems, social care, education, housing, the justice system, and the wider economy. On the other hand, the economic benefits of mental well-being are broad, far-reaching, and can be experienced at many levels, from individuals, families, kinships, and society at large.

In any given society, there are likely to be levels of inequality that will be strongly influenced by political factors, such as policies based on political ideologies, taxes, and burdens. In theory, virtually every member country of the United Nations has signed on to the United Nations Convention on the Rights of Persons with Disabilities, but in reality, there are major variations. As described in chapter 1, while studying the laws of equality as applied to the rights of persons with mental illness (Bhugra et al., 2016a, 2016b, 2016c; Nardodkar et al., 2016). less than half allowed all basic rights. As mentioned before, a major role for health professionals in general and for mental health professionals in particular is taking on the roles and responsibilities of advocacy. There is no doubt that almost universally, mental health services are not only underfunded, but they also lag behind physical health services and research. Stigma produces discrimination in law that can be addressed by changing the laws accordingly. The key solution is to eliminate discrimination through legal approaches.

It has been shown that every dollar invested in early intervention can, after one year, yield a return of $12 for parents of children with conduct disorder and $20 for psychosis (Department of Health [DoH], 2011; Knapp et al., 2011). There is no doubt that effective interventions for children who are at risk show cost-effectiveness over time. The savings accrued come from better social functioning, greater contributions to taxes and to society, and lower rates of imprisonment, among other factors. The Department of Health (DoH, 2011) strategy concluded that for every $1 spent, the returns can be truly impressive, ranging from $10 to $100. Investing in mental health in the workplace can produce gains nearly ten times that of the initial investment (Knapp et al., 2011). Improved mental health in children can lead to a reduction in behavioral problems, violence and crime, teenage pregnancies, drug and alcohol misuse, as well as improved cognitive and academic achievements, thereby contributing positively to the well-being of the community and the population.

Role of Doctors in Public Mental Health

Psychiatrists as mental health specialists play a crucial role in public mental health advocacy by shaping policy, promoting anti-stigma initiatives, and ensuring equitable access to care. The World Psychiatric Association (see appendices 3 and 4) has emphasized psychiatrists' responsibility to advocate for mental health parity in health care systems (WPA, 2017; 2019a). Additionally, psychiatrists can contribute to public awareness campaigns aimed at reducing stigma and discrimination against people with mental illness (Henderson et al., 2013).

A key responsibility that doctors carry as medical experts is that of advocating for our patients, whether it is for prevention, treatment, cure, or support. Advocating for population mental health and public education can be seen as key components of this responsibility. Although public health physicians have a specialist role in managing population health, the responsibility of both primary care and specialist physicians should be recognized and supported. Having the scientific knowledge base, doctors are aware of recent advances in our understanding of causality and therapeutic interventions. As long as physicians remain highly trusted professionals, they have a responsibility to support prevention and health promotion strategies, engage with policymakers, and share their clinical and scientific expertise for the wider good.

In many countries, especially low-income ones, the focus of public health is understandably on common local health issues such as communicable diseases. Laudable as it is, that emphasis tends to ignore the mental health implications of infectious diseases—for example, the stress experienced by family caregivers, those who survive the infection, and the professionals who look after those who are experiencing the infections. In many countries, health outcomes are often measured by simple reductions in the rates of infection. This is perhaps easier to measure compared with mental health outcomes. There is clear evidence that reductions in infection, along with increased awareness of other factors such as hygiene, clean water, improved diet, reduced pollution, smoking bans, and price increases on alcohol, have contributed to better health in many countries.

Social inequalities contribute to health inequalities, and once again doctors are well placed to advocate for reduction in social inequalities. Doctors should be aware of all levels of prevention. These strategies need to be embedded in the personal and social lives of patients, their carers, and their families while working with key stakeholders including policy workers.

Supporting the role of patients as advocates is a clinical skill and needs to be taught from the undergraduate level. Although health care systems vary widely, the basic principles of public mental health remain the same. Doctors, whether they work in public health or not, have responsibilities as leaders, co-producers and partners, advocates, and evaluators.

Public mental health action must cover these key areas:

1. All policies must include a mental health impact assessment. This assessment must examine and ensure that the specific impact on the individual's health and population mental health is considered.

2. Appropriate and adequate funding must follow, not only for mental health services on an equitable basis with physical health services but also for public health, including public mental health. It is important to reduce rates of communicable diseases while also ascertaining their impact on the mental health of patients, their carers, and families.
3. Public mental health policies require a life course approach from birth to death: from pre-pregnancy advice to parenting skills, school mental health and university mental health, and mental health in the workplace and later life.
4. Prevention of mental illness and promotion of mental health are at the core of any health care system. In settings where health care is largely or exclusively private, it is the government's moral obligation to invest in public health, including public mental health.
5. There is solid research and policy evidence that inequalities create more psychiatric disorders. Policymakers must ensure that social determinants are considered and, where needed, eliminated.
6. Mental health must form an integral part of health care, and appropriate adequate resources must be made available for research and health care delivery and training.
7. A comprehensive public mental health approach—one that reduces stigma against mental illness and those who experience mental illness, helps prevent future mental ill-health, and focuses on vulnerable groups in the context of overall health improvement—therefore requires prevention and health promotion strategies.

Conclusion

Risks and protective factors for population as a whole and for vulnerable individuals must be identified, recognized, and balanced using multiple strategies. Reducing inequalities where they exist is the first step. To facilitate better childhoods, an early positive start must be encouraged and supported. Promoting prenatal care, perinatal teaching, and parenting skills, helping develop personal mental well-being, and promoting physical exercise and activity are essential components of mental health promotion. Preventing domestic violence, drug and alcohol abuse, and interpersonal violence are important steps in creating a safe environment in which infants, children, and young people can prosper. The population must be encouraged to develop resilience through stability and prosperity of the community in which everyone has a stake and a sense of belonging and purpose. Communities need to remain interconnected, and urban environments must be created in order to facilitate these qualities. Furthermore, reducing stigma, on the one hand, and creating green and blue spaces, on the other, will enable and improve connectedness. Linking physical and mental health to behavior change (e.g., stopping smoking, reducing alcohol intake, reducing obesity) can pay huge dividends. Relaxation activities, physical exercise, participation in the arts, and social prescribing can be used to improve well-being. Reducing insecurity in housing as well as job settings can help further. Adulthood needs for well-being and resilience may vary from those required by the younger age group and the aging population. Furthermore, loneliness in older adults must be tackled, and various options at the street, local community, and regional levels should be made available. This needs to be accompanied by ease of access to facilities through better affordable public transport. Sharing time, use of time banks through volunteering, and community activities can help.

7 Caring for a Community

Introduction

In the past 40 years or so, in many parts of the world, psychiatric asylums and institutions have been closed and services moved into the community. In the UK for past few decades, there has been a shift toward more specialized services such as home treatment and developing services like crisis support and intervention and community rehabilitation. Crisis houses have been set up where patients can be admitted for short periods. The role of psychiatric services is to provide prompt, appropriate assessment and offer evidence-based interventions.

Irrespective of the resources, a comprehensive mental health service should provide affordable, accessible, culturally sensitive, and prompt services to those who need it, in a partnership between specialist psychiatric services, other medical specialties, primary care physicians and staff, clinical psychologists, nurses, social workers, social services, occupational therapists, physiotherapists, voluntary organizations, and patient groups. A major function of clinical psychiatry is to provide specialist assessment and investigations along with those treatments that fall in its specialist purview. Psychiatric disorders are often caused by biopsychosocial etiological factors and thus require the biopsychosocial interventions, but psychiatrists in addition to being experts in medical (i.e., biological) interventions must be cognizant of social and psychological factors. This allows them to seek appropriate advice and provide suitable therapeutic interventions, including medical psychotherapy. Furthermore, psychiatrists can advise other professionals and work with them to provide shared management according to an individual patient's needs. A comprehensive mental health service depends on efficient and effective use of available resources with clear and agreed-on outcomes.

Community mental health care must be seen in the context of treatment, rehabilitation, and support that the social milieu can accept and support. Community care reflects on the individual's social situation, its relationship with the illness, and how the individual patient and their carers and families cope with it.

A small minority of patients with psychiatric diagnosis will need safe containment in order to recover, whereas others will stretch their social networks, creating further tensions within their families and circle, perhaps leading to rejection.

Principles of Caring for a Community

1. Between those planning, designing, and delivering services to the community and other stakeholders (e.g., policymakers, funders, community leaders, clinicians, educators, social care professionals), there must be a clear acknowledgment and agreement on what is meant by caring for a community. It may be that a range of services are needed and made available—for example, from primary care to generic community mental health teams to specialized community treatments such as home treatment, crisis intervention, and continuing treatment and rehabilitation.
2. Comprehensive mental health services should be made available in the community in a coordinated fashion. Wherever possible, social care and health care should be integrated and delivered in a coherent manner. As services can be provided by any number of providers, working across boundaries, such as with voluntary agencies, is important. Respective roles and lines of responsibility, along with clinical management, must be clarified. Co-creation with communities is essential for optimal service design and implementation which will help reduce stigma.
3. Information-sharing, while maintaining confidentiality, is essential for integrated care. Patients should be given appropriate information and their own case notes so that they can share them with other health and social care providers. Patient information could be shared in the form of password-protected USB sticks, shared electronic records, or written notes.

4. There need to be clear lines of clinical and medical responsibility, especially related to primary, secondary, tertiary, and social care. Irrespective of the health care system, there should be bidirectional links between primary and specialist care services, allowing for information-sharing, clinical support, and smooth transfers of care.
5. Health care resources need to be dedicated to the patient's needs.
6. Services must be efficient, effective, appropriate, accessible, sensitive, and safe.
7. Staff at all levels must be comprehensively and properly trained. They should be able to recognize the changing needs of patients and act accordingly and appropriately. They should also be fully cognizant of local mental health laws. They should be able to assess and manage risk to the patients and others.
8. Trauma-informed care (TIC) enhances care delivery and improves patient outcomes. TIC emphasizes safety, trustworthiness, empowerment, and cultural sensitivity in service delivery (Harris & Fallot, 2001). This approach reduces re-traumatization and increases treatment adherence in psychiatric populations (Goldstein et al., 2024).
9. Ethical considerations in psychiatric practice revolve around patient autonomy, informed consent, and balancing clinical responsibilities. Psychiatrists and other staff must be trained in managing ethical dilemmas such as involuntary hospitalization, medication refusal, and confidentiality breaches in high-risk cases (Beauchamp & Childress, 2013). Informed consent is a cornerstone of ethical practice, ensuring patients understand treatment risks and benefits (Appelbaum, 2007).
10. Clear quantitative outcome indicators must be used that consider a person's strengths, resilience, abilities, attitudes, and available support.
11. Confidentiality carries different values in different cultures. However, within the regulatory framework, confidentiality must be maintained.

Community Psychiatric Services

Community psychiatric services must be comprehensive. In addition, the members of the team should coordinate services. Comprehensiveness in this context has two related meanings—first, complete coverage of mental health needs, which may require some prioritization and focus, and second, providing total care for an individual's needs. For services to be comprehensive, they require the following:

a. Appropriate infrastructures and resources
b. Access to a range of effective interventions
c. Attention to hidden and complex comorbidity
d. Alliances with other community agencies
e. Accord with other professions and professionals
f. Attention to the needs of carers and families

In addition, they must be affordable and accessible. Affordability applies both to the service providers and to the individuals who may have to pay for the services directly or indirectly. The range of psychiatric services must include public mental health, primary care, secondary and tertiary care, but also care in and for the community across all ages, genders, religious affiliations, sexual orientations, and other variables and vulnerabilities.

It is worth noting again that a mental disorder or mental illness is a behavioral or psychological syndrome consisting of a cluster of symptoms (related to mood, thought, or behaviors) and observed psychopathology that causes distress to the individual or to others around them. Both objective and subjective distress, when it occurs, is likely to influence social functioning. A diagnosis based on the set of symptoms and syndromes may be required to ensure targeted therapeutic interventions and outcomes. This is no doubt that often syndromes may overlap and thereby create difficulties in reaching a diagnosis and managing patients. Furthermore, most diagnoses are based on duration and description (both subjective and objective) and may also be associated with certain age groups or stages of the life cycle. The disorders will vary according to severity, organicity, prodrome, type of onset, duration, course, and outcome. The prevalence of disorders will breed familiarity with the illness. Some disorders may be acute while others are chronic; some disorders will be episodic or recurring whereas others are enduring and persistent. Psychiatric disorders may cause social and medical disabilities. Social disabilities refer to the extent to which an individual is unable to perform social roles and tasks using their premorbid skills. Such functional disablement or limitation will prevent the patient from actively taking part in social activities, contributing to social exclusion. These circumstances may affect self-care and impact relationships and the social roles that all human beings are expected to perform, including marital, sexual, and parental roles and occupational and professional activities. The nature, duration, and severity of these activities will contribute to poor self-hygiene, self-neglect, squalid living conditions, and a downward drift. Associated comorbidities with physical illnesses will be of great importance in many cultures. Some individuals will find it easier to seek help for physical problems from physicians. Caring for a community means that looking after the community's members from birth to death, with care provided as close to home as possible or even in a home-like environment. For individuals with mental illnesses, normalization and integration are key to improving social functioning. Furthermore, caring in the community is about a preference for small over large, with a clear preference for local services. In addition, the community and its members also have a responsibility as part of their social contract with psychiatry. This responsibility involves looking after their own health (physical and mental) and ensuring that health resources are not misused but are used appropriately and cautiously.

Community mental health services need to be accessible, acceptable, and accountable. Accessibility is both geographical and emotional—the latter, in the sense that those who need services feel welcome in a non-stigmatizing manner. Geographical access is about not only traveling distances but also availability outside normal hours, physical access (e.g., wheelchair access), cost, and cognitive acceptability. As mentioned earlier in this volume, the social contract is a three-way agreement between patients and health care staff, between health care staff and the government, and finally between the government and the patients. In addition, a contract also exists between the individual clinicians, their employer, their regulator, team members and the community. Continuity of care depends on a variety of factors. It is likely that community care will provide better continuity based on mutual trust and a therapeutic alliance between patients and health professionals in a secure, reliable, and dependable manner. This can help identify early signs of relapse, leading to appropriate early interventions.

The design, development, and delivery of mental health services need to be supported by the community so that individuals feel confident using them. This will also help reduce stigma. Thus, the range of services and partnerships across stakeholder groups and disciplines is crucial in ensuring that services are not only accessible but also affordable. Depending on the explanatory models followed by the population at large, services need to engage with others in the design of those services. Working with religious leaders and healers (as explained in appendix 12) may be helpful. The service designers and developers also need to examine the pathways into care that individuals use after noticing their symptoms. The role of primary care physicians in making an early diagnosis, starting early intervention, and providing ongoing support cannot be underestimated. In many health care systems, primary care physicians tend to act as gatekeepers to secondary care, whereas in other systems, patients may be able to access specialist secondary care directly.

Task-Shifting

As mental health systems globally pursue cost-effective, scalable solutions, task-shifting has become crucial to closing the treatment gap, particularly in underserved populations (Patel et al., 2018). Task-shifting in mental health is a strategy that reallocates specific mental health care responsibilities from specialized professionals (e.g., psychiatrists, psychologists) to trained nonspecialist health workers (NSHWs), such as general nurses, community health workers, and peer supporters who are typically based in the community. This approach has been widely adopted to address the global shortage of mental health professionals, particularly in low- and middle-income countries (Bolton et al., 2023). The WHO has endorsed task-shifting as a key approach for expanding access to mental health services in primary care and community settings where specialists are scarce (WHO, 2021c). Research demonstrates that trained nonspecialists can effectively deliver interventions such as cognitive behavioral therapy (CBT), brief psychological interventions, and psychoeducation, with outcomes comparable to those of specialist-delivered care for depression, anxiety, PTSD, and alcohol, nicotine, and opioid use (Abba Hassan et al., 2024; Connolly et al., 2021). Task-shifting is especially effective in integrated care models, where NSHWs collaborate with primary care physicians to provide stepped care interventions, ensuring that patients receive appropriate support according to severity (Lange, 2021). Examples of task-shifting include Friendship Benches (Zimbabwe), "Aunties" (Cameroon), and lay "Lady Health Workers" offering support to women with postpartum depression (Pakistan) (see appendix 12 for more examples).

Despite its benefits, task-shifting encounters challenges such as variable training quality, gaps in supervision, and the risk of burnout among non-specialist health workers (NSHWs) (Jain & Koon, 2022), and these factors need addressing—not as cheaper alternatives but proper community engagement. Maintaining treatment fidelity and ensuring that task-shifted interventions align with evidence-based practices necessitates ongoing supervision, structured protocols, and adaptation to local cultural contexts (Rabie et al., 2023). Furthermore, while task-shifting enhances service delivery, it does not entirely replace the need for specialist care, particularly for individuals with severe mental illnesses (e.g., schizophrenia, bipolar disorder) who frequently require medication management and intensive interventions (Bolton et al., 2023), sometimes against their will. Scaling up task-shifting approaches demands investment in NSHW training, supportive policies, and integration within national health systems to guarantee long-term sustainability and effectiveness.

Nonprofits and Nongovernmental Organizations

In many countries, not-for-profits and nongovernmental organizations (NGOs) play a critical role in community mental health by filling gaps in care, advocating for policy change, and providing culturally tailored interventions. These organizations offer mental health education, crisis intervention, peer support, and affordable treatment services, particularly in underserved areas where government health care infrastructure is weak (Thara & Patel, 2010; Doshmangir et al., 2025). NGOs also spearhead task-shifting initiatives, training lay health workers to deliver basic mental health interventions in low-resource settings (WHO, 2022g; see also appendix 12 for more on task-shifting). Many nonprofits focus on harm reduction, suicide prevention, and trauma-informed care, often addressing social determinants such as poverty and housing instability (Padgett et al., 2016). Additionally, NGOs influence policy and funding allocation by conducting research and mobilizing grassroots advocacy (van Voren & Keukens, 2014). Their flexibility and community-driven approaches make them essential to strengthening integrated, equitable, and sustainable mental health systems worldwide.

Primary Care Services

Primary care physicians are also known as family doctors or family physicians because they may well be looking after the whole family. They are well trained, specialist in primary care, readily accessible, and take a holistic approach while attempting to manage frontline risk. They provide continuity of care in many settings and manage complex comorbidities, including the interplay between mental and physical health. One of the major changes that can bring out a major benefit is establishing family medicine centers or community health centers or hubs run by primary care physicians and nurses, but with input from a specialist on a regular basis.

Primary care is the backbone of any health care system, although in many countries it is not recognized as such. Doctors and staff working in primary care settings are often the first point of contact in the community. Yet in many, if not most, countries they are likely to be underappreciated. Often, this is because primary care physicians are (incorrectly) not viewed as specialists. Primary care physicians see a vast number of cases of increasing complexity, and at least one-third of their caseload is likely to be purely psychiatric, with a significant proportion of other cases likely to have a psychiatric overlay.

In many countries, individuals with mental illnesses are seen first in the primary care settings. These individuals fall into three main categories: (1) those with common mental disorders such as depression, anxiety, and phobias, who may present with or without physical (somatic) symptoms; (2) those who present with obsessive compulsive disorders, eating disorders, and substance use disorders; and (3) those who present with symptoms of psychosis. All these individuals may also have comorbid physical symptoms, or both conditions may affect each other.

One of the major advantages of psychiatric care occurring in primary care settings is that it takes place locally in an accessible and less stigmatizing environment. Such care can integrate physical and mental health. Psychology and nursing services can be based in the community. Joint consultations with mental health specialists may support primary care physicians and further empower them to manage individuals with mental illness, reducing demands on secondary care.

As mentioned in chapter 2, in many countries, the shortage of doctors means that healers trained in traditional medicine (TM) systems (e.g., traditional Chinese medicine, Ayurveda, or homeopathy) may well be the first frontline professionals to be consulted. In many countries, these professionals have been trained in or are allowed to prescribe allopathic medication as well. Often, they are an underutilized resource, and improved coordination between systems could improve overall care for the mentally ill. In South Africa, where an estimated 80 percent of the population use TM, traditional healers are now regulated similarly to allopathic physicians, and initiatives supporting knowledge-sharing and inter-referrals are ongoing (Mothibe & Sibanda, 2019).

This interaction between psychiatrists and primary care physicians is of great importance. The association can be advisory, collaborative, a partnership, or simply liaison support. The advantages of such a collaboration are many, with family physicians providing the following:

1. *Accessibility of care:* Not only are family physicians normally the first point of contact, but in many health care systems, including private ones, they are also more likely to cost less, whether the charges are paid for by the individual from their own pocket or by the insurance companies. They provide easy, equitable, and timely access to all patients for diagnosis and treatment. They are also more likely to be found in many geographical areas. They can provide initial assessment and appropriate referral, if needed.
2. *Continuity of care:* In many countries, they provide care for a considerable period, from childhood to death or from the onset of a disease to its resolution. They may have provided both prenatal and perinatal care and pediatric interventions. They get to know their patients and their families and caregivers, and by forming close bonds with individuals, they can respond appropriately to changes in the patient's circumstances or to their physical, psychological, social, and cultural background.
3. *Whole family approach:* It is quite likely that the whole family may seek treatment from the same family physician. As a care provider, they will be fully aware of any changes in family circumstances and will thus provide a true community service. This approach may also lay a strong foundation for some public mental health interventions and support, allowing for the recognition and correction of some types of mental health inequality, as well as more appropriate access to secondary care and the management of complex comorbidities.

4. *Complex comorbidity care:* Because primary care physicians are on the front line, they can recognize and learn to manage complex comorbidities. This is particularly important and useful in comorbidities between physical and mental health. Physical ill-health can contribute to development and perpetuation of mental illnesses, and individuals with a mental illness have higher levels of physical morbidities and are likely to die younger than their healthy counterparts. Family physicians can reach appropriate decisions and learn to manage risk in the community.
5. *Holistic approach:* Because they are based in the community, they are also more likely to be aware of local resources and can work across boundaries providing care over the individual's lifespan. They are aware of a wide range of problems and diagnoses and can provide preventive care, early diagnosis and intervention for individuals who may have more than one chronic condition.
6. *Coordination of care*: Family physicians are best placed to coordinate care across medical and nonmedical specialties and navigate the health care system, not only on behalf of their patients, but also with them recognizing when they should intervene and when they should step back. They coordinate care with other professionals to make sure that patients get the best care and that their health and social care needs are met.
7. *Cost-effective care*: In many countries, they see 90 percent of first medical contacts and treat a variety of problems, thus controlling the number of unnecessary investigations and inappropriate interventions. They can reduce health care costs in hospitals.

Specialist Care Services

Secondary care services or hospitals are often not able to select who they provide care to, so they may need to design, develop, and deliver a range of services for a range of conditions across the lifespan. For people with mental illnesses, services need to take risk assessment into account while evaluating the needs of the patient. The links between secondary care services and community mental health teams are incredibly important and need to be wide-ranging with other stakeholders. Secondary care often means specialist care, and the range of services must include short-term admissions on a crisis basis so that once the crisis has passed, patients can be discharged home. In addition, acute care, ongoing care, and supported accommodation will be needed, which will require staff and other resources. Day hospitals, day centers, or sheltered/supported employment may be needed, depending on the needs of patients. Whether in secondary care or in the community, delivery of care relies on multidisciplinary and intersectoral care and approaches though this may not be possible but should be strived for. Diverse team members bring different sets of skills and expertise as well as experience to ensure that the biopsychosocial–spiritual model of mental illness management is followed and delivered. These workers will need appropriate training and clearly identified and agreed-on responsibilities but also support.

No service can be expected to meet the needs of everyone with mental illnesses unless it is also able to provide a safe haven (and asylum in the true sense of the word) for those requiring care in both the hospital and the community, with full support. Those who are severely and persistently ill and incapacitated may need a range of options in which they can be cared for, recover, rehabilitate, and return to the community. One way of designing, developing, and delivering services is to focus on specific geographical catchment areas that could be administrative districts. Each district can focus on the needs of a set population, with extra attention paid to vulnerable individuals, those with special needs, and transitory populations. Thus, a range of inpatient activities, wards, crisis homes, respite care, halfway houses, day hospitals, and day centers will be required, although the actual number of facilities can vary.

For all services, electronic care records and modern information technology are likely to play a major role. Within any country, it is a good idea to use the same system across territories if at all possible. The datasets need to be fit for purpose to ensure confidentiality, utility, and data quality so that accurate levels of morbidity are known in order to develop appropriate services, evaluate them, and modify them if needed. Furthermore, many but not all services can now be delivered online or as hybrid "online and in person" models. The benefits and risks of tele-mental health and e-mental health are further discussed in chapter 10.

In any given district (geographical or administrative), the following components should be considered, with services ranging from adult psychiatry to outpatient services to (medical) psychotherapy, among others.

Adult Psychiatry

This service can be available to those over the age of 18; however, while an upper age limit may be established, the focus should not be on an arbitrary age cutoff but rather on the needs of the patients. Continuity of care is important. The number of beds required for such care can be adjusted according to needs, but close collaboration with social care, primary care, and other agencies, such as employment services, should be encouraged. Within the broad scope of adult psychiatry, rehabilitation and recovery services that focus on integrating those with severe mental illnesses must provide varying and tailored levels of support. This support may be ongoing and long-term but should remain proactive; often, NGOs may be better suited to meet these needs, hence local collaborative partnerships are important.

The relationships between primary care, community teams, community care, and secondary hospital care must be clear and seamless. Community teams may be based in primary care, operate as independent centers (such as mental health resource centers or community hubs), or be located within hospitals. In any setting, the team must have easy access to both primary care and hospital care without barriers. Community teams may create obstacles if they are divided into functional teams. It is always vital that the referral of patients across teams is as smooth as possible.

For adult services, access to urgent and immediate services is important. In many countries, there are separate psychiatric emergency rooms; by and large, individuals with mental illnesses present to emergency rooms and are assessed by psychiatric teams. It has been shown anecdotally that individuals presenting with mental illnesses, if aggressive or violent, may be perceived as disruptive and may find a more stigmatizing environment outside these settings. These services must be readily available and should be known to families, patients themselves, their caregivers, and the community. There are two types of crises that individuals with mental illnesses may face—life-threatening crises, which involve the danger of self-harm or harm to others, and non-life-threatening crises. Thus, it is important to have access to "safe spaces" where individuals can be looked after. Appropriate interventions need to be put in place when there is the danger of self-harm, suicide, and risk to others. Safe spaces allow individuals in crisis to withdraw from their normal social roles in order to manage their stress before returning to their usual environment.

Under these circumstances, supportive care and psychotherapy may help them to recover.

People with a short illness with rapid onset, those who have been destabilized, or those in acute psychosocial crisis may require crisis homes or safe spaces for a specified time period. In addition, emergency services may include telephone or video counseling and assessment (which can be provided by volunteers or NGOs—also see chapter 10 on telehealth), walk-in services, short stays for assessment at day centers, and inpatient access. Families and carers may need support and in certain situations may approach police or emergency services, so regular liaison work with these entities will be important. Crisis intervention teams can be helpful sometimes to avoid admission so that individuals can be looked after at home; however, this option requires elevated levels of support. Domiciliary visits and assessments at home can be extremely helpful in understanding the levels of functioning and circumstances in which individuals are living. They also allow the assessors to determine the patient's available levels of support. It is not always possible to call on crisis intervention teams, though, as they are costly and require close collaboration with inpatient units for those patients who cannot be safely or therapeutically helped in the community. It may also be worth considering establishing specialist peripatetic support teams dedicated to those with long-term needs. Emergency services require close collaboration with mental health teams so that stays or contacts with emergency services can be as brief as possible. Short-term services refer to day hospital admissions, attendance at day centers, primary care settings, or outpatient services.

Outpatient Services

Outpatient services can be provided in primary care settings, community mental health centers (mental health resource centers), hospitals, or voluntary agency or social services premises. In some settings, psychiatric nurses or other mental health professionals provide initial assessments, whereas in others it may be the psychiatrist.

Day Centers/Day Hospitals

Day hospitals provide assessment and treatment, whereas day centers can offer rehabilitation and training for employment. In many places, day hospitals are run by nurses and day centers by occupational therapists. Both facilities provide structure to individuals who need it.

Day hospitals can be used for avoiding inpatient admission; they provide assessment and medical supervision and serve as sites for brief intervention or long-term support. Day centers provide medium- to long-term facilities to engage individuals with chronic mental illnesses, personality disorders, and severe nonpsychotic disorders, offering support and training.

Inpatient Units

There is no doubt that some patients, because of the severity of their illness or for assessment purposes, will require inpatient admission. Admissions can be urgent or routine, emergency or planned, short or long. The number of beds required can be calculated according to the population and their needs. It is critical that the wards are therapeutic environments where patients can feel safe and recover with suitable therapeutic alliances. The wards must be welcoming and calm places with adequate staffing. The teams need to be multidisciplinary, and ward rounds should accordingly offer biopsychosocial models of management. Occasionally, intensive care units may be needed. Acute care wards, long-stay wards, and intensive care require different philosophies. The wards should be small with options for privacy. Occasionally, the inpatient units can be located in acute medical/surgical hospitals. Confidentiality remains paramount, and close collaboration across various facilities is important. The needs for physical health care may require liaison physicians and initiating treatment in the wards, but transitioning care to the community is a must.

Outreach Services

In many countries, outreach services provide material resources (e.g., food, shelter and clothing), cognitive resources (e.g., rehabilitation, coping strategies, motivational training), and medication (e.g., long acting or monitoring medication with appropriate support and education). Resources in the form of trained or voluntary personnel are also required for delivering these services.

Long-Term Care

Long-term care will be needed for some individuals who have chronic psychiatric conditions, whereas others will benefit from day care. Specific, targeted, and tailored interventions are better for therapeutic engagement and outcomes, but they may be more expensive. Thus, rehabilitation should be viewed as the process through which individuals with mental illnesses can acquire skills and improve their functional abilities, leading to improvements in their latent strengths and capabilities to overcome or minimize any deficits they may be experiencing as a result of their illness. There is no doubt that one size does not fit all, but these core principles must apply to all:

- Prevention or reduction of impairments and social disabilities
- Improvement of strengths and resilience by enabling individuals to perform roles according to social needs and expectations
- Enhancement of well-being in order to minimize the burden on caregivers, whether professional or social/informal carers

Rehabilitation

The aim of rehabilitation is to slow down any deterioration and maximize levels of functioning so that an individual can achieve their best potential. Individuals with a severe mental illness, including organic brain disorders, can benefit from rehabilitation if appropriate levels of intervention are instigated. With specific targeted services, individuals may live in sheltered or supported accommodations, moving up or down the scale according to their needs and their response to rehabilitation. Rehabilitation therefore needs to focus on daily living, employment opportunities, and recreational activities—each requiring specific levels of support. Some of these services will be provided by health care professionals and others by social care or nongovernmental agencies.

Community-based rehabilitation for schizophrenia includes assertive community treatment (ACT) and supported employment programs. ACT provides intensive, multidisciplinary support to individuals with severe mental illness, reducing hospitalization rates and improving social functioning (Bond & Drake, 2015; Kim, et al. 2015; Marshall & Lockwood, 2000).

Some individuals who require rehabilitation may need community-based accommodations from hostel wards (for those needing 24-hour care) and group homes; they may require sheltered support accommodation, sheltered single accommodation, independent accommodation, or family accommodation. However, patients must be encouraged to express their choice and control over their living environment. Peer support and patient advocates can facilitate assisted living decisions. Team members, too, can act as brokers and advocates. Self-help groups and peer support should be encouraged, if needed. Counseling and training for employment, consumer-run housing facilities, peer-support workers, and educators can all help engage the community. The health services need to build links with local employers to help develop a range of sheltered employment, training opportunities, vocational services, and full-employment opportunities for finding placements that match individual needs and abilities. Such activities and developments must be protected and ring-fenced, especially during periods of high unemployment or economic recession. Employers, schools, and religious institutions can all help to ensure that sheltered employment opportunities are available that work for the betterment of individuals with mental illness.

Supporting Carers

Informal carers play a vital role in helping to look after individuals with severe mental illness, but very often, they do not get any support or even acknowledgment. They must be part of the management process and strategy. Involving and engaging them and providing them with information about the illness, the warning signs of relapse, and the side effects of medication and other drug interactions can help reduce the likelihood of relapse and improve better engagement. Improved engagement and involvement of carers (see appendix 10) may well lead to their increased satisfaction and potentially lower rates or the need for admission.

Often in low- and middle-income countries, relatives are the frontline caregivers, but they may not know about relapse signs, access to services, and the role of medication. Engaging with the community and educating them is important. Families and carers should not be blamed; if needed, they should be encouraged to participate in family therapy. A range of activities, from simple education to involving informal carers in managing individuals with mental illness through counseling and practical support, should be provided at both the individual and community levels. The aim is to empower informal carers to cope with long-term disabilities, including providing respite care if needed. Caregiver involvement in service design and education is helpful and should be encouraged. Appropriate support may be required to ensure their participation.

Services for Children and Young People

These services must consider the educational needs of children and young people as well as the needs of their families. The very nature of children and their developing inner worlds and external contacts makes it essential that services are linked with families, schools, special needs, and social services in a cogent and accessible manner. In most countries, school education is compulsory, thereby creating an easily approachable population. School-based mental health services are discussed in chapter 8.

WHO (2022a) offers overview of Child and Adolescent Mental Health Services (CAMHS). These services in high-income countries such as the UK, offer a model with four tiers. The first tier includes school nurses, health visitors, and similar professionals. Tier two comprises primary mental health workers who provide support to other professionals regarding child development. Tier three is made up of specialist multidisciplinary teams, while tier four includes specialized day and inpatient units where individuals with more severe mental health issues can be assessed and treated. Depending on the population and its needs, a number of beds will be required for inpatient treatment. Special schools might be necessary alongside mainstream education, even though efforts to integrate schools are underway. In many settings, children may be looking after parents who have a mental illness. As many of these individuals will be in touch with adult psychiatric services, it is crucial that closer links across services are maintained. Children who may have other comorbidities, are in social care, or have intellectual disabilities will require more specific and better targeted services.

For young people, the use of social media is increasingly relevant, and it may be used in a more focused and productive way as described in chapter 10 (on tele-mental health and e-mental health).

Services for Older Adults

In the past half century, there has been truly astonishing progress in increasing the longevity of populations around the globe, although these advances are beginning to stall in many high-income countries. However, people living longer has also meant that rates of dementia and other complex comorbidities are rising. Some individuals develop mental illness in adulthood and live to old age and therefore require appropriate services. However, social and economic determinants of mental illnesses in old age and comorbidity between physical and mental illnesses also contribute to higher rates of psychiatric disorders among older adults. Primary care, social care, and geriatric physicians together are an inherent part of psychiatric services for older adults. Specialist services for older adults should also champion services for older individuals with mental illness.

Psychiatric services for older adults are best located in the community. Local needs must determine whether the distinction is based on age or needs. For example, some services cater only to individuals with dementia, whereas others care for everyone over the age of 65. This age cut-off can be purely arbitrary. Services need to work closely with primary care physicians, other secondary care specialists, social care, community agencies, and NGOs. Acute services may be community-based but need to be fast, flexible, and close to the population they serve. Rapid assessment by a trained individual, irrespective of the discipline, is a must. Crisis interventions conducted at home, day centers, day hospitals, acute medical settings, and other appropriate locations are important. If at all possible, crises should be avoided through preparedness to implement suitable and appropriate actions. It is likely that older adults will require acute beds, continuing care beds, day hospital placements, and outpatient services. Electronic case notes can help trigger "red flags" to warn the team about impending crises.

Consultation Liaison Services

General hospital psychiatry, or consultation liaison psychiatry, is an important specialty within the field. A significant number of patients with physical disorders are likely to have psychiatric disorders, usually common mental disorders such as anxiety or depression. The services may be based in acute hospitals or in the community. The service must comprise a range of psychiatric, psychological, nursing, and social work skills and expertise. Various models, from simple advice to joint ward rounds and joint working, can be used. Services should extend to emergency rooms where suitable interview spaces are available so that individual patients can be interviewed in peace and quiet. Assessing patients for compulsory treatment can be an important aspect of liaison services. Team members must be trained in brief psychotherapies as well as family and couples counseling.

Depending on the needs of the population, neuropsychiatrists may, for example, work with diabetes specialists or gynecological or other specialties in order to deliver suitable and appropriate services. Whether funding of these services comes from mental health services or acute care will depend on the local needs and local health care systems, but it is essential to ensure adequate resources and staffing.

Forensic Services

Offenders with a mental health disorder often end up inappropriately in prisons. Health resources may not be available to look after these individuals in health care systems. A majority of therapeutic work with these individuals is carried out by general psychiatrists rather than specialized forensic psychiatrists. Thus, there must be a close working relationship between general psychiatric services, prisons, forensic facilities (if they exist), and special hospital services in order to provide a spectrum of services, from special hospitals to secure units to locked wards to open wards. Again, depending on needs, high-, medium-, or low-security units must be developed. These will have to be at a regional or supra-regional level. The secure units are required to deliver a range of services, including rehabilitation. Pre-discharge units may help prepare individuals for smoother reintegration into the community. The delivery of psychiatric care in prison has its own set of imperatives. Issues such as confidentiality, as well as urgent and ongoing treatments, need to be addressed. Liaison with the police and court division schemes may be beneficial. Again, multiagency collaboration is critical.

For example, over two-thirds of prisoners in US jails are said to have psychiatric disorders. These prisons have been called asylums without treatments. The Los Angeles County jail is reported to serve more people with mental illness than any single mental health facility in the US, although local programs, such as court diversion schemes, have been initiated. These prisons accommodating individuals with mental illness have been described as nothing short of a public health crisis (Haneberg et al., 2016). These authors suggest that local leaders should plan and allocate funds with well-defined lines of responsibility. They propose that a clear definition of mental illness as well as severe mental illness be agreed on and applied. Similarly, a system-wide definition of substance use disorders should be agreed on, with valid assessment tools and clear lines of communication and information-sharing. Salt Lake City, Utah, has an interesting framework in place that looks at criminogenic risk, which can be applied to the likelihood of criminal activity, developing substance use disorder, and developing mental illness. Haneberg et al. (2016) also go on to emphasize the importance of establishing clear definitions of recidivism within the prison system. Coordinated planning of services with community partners and other stakeholders is essential, and outcomes need to be clearly defined and agreed on.

Substance Use

Individuals who have problematic substance use have similar needs to those with mental illnesses. The type of dependence and the preferred substance will vary across cultures and geographies. Increasing decriminalization and legalization of certain substances has raised issues related to rates of dependence. Education about substance misuse and prevention strategies is incredibly important. Comorbidity with mental illnesses is well recognized. Many individuals with mental illnesses will use substances such as tobacco or cannabis to dampen their symptoms, although cannabis use is strongly associated with psychotic disorders in vulnerable individuals (Di Forti et al., 2019). Substance misuse reflects mental health in general. Community care for substance use in many high-income countries has been delegated to primary care, but in many other cases, specialist interventions will be needed. A small proportion of individuals will need short-term inpatient care or longer-term residential care. Sometimes day hospitals, day centers, and opiate substitute treatment clinics may be more effective. Managing substance misuse in the community also has major challenges considering legal issues, psychiatric comorbidities, the stigma around drug use, and variable engagement by patients. Furthermore, high rates of substance misuse in prisons raise special concerns, particularly the higher risk of drug overdose after release due to reduced tolerance. It is essential that all mental health professionals are trained in managing substance misuse. Alcohol dependence is also associated with higher levels of physical morbidity. Certain steps can be taken at the policy level—for example, alcohol pricing and the legal age for purchase—but other interventions will need to occur at the local or clinical level. Other addictions such as gambling must be acknowledged and treated.

(Medical) Psychotherapy Services

Some individuals with mental illnesses will require (medical) psychotherapy of any number of types: psychoanalytic, cognitive behavioral, behavioral, family, couple, or dialectic. These services should be available in primary care settings or in community mental health centers. District-wide psychotherapy teams may be formed. It is entirely possible that in many countries, owing to the lack of training opportunities and resources, the access to psychotherapy may be limited and difficult. District teams can help develop psychotherapy skills in community mental health teams, in primary care, in day care, and in other community settings with NGOs and religious or community leaders. It is essential that district teams screen psychotherapy referrals and that those accepted should be pointed in the right direction. They should be able to provide specialized psychotherapy services and therapeutic support. They should also deliver supervision and education. In improving access to psychological treatments, a number of therapists can be trained and supported. In some countries, community workers or religious leaders have been trained to offer psychotherapy services. Based on need and demand, inpatient psychotherapy units such as therapeutic communities may be needed. Even in high-income countries, the number of psychotherapists is low, therefore delivering services through other trained individuals may be the best way forward in delivering services.

Vulnerable Groups

As mentioned before, many vulnerable groups show high rates of psychiatric disorders for any number of reasons. Only some are discussed below.

Homeless People

Globally, homelessness is an increasing problem. Sometimes, individuals with mental illness can lose their homes or security of tenure, while those already homeless may develop psychiatric disorders. It is estimated that up to half of all homeless individuals may have a psychiatric disorder. In addition, they are also likely to have coexisting physical or infectious illnesses. Many migrate to big cities or places with better weather, placing further pressure on existing services in those communities. It is important that services conduct outreach in the community, either directly or indirectly through shelters and hostels for the homeless, with close collaboration between NGOs and primary care services. Homeless individuals are also highly likely to have addiction problems and may thus require these services as well.

Veterans

After leaving the services, many veterans develop various psychiatric disorders and are homeless, which makes it complicated to deliver health care to them in spite of veteran administration facilities being available around the country. Similar observations have been made from other countries. Veterans often have higher rates of conditions such as depression, substance misuse, agitation, and post-traumatic stress disorders which will require specialist interventions. Their health care needs can be provided in civilian settings, but clear coordination is necessary with military facilities to ensure proper handover and follow-up, which must include accommodation, if needed, and rehabilitation services.

LGBTQ+ People

Ensuring legal equality for LGBTQ+individuals can lower the rates of mental health concerns in this population. Hatzenbuehler (2012) found that LGBTQ+mental health outcomes improve in jurisdictions with protective legislation. Bhugra et al. (2022) emphasize the need for affirmative therapy and legal protections to counteract the psychological toll of discrimination. Advocacy for policy change is thus essential. The question whether LGBTQ+individuals should have separate services raises challenging issues about generic versus specialist services. In countries where such behavior is illegal, individuals are more likely to hide their sexual orientation and therefore may not seek psychiatric help at all or, if they do, they may share only partial information about themselves. Mental health care staff need to be trained to be sensitive in their approaches and to be aware of their own prejudices and weaknesses.

People with Intellectual Disabilities

Individuals with intellectual disabilities are also likely to have comorbid psychiatric disorders across different age groups. Furthermore, they are more vulnerable to abuse and exploitation. Thus, services need to cater to several needs at once. Individuals with intellectual disabilities are more likely to have sensory or motor impairment and high rates of self-harm, autism, challenging behaviors, epilepsy, and other organic conditions. Hence, services must to be prepared to cater to a range of needs. Services must include education and social care in addition to health care. In these circumstances, working with voluntary agencies can be fruitful. Supporting services for families, teachers, and informal carers must also be part of health care. Genetic counseling and advice, along with screening options, are important and, wherever possible, should be made easily accessible. A range of options—from outpatient services to day centers, day hospitals, respite care, and inpatient units—should be developed. There may be specialized services, but the movement across services must be seamless.

Black and Indigenous People of Color (BIPOC) and Minority Ethnic Groups

The needs of people of color and minority ethnic groups must be emphasized. The rates of psychiatric disorders are higher among these groups for many complex reasons as described in chapter 5. They may delay help-seeking due to different explanatory models of mental illnesses, different levels of awareness and knowledge about health care systems, and also stigma against mental illness. Language and lack of access to interpreters may prove to be barriers, too. It must be emphasized that communities are heterogeneous, and their characteristics and needs will vary. Monitoring of ethnic groups can help providers plan services in a more focused and targeted manner. Culture brokers or culture mediators may facilitate knowledge and interactions between service providers and communities. Ethnic matching of therapists and individuals needing health care may not always lead to better therapeutic adherence or alliance. Some individuals may feel that by presenting to the services they are showing weakness and letting their culture down. Trained interpreters should be used whenever possible.

Cultural sensitivity and humility training for anyone working with BIPOC and ethnic minority groups is essential. It is good clinical practice for health care practitioners to be aware of their own prejudices and cultural biases as well as the sociocultural strengths and weaknesses of their patient's culture. Practitioners need to be aware of cultural norms and values of the patient they are looking after. Similarly, the role, importance, and expectations of medication and psychotherapy vary across cultures. Ego-based therapies, for example, may not work in sociocentric individuals.

A community is formed of a group of people based on some common features. However, communities are heterogeneous; individuals will have a common template, but their responses, expectations, and engagement with health care will differ. Community mental health services or mental health resource centers need to be engaged in and with the community. These services require different levels and varieties of activities for patients, their carers, and their families. Furthermore, community mental health services can be based in primary care, in independent settings, in partnership with nongovernmental organizations, and in hospitals. However, these services must be accessible, available, and appropriate to meet the needs of the community they are expected to serve. Working with the community and other stakeholders in designing, developing, and delivering services is crucial. Ownership by the community will lead to better therapeutic engagement. Service delivery needs to consider all the vulnerable groups that may require more targeted and specialist interventions.

There are good examples of partnerships in providing care in the community in Los Angeles. By partnering with safety net partners, Community Partners in Care (CPIC, 2016) was able to target low-income Latino and African American communities, focusing on depression. The results were fewer behavioral health hospitalizations, reduced homelessness, and increased use of faith-based depression services. According to CPIC, community coalitions across multiple service sections should be engaged to develop effective strategies to improve health and social outcomes for depression in under-resourced communities. Their second observation/recommendation is that mental health disparities can be addressed through direct partnerships with community stakeholders, collaborating in evidence-based strategies adapted to the community context (CPIC, 2016). This model works especially as a vast majority of individuals with depression are treated in the community. It is vital that communities take ownership of such innovation rather than having it imposed from above. For deeper explorations of race, ethnicity, and mental health, the interested reader is referred to Fernando (2010) and Moodley and Lee (2020).

Refugees, Asylum Seekers, and Migrants

People who seek refuge or asylum or migrate are particularly vulnerable to poor mental health as they face multiple stressors before, during, and after migration, as well as the factors described in the previous section on BIPOC. Many have experienced conflicts, war, persecution, violence, or natural disasters, leading to high rates of post-traumatic stress disorder (PTSD), anxiety, and depression (Silove et al., 2017). Forced displacement and loss of home, loved ones, and identity further contribute to grief and emotional distress (Fazel et al., 2012). Uncertainty regarding legal status, work rights, and potential deportation creates chronic stress and anxiety (Lindert et al., 2009). Economic hardship, limited job opportunities, and barriers to social support exacerbate financial and psychological strain (Priebe et al., 2016; Reibling et al., 2017). Language difficulties and cultural differences can result in social isolation and hinder access to health care (Bhugra & Becker, 2005). Additionally, discrimination, racism, and exclusion increase distress and feelings of hopelessness (Abebe et al., 2014). Many migrants are also separated from family members, leading to loss of support, prolonged psychological distress, and difficulty integrating into new societies (Miller & Rasmussen, 2010). Addressing these challenges requires appropriately targeted, culturally sensitive, and competent mental health services, legal protections, and social integration policies to support the well-being of displaced populations (see Bhugra et al., 2010; Bhugra & Gupta 2010; Cossu et al., 2018).

As the first Western-trained psychiatrist in Africa, Thomas Adeoye Lambo established the Aro Village system in Nigeria, a pioneering approach that placed patients in therapeutic communal settings resembling their home environments. This model facilitated the combination of conventional medical treatments with traditional healing methods, effectively reducing stigma and improving patient outcomes (Heaton, 2018).

Experts in many countries have developed culturally aligned innovations to improve mental health, some of which are presented in appendix 12.

Types of Services

Psychiatric services in the community should be accessible 24 hours a day. If that is not possible, then training should be mandatory for emergency room staff to provide psychiatric assessments and urgent intervention. It is important to draw a distinction between 24-hour routine and 24-hour emergency services. These should be configured according to local needs. When a range of services are provided, it is critical that the borders between services are permeable for the patients. Community services must include various forms of accommodation, including crisis homes and various types of employment (e.g., sheltered, independent, assisted).

Social structures and epidemiological data should guide the types of services provided, based on population needs. Wherever possible, primary care teams and the community mental health team must work collaboratively. While it may not always be possible to establish specialized services (e.g., age-based services), it should be possible—and indeed encouraged—for individuals to develop specialized skills. Then, for example, even if they are working within adult services, some staff can be trained to look after young people, while others manage older adults or individuals with learning disabilities.

Secondary care services must be encouraged to devote time and resources to education, partnerships, training, and after-discharge support, including working with local employers for sheltered employment, if needed.

For children and young people (adolescents), clinical services should have close links with schools, teachers, school nurses, and pediatricians. Admission and assessment beds may be needed. For young people, early intervention services, rapid assessment, and support for education as well as employment must be made available. Services must be provided for children, young people, and younger and older adults with intellectual disabilities. Furthermore, working with families is a core part of service delivery. Again, facilities ranging from acute intensive care, at one end of the spectrum, and independent living facilities, at the other, must be available and supported. A range of secure facilities may be needed. The specific needs of children with intellectual disabilities must be met.

For adults, a range of services (e.g., consultation liaison psychiatry, substance abuse, psychotherapy, prison services, rehabilitation services, perinatal services) should be available. Adults should have access to specialist neuropsychiatry and services for eating disorders. Team members should be supported and encouraged to have specialist training in selected fields. Inpatient services should include intensive care and acute care, but day centers and day hospitals are needed, too.

Services for older adults must ensure access to different assisted living options, coordinated across different areas and with accessibility to hospital beds. The number of beds needed will depend on the needs of the local population. Inpatient units must include acute beds, continuing care beds, day hospitals, day centers, and outpatients services. Integrated medical and social care is critical for the effective delivery of services for older adults.

Conclusion

Caring for communities is at the heart of psychiatric services. There can be basic models, but they must meet the mental health needs of local populations. Good epidemiological data, regular audits, and evaluation of services are important aspects of service delivery. Services must be accessible and supportive. Services must be able to offer rapid assessments to all age groups, but especially vulnerable groups. Triage services may be needed, whereby services are set up in community hubs, places of worship, schools, and universities. Working closely with primary care physicians, social services, prison staff, and others such as community and religious leaders can help reduce stigma and improve engagement. It may not be possible to have specialized services due to resource constraints, but efforts must be made to encourage teams to develop specialized skills in looking after vulnerable groups.

Acknowledgments

This chapter relies heavily on *Caring for a Community* by D. Bhugra, K. Bridges, and C. Thompson (1998), Council Report CR36, Royal College of Psychiatrists, London.

8 School Mental Health

Introduction

Mental health of children and young people is often overlooked for reasons ranging from a lack of understanding to stigma and insufficient resources with poor accessibility to specialized services. Teachers may frequently observe difficulties but expect parents to respond and behaviors may vary between home and school, which can further complicate identification and therapeutic interventions.

Mental health disorders in children and adolescents are not uncommon. They affect 10–20 percent of children and adolescents globally, impacting academic performance, social relationships, and long-term well-being (Kieling et al., 2011). An estimated 13–20 percent of children worldwide have a diagnosable psychiatric disorder (Polanczyk et al., 2015), yet only around half of affected children receive any mental health intervention (Whitney & Peterson, 2019). In low- and middle-income countries, these figures may well be lower. Schools are critical access points for mental health services, particularly in low-resource settings, where community-based care is limited (Layard, 2018). As emphasized in previous chapters, early intervention is essential, as 50 percent of mental illnesses in adulthood begin by age 14 (Kessler et al., 2005). Randomized controlled trials of school-based interventions yield mixed results. In a meta-analysis, Sanchez et al. (2018) showed that school-based interventions have a small to moderate long-term effect on reducing mental health issues, with targeted interventions demonstrating the most significant impact, particularly those integrated into the curriculum.

Prevalence Rates

The global prevalence of mental disorders among children and adolescents is a significant public health concern. The World Health Organization (WHO) reports that 8 percent of children and 15 percent of adolescents experience mental disorders globally (WHO, 2022a). Similarly, UNICEF estimated that one in seven adolescents (aged 10 to 19), or approximately 166 million individuals, were living with a mental disorder in 2019 (UNICEF, 2021). These figures predate COVID 2019 pandemic. A systematic review examining high-income countries found that the overall prevalence of any mental disorder in children was 12.7 percent, with anxiety disorders being the most common (5.2 percent), followed by attention deficit hyperactivity disorder (ADHD) (3.7 percent) and oppositional defiant disorder (3.3 percent) (Polanczyk et al., 2015).

A Whole School Approach

A mentally healthy school is one where the policies and actions support children and young people, allowing them to flourish, learn, and succeed by virtue of access to opportunities with or without caregiver support. Positive mental health and well-being (physical, mental, or emotional) are critical components in the school's mission, values, and cultures and affect not only the children and young people but also teachers and other staff. A whole school approach is needed with partnerships between teachers, pupils, parents, school governors, the community at large, and nongovernmental organizations (table 8.1). The whole school approach integrates mental health into policies, curriculum, staff training, and parental involvement. Schools that adopt this approach show better mental health outcomes and improved academic performance (Weare & Nind, 2011; Goldberg et al., 2019).

The key components of a whole school approach include the following:

- Staff training—equipping educators with youth mental health first aid (YMHFA) skills (see appendix 13)
- Student involvement—encouraging peer-led mental health initiatives.
- Family engagement—providing parental education programs on emotional well-being

Well-being encompasses access to nutritious and affordable food, physical activities, and the cultivation of resilience, empathy, and positive peer relationships. Addressing potential aggression and behavioral issues at an early stage can also enhance well-being. Integrating emotional literacy, social skills, spiritual development, and play-based individual or group therapies—along with improving teacher competencies in managing distressed children and employing role-play—can effectively tackle a variety of challenges. School curricula must therefore address well-being, resilience, early-warning signs of stress and distress, early access to help if needed, and clear pathways to sources of help and safe spaces.

Principles for School Mental Health Interventions

School mental health encompasses public mental health, educational psychology, and related aspects of health and well-being. Randomized controlled trials of school-based interventions yield mixed results. Sanchez et al. (2018) conducted a meta-analysis showing that school-based interventions have a small to moderate long-term effect on reducing mental health issues, with targeted interventions demonstrating the most significant impact, particularly those integrated into the curriculum. Effective strategies should consider the varied learning needs of children, young people, parents, and teachers.

Public Health England (PHE, n.d.) has created a toolkit to help schools measure and monitor student well-being, emphasizing the importance of a systematic approach to support students through appropriate assessment and evaluation. PHE stresses that evaluation should be central to the process, enabling the identification of effective areas as well as those requiring intervention. PHE outlines seven steps for implementing mental health and well-being measurement in educational settings:

1. Why is the approach being taken?
2. What needs to be measured?
3. Who provides the information?
4. When is the information collected?
5. Where is the information collected?
6. How is the information collected?
7. What next?

While variations in school mental health approaches will exist across countries, it is feasible to enhance knowledge about mental health, stress management, early issue recognition, and guiding individuals and families through care pathways. Establishing strategic partnerships for educational activities is essential. Despite limited resources, training can be offered to students, teachers, and community members to recognize mental ill-health, early signs, and ways to seek help. Mental health literacy can be taught through a variety of methods.

Levels of Mental Health Service Delivery in Schools

Schools vary in their mental health service models, ranging from universal prevention programs to targeted clinical care. The tiered model of school mental health, often referred to as multitiered systems of support (MTSS), is a structured framework used in schools to deliver mental health services at three levels of increasing intensity, ensuring that all students receive appropriate support based on their needs (Fazel et al., 2014). This model (table 8.1) is widely adopted in high-income countries and serves as a foundation for integrated school-based mental health systems (Nitz et al., 2023). Such multitiered models improve access to care and reduce symptom severity by 30–50 percent when effectively implemented (Fazel et al., 2014). A study by Walter et al. (2019) evaluated a school-hospital partnership that implemented an MTSS model over three years in urban schools. The findings indicated that such a model is feasible, valued, and effective in improving students' mental health status and enhancing schools' capacities to provide mental health services (Walter et al., 2019).

Box 8.1
The Whole School Approach

1. Identifying and building resilience
2. Identifying sources of support
3. Early recognition and management of stress
4. Early assessment if needed
5. Working with children and young people
6. Working with parents
7. Working with the community
8. Destigmatizing approaches
9. Identifying and eliminating bullying
10. Supporting and protecting vulnerable children and young people

Table 8.1
Three-tiered structure of MTSS

Tier	Target population	Key features	Example interventions
Tier 1: Universal (whole school approach)	All students	• Focuses on mental health promotion and prevention • Incorporates mental health literacy into curricula • Reduces stigma and promotes help-seeking behaviors	• Social and emotional learning (SEL) programs • Anti-bullying policies • Mental health awareness campaigns
Tier 2: Targeted (early intervention for at-risk students)	Students identified as at-risk for mental health issues	• Provides small-group interventions • Uses teacher referrals and screening tools to identify at-risk students • Addresses mild to moderate emotional/behavioral concerns	• Small-group therapy (e.g., anxiety management) • Teacher-led cognitive behavioral strategies • School counselor check-ins
Tier 3: Intensive (specialist mental health support)	Students with severe and complex mental health needs	• Offers individualized interventions for students with diagnosed mental illnesses) • Involves school psychologists, social workers, and external mental health professionals • Ensures referral pathways to specialized care (e.g., CAMHS).	• One-on-one counseling and therapy • Collaboration with external mental health services • Individualized education plans (IEPs) for students with psychiatric conditions

Note: CAMHS, Child and Adolescent Mental Health Services; MTSS, multitiered systems of support.

Evidence-Based School Mental Health Interventions

There are proprietary programs for school mental health that go over the whole school period and may include simple measures such as media exposure training, stress management, and sex education but also more complex teaching about resilience and parenting skills (Gillham et al., 2007; Brunwasser et al., 2009; Layard et al., 2018). In many countries, these programs may be hard to deliver, but every effort must be made to prepare future generations to take care of their mental health and well-being.

Mental Health Literacy in Schools

Mental health literacy programs teach students to recognize symptoms, seek help, and practice self-care. Studies demonstrate that school-based mental health literacy programs enhance knowledge, attitudes, and help-seeking behaviors (Mori et al., 2022). Furthermore, increased mental health awareness reduces stigma and improves mental health literacy (Perry et al., 2014).

Peer Mental Health Education

Peer-led interventions among school students have been shown to enhance help-seeking behavior and reduce stigma associated with mental health issues. For instance, a study by Wyman et al. (2010) evaluated the "Sources of Strength" program, a peer-led suicide prevention initiative implemented in high schools. The findings demonstrated that the program improved peer leaders' connectedness to adults and increased the likelihood of students seeking help for distress, thereby contributing to reduced stigma and enhanced help-seeking behaviors. Hamwaka (2015), in a study in Malawi, demonstrated that peer mental health education may improve youth mental health through improved (and perhaps better) education and positively impact overall community mental health literacy by connecting peers with communities and schools. Therefore, involving peers may lessen stigma and enhance help-seeking behaviors. Peer health education can therefore be a vital resource in education.

Managing Bullying and Cyberbullying

Bullying is a significant risk factor for mental health issues among adolescents, with victims being twice as likely to develop anxiety and depression (Arseneault, 2022). Over a period of three years, Bonell et al. (2018)

demonstrated that for an additional cost of $75 per pupil in intervention schools, there was a significant reduction in bullying but not in aggression. Research indicates that comprehensive anti-bullying policies implemented throughout the entire school can lead to a reduction in bullying incidents and victimization, although effect sizes are modest (Gaffney et al., 2021). Family training and bystander training improves students' ability to cope with cyberbullying (Chicote-Beato et al., 2024). Moreover, restorative justice approaches reduce violence, improve emotional well-being, and promote socio-emotional skills (Alonso-Rodriguez et al., 2025).

Parental Education Programs

Parental involvement in school mental health enhances early identification of issues and treatment engagement. Scott et al. (2010), in a randomized controlled trial, demonstrated that educating parents of six-year-olds on managing a child's aggressive behavior effectively reduced and improved the management of such behavior. Baker-Henningham et al. (2012) demonstrated in a randomized controlled trial conducted in Jamaica that training teachers can also reduce aggressive behavior in children, thereby confirming the third aim of the school mental health programs. Other effective models include the Triple P (Positive Parenting Program), which has been shown to reduce conduct disorders and improve child emotional regulation (Sanders, 1999), and the Family Check-Up Program, which effectively lowers rates of adolescent substance use and depression by approximately 30 percent (Stormshak & Dishion, 2009).

Digital Mental Health Tools

Digital mental health tools have become increasingly integrated into school-based interventions, offering students accessible and scalable mental health support. Online counseling services and AI-driven chatbots such as Woebot may reduce depression scores and appear to be a feasible, engaging, and effective way to deliver cognitive behavioral therapy (Fitzpatrick et al., 2017). Applications such as Calm and Headspace have been shown to reduce stress levels in college students (Huberty et al., 2019; Pierce et al., 2024). These apps require further exploration to assess their feasibility and success rates, as a recent meta-analysis did not show that school-based universal e-mental health interventions improved anxiety, depression, or well-being; additionally, a high risk of bias and low-quality studies were noted (Miller & Thabrew, 2024).

Personal, Social, Health, and Economic Education

Layard et al. (2018) conducted a thorough global review of the literature on school-based mental health interventions, exploring crucial areas such as resilience, social and emotional learning (SEL), relationships and sex education, healthy habits, social media awareness, and parenting. Their research underscored the significance of early intervention and structured well-being programs in schools to promote long-term psychological resilience and life skills.

Based on their review, these authors developed a four-year structured curriculum for mental health and well-being aimed at schools. The "Healthy Minds" course was conducted over four years for students aged 11 to 15, featuring one hour-long session each week that covered evidence-based psychological, social, and emotional skills to enhance student well-being. The contents of the course are detailed in table 8.2. The program aimed to equip students with lifelong coping strategies and reduce the risk of mental health disorders through preventive education and skill development. The course was evaluated in a randomized controlled trial that measured global health, life satisfaction, physical health, behaviors, and emotional health (London School of Economics [LSE], n.d.). Significant improvements were observed across all these domains, with a 10 percent increase in global health. However, in the case of emotional health, the sample size was deemed too small for the effect to be considered significant. The primary outcome measure revealed an effect size of 0.245 for general health improvement, indicating that the average Healthy Minds student's health surpasses that of 60 percent of students not participating in the program. This course was developed and evaluated at government-funded schools in the UK and therefore is likely to require local adaptation.

Looked After Better: Examples of Good Practice for School Mental Health in High- and Low-Income Countries

Examples of effective practices in school mental health from both high- and low-income countries are illustrated in table 8.3. These models should not be applied indiscriminately across all nations; they may require adaptation to suit local cultures, needs, and resources.

Table 8.2
Components of a four-year school "Healthy Minds" curriculum

Year (age)	Contents	Number of lessons
7 (11 to 12)	Penn Resilience Program*	18
	Media navigation (critical thinking around media)	6
	Breathe (stress management)	6
8 (12 to 13)	School to life (life skills for after graduation)	9
	Unplugged part 1 (substance use/ misuse)	4
	Media influences	8
	Sex education part 1	4
	Relationships	4
	Review and connect (reflection, personal growth, integration)	2
9 (13 to 14)	Relationships continued	8
	School health alcohol harm reduction	6
	Sex education part 2	6
	Resilient decisions (effective decision-making)	4
10 (14 to 15)	Mental illness (mental health literacy)	6
	Unplugged part 2 (substance use/ misuse)	8
	Parents (child development, mental health, positive parenting)	10
	Resilience (emotional strength, problem-solving, stress management)	4
Total		113 (over 4 years)

Source: London School of Economics (LSE), n.d.

* The Penn Resilience Program (PRP) is grounded in cognitive behavioral theory and stresses problem-solving, goal-setting, mindfulness, emotional regulation, and connection and social support skills as well as real-life application and practicing the skills (Gillham et al., 2007; Brunwasser et al., 2009).

Table 8.3

Examples of good practice in school mental health in high- and low- income countries

Country	Model/approach	Key features
Canada	Pathways to care model (Wei et al., 2015)	Integrates mental health promotion, early identification, triage, referral, and continuing care. Involves teachers, school staff, families, health providers, and policymakers. Transitions program for final-year secondary and first-year postsecondary students to enhance mental health literacy and help-seeking behavior.
Ireland	WHO tiered model for school mental health promotion (Clarke & Barry, 2015)	Three tiers: (1) universal support for all students, (2) targeted support for at-risk students, (3) intensive support for students with complex emotional needs. Health-promoting initiatives integrated into the curriculum. Emphasizes belonging, self-management, relationships, emotional health, and decision-making.
Japan	Limited mental health education (Ojio et al., 2015)	Schools are required to have 1–2 full-time nurses for student health. A two-lesson intervention showed students could learn about mental illness outcomes effectively when delivered by researchers or mental health professionals.
Australia	Linking school mental health with educational change (Rowling & Mason, 2005)	Focuses on teacher awareness of mental health and its link to academic achievement. Uses a public health approach for mental health promotion. Sustainability depends on partnerships, resources, teamwork, and institutional support.
New Zealand	Whole school approach (Dickinson & Peterson, 2015)	Framework includes preparation, discovery, initiatives, skills development, and professional training. Promotes personal and social skills, targeted support for vulnerable children, and school-wide mental health policies. Core principles: (1) connect with people, (2) be active, (3) take notice, (4) learn, (5) give, (6) stepwise support.

Country	Model/approach	Key features
Singapore	REACH Program (early assessment and intervention) (Xie et al., 2015)	Early detection and intervention for mental health issues. Enhances schools' and communities' capacity to manage mental ill-health. Develops mental health support networks with community stakeholders.
Brazil	Teacher-led mental health awareness and skills for life program (Estanislau et al., 2015; Romanoa et al., 2025)	Mental health programs evaluated in schools. Teacher training in mental health awareness to improve identification of early issues. Teachers not seen as replacements for mental health professionals but as first-line identifiers of mental health concerns. "Skills for Life" program enhances emotional resilience and stress management.
China	Mental health education and teacher training (Deng & Fang, 2015; Qu, 2024)	Mental health education integrated since the 1980s. Focuses on public awareness, psychological counseling, and life skills education. Emphasizes teacher training and participatory education.
Ghana	University-community mental health partnerships (Lee et al., 2015)	Mobilization of mental health professionals and health workers to run school clinics. University-led mental health education initiatives. Locally developed interventions tailored to regional needs and resources.
India	School mental health program and early intervention (Kumar et al., 2015; John & Rajiv, n.d.; Shinde et al., 2018)	School education is highly variable by state and funding. Focus is on teacher-led short-term programs. Common challenges include stigma, lack of trained staff, and integration issues. Addresses learning disabilities, ADHD, autism, and emotional disorders. Family education and structured multisensory programs are recommended.

(*continued*)

Table 8.3
(continued)

Country	Model/approach	Key features
Turkey	Public-private partnerships in school mental health (Yazgan & Karacau, 2015)	Joint government and private-sector delivery of mental health programs. Uses trained professionals and consultation models. Data-driven interventions tailored to students' needs. Family and multidisciplinary professional involvement. Regular monitoring and assessment of progress.
Ukraine	School-based psychological services (Zhabenko & Zhabenko, 2015)	Strong emphasis on mental health promotion since 2011. School services include diagnosis, behavior correction, rehabilitation, and prevention. Programs address aggression, anxiety reduction, and deviant behaviors. Focus on training health and mental health professionals.

Note: ADHD, attention deficit hyperactivity disorder; WHO, World Health Organization.

Policy Implications

While schools provide the basic foundations for education and subsequent successful living, parents, teachers, and governments play key roles in nurturing healthy children.

a. Parents and caregivers should offer their children opportunities for healthy living and exercise while fostering responsible attitudes toward smoking, alcohol, addictions, sexual health, and relationships. Collaboration between parents and teachers is vital for the success of these efforts.
b. Teachers and schools should develop specific teaching activities to address stress and bullying. They ought to promote physical activity and healthy eating, recognize and manage stress and bullying, and foster an environment conducive to the emotional well-being of children and young people.

c. Governments have a moral and ethical responsibility to invest in the physical and mental health of children and young people. They must set high standards for educational attainment, teaching, and safe learning environments and accompany these standards with appropriate resources.

Many countries lack adequate mental health support in schools, both in terms of policy and practice. Policymakers ought to develop mental health policies that are sufficiently resourced, including training and community collaboration. Continuing evaluation of implementation, support, and evidence-based practices is crucial, as is involving children and young people. Using social media for communication can also encourage positive emotional and social functioning, although policymakers should remain mindful of the increasing concerns about social media use among young people (see chapter 10 and the section on social media).

School mental health should be prioritized alongside physical health within public mental health. It must focus on promoting well-being, resilience, and preventing mental health issues. Early intervention, recognition, and collaboration with community resources are essential for a comprehensive school mental health strategy. In low- and middle-income countries, limited resources for mental health and education complicate these efforts.

Public Health England (PHE, n.d.) emphasizes the importance of adopting a whole-system approach to student well-being, which helps identify the strengths and needs of entire cohorts. PHE defines mental well-being not merely as the absence of mental illness but as a broader measure that encompasses emotional, social, and physical wellness. This includes children's happiness, life satisfaction, and positive functioning, influenced by individual factors (such as physical health and social skills), family dynamics (including parents' health and relationships), and community elements (like social support and neighborhood safety) that shape their learning environments.

Implementation Challenges

Approximately 40–50 percent of teachers report experiencing burnout, which adversely affects their ability to support student well-being (Skaalvik & Skaalvik, 2016). Regular mental health training for teachers boosts their confidence and enhances student outcomes (Jorm et al., 2023); however, it is vital to address the root causes of burnout, which fall outside the scope of this book. Chronic underfunding in numerous countries restricts access to school-based mental health care (Fazel et al., 2012). Furthermore, stigma may impede students from seeking help (Rickwood et al., 2005). Anti-stigma campaigns have been demonstrated to increase help-seeking rates among students (Yamaguchi et al., 2013). Nevertheless, multi-sector partnerships (e.g., government, NGOs, private-sector funding models) can sustain programs that provide effective and cost-efficient mental health initiatives in schools (Heinrich et al., 2023).

Conclusion

Schools can be stressful environments, particularly in competitive cultures, leading to issues such as bullying that leave children feeling isolated. Domestic violence, parental mental health issues, substance misuse, poverty, overcrowding, and malnutrition further affect children's mental health. Vulnerable groups, including children in care, young carers, those with disabilities, migrants, and refugees, face heightened risks of distress and its consequences. School-based mental health programs enhance student well-being, improve academic outcomes, and reduce the long-term burden of mental illness. Effective strategies include multitiered mental health service models (universal, targeted, specialist care); whole school approaches that integrate mental health into curricula and policies; peer education, anti-bullying, and parental engagement programs; and mental health literacy initiatives to reduce stigma and promote help-seeking. Overcoming barriers such as funding shortages, stigma, and teacher burnout is essential for scaling sustainable mental health services in schools worldwide.

9 Mental Health in the Workplace

Introduction

Mental health in the workplace is a crucial aspect of any health care policy. Most people of working age will spend one-third or more of their day at their workplace, and yet until relatively recently, very little attention has been paid to the issue. There is no doubt that employment by itself provides social support, improves self-esteem, creates opportunities for social interaction thereby reducing loneliness and isolation, allows one to use their skills, and at the same time provides economic stability. It gives structure to the day, which helps with functioning.

In addition to prevention strategies, there are two key aspects to mental health in the workplace: first, to support those who develop mental illnesses while employed, and second, to engage with those who have developed mental illnesses, then dropped out and need to be brought back into employment. It is well recognized that the rates of psychiatric disorders are much higher among those who are unemployed. It is also extremely likely that those who develop psychiatric disorders during the period of employment are likely to lose their jobs, thereby adding to their distress and stress. Suitable work with appropriate remuneration is good for people's mental health and well-being (WHO, 2017).

A Deloitte Monitor report (Hampson & Siegel, 2017) points out that the mental health of any employee can fluctuate between thriving and struggling. Several factors are at play in this case. It is very likely that if a job is stimulating and fulfilling, the satisfied and contented employee may feel well and be able to cope with stressors that the work environment may throw at them. The work environment itself, in combination with relationships with peers, supervisors, and others, can lead to stress.

If employers are sensitive to the possibility and likelihood of stress due to work, they may put preventive strategies in place. The authors of this report estimated that in the UK, the cost of mental health–related presenteeism to the employers is between £16.8–£26.4 billion (roughly 22 billion to 35 billion US Dollar) per annum. In addition, the cost estimated due to mental ill-health and absence is an additional £7.9 billion (roughly $10 billion). There are additional differences related to public versus private sectors. In addition, turnover cost is £7.9 billion, and self-employed absence cost of £0.9 billion ($1.2 billion approximately) has been estimated. Although overall sickness absence rates per worker have been trending downward in the past 12 years, 11 percent of these absences are caused by mental illness, although it is quite likely that physical illnesses may be influenced by or accompanied by mental illnesses.

Presenteeism is of particular interest. The Deloitte report (Hampson & Siegel, 2017) defines presenteeism as attending work while ill and working at reduced productivity. Presenteeism is not always easy to detect, and its links with absences need to be considered. It is possible that individuals, even when ill, continue to work—often because of worries about job security or expectations tied to remote work flexibility. Zero-hour contracts may further encourage individuals to be present in body even if they are not able to function fully. It is quite likely that the rates of presenteeism and absenteeism will vary across different sectors.

If an employee develops a psychiatric disorder and exhibits signs of "presenteeism," it creates further problems as they may feel stigmatized for seeking help and may believe that a public acknowledgment of their illness could affect their chances for promotion at work. Alternatively, they might choose to take time off, which could place additional pressure on them and their families. Some may be genuinely experiencing physical illnesses, but the added stigma can complicate matters even further. The cost of presenteeism is 2.5 times that of absenteeism (Centre for Mental Health, 2007).

In a survey of 9,500 respondents, 69 percent reported poor mental wellbeing, but only 29 percent took time off (Mind Wellbeing Index, 2016). Those employed in the private sector are less likely to take time off compared to those in the public sector, while the third sector (local small businesses and community organizations) falls in the middle. This survey also revealed an interesting and unusual finding: rates of mental illnesses vary across sectors. For example, the public sector has the highest rates, followed by the financial sector, while transportation and media rank among the lowest. Those experiencing mental ill-health are also likely to change jobs frequently, which contributes to stress and further alienation. This is an intriguing phenomenon that warrants further exploration. Self-employed individuals are less likely to take time off due to illness, mainly because of the risk of losing income, but they may also be able to work in a more flexible manner. The Deloitte report estimated that the cost of poor mental health among self-employed individuals in the UK is £0.86 billion (approximately $1.1 billion). Most people opt to become self-employed for personal lifestyle and family reasons.

Workplace mental health programs have demonstrated strong cost-benefit outcomes. A meta-analysis of workplace mental health interventions found a return on investment (ROI) of $4 for every $1 spent due to reduced absenteeism and improved productivity (Knapp et al., 2011). Furthermore, mental health-supportive workplaces report lower turnover rates and increased employee satisfaction (Goetzel et al., 2018).

Strategies to support individuals with mental illness in the workplace must encompass assistance for those seeking employment to secure appropriate positions. This may involve sheltered or supported employment alongside gradual reintegration when necessary. Additionally, it is crucial to help employed individuals with mental health difficulties maintain their roles according to their capabilities and skills. Productivity can improve through enhanced support, as this reduces stress—deemed a primary intervention—while addressing individual needs. By helping and supporting individuals with mental health issues at work, absenteeism due to illness can be reduced.

Promoting well-being in the workplace is a vital preventive strategy. Establishing stronger connections and a coordinated approach between government health and employment /labor departments can convey clearer and more consistent messages about the importance of employment for mental health and well-being.

The mental health and well-being of the individuals working in any organization depends on the individual themselves, their personal strengths and vulnerabilities, and various societal, familial, and environmental factors that may cause stress and lead to mental illness. Vulnerabilities may also be systemic by the person as described in chapter 5 on the epidemiology of mental illness (in the section on other vulnerable groups). These factors may all interact with each other (figure 9.1).

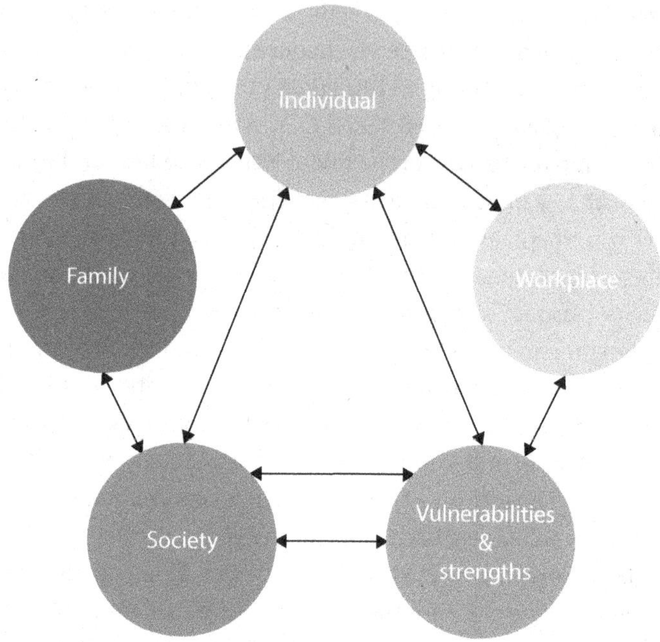

Figure 9.1
Larger societal factors affecting mental health and well-being.

People do not live or work in a vacuum. Other individuals around them, including supervisors and managers, can and often do contribute to stress; similarly, family members and demands from society at large can further add to stress and contribute to mental ill-health. Thus, any actions to improve mental health in the workplace can be and must be seen in the broader social context as well. Workplaces are important because this is where we tend to spend at least one-third of our working years. To develop mentally healthy workplaces, several steps are indicated.

The Global Agenda Council World Economic Forum (2017) outlines seven steps for developing a mentally healthy organization (box 9.1) and provides examples of best practices from several large companies that not only assess stress and mental ill-health but also focus on psychological well-being and resilience. A list of various assessment tools constitutes a vital part of the report. The report highlights that presenteeism due to stress or mental ill-health must be taken into account. Engaging with

Box 9.1
Seven Steps to Better Mental Health in the Workplace

1. Be aware of the workplace environment:
   - Understand benefits of mentally healthy work environment.
   - Understand the landscape from stress.
   - Understand how to intervene to create a healthy workplace.
   - Take action.
2. Learn from the motivations of organizational leaders and employees who have taken action.
3. Be aware of other companies' actions and lessons.
4. Understand the opportunities and needs.
5. Take practical steps for the organization.
6. Have a list of resources available.
7. Make a start.

employees can also enhance customer satisfaction. Furthermore, there are instances of best practices from a number of large employers. One excellent example from BT (British Telecom) in the UK is detailed in appendix 9.

Responsibility for the Mental Health of the Workforce

Interventions for a mentally healthy workforce are not only the responsibility of employers and the government but also of civil society as a whole. These interventions include protecting mental health by reducing work-related risk factors and providing education for maintaining well-being, promoting mental health by developing the positive aspects of being able to work, and helping to build strength and resilience, as well as fostering a supportive atmosphere in the workplace. Employers, regardless of size of the work place, must have resources in place or accessible to address mental health issues among their employees, irrespective of the cause. Policymakers must create provisions for those with mental health challenges to find suitable sheltered employment, with a gradual increase in responsibilities, accompanied by adequate support and assistance.

Employers have a moral and ethical responsibility for the mental health of their workforce, but this requires partnerships with employees and the government.

a. Employees need to be aware of health and safety regulations and work toward developing a healthy working environment. Psychological first aid should be made available in a way similar to physical first aid (see appendix 14). Employees should provide support to colleagues who need help and also enable those returning to work after illness in a supportive manner.
b. Employers must support employees who develop a mental illness and encourage and enable their return in a flexible manner. They must make every effort to support healthy lifestyles (e.g., by offering a nonsmoking environment, following high standards of health and safety management, and making affordable nutritious food available). The working environment should be supportive and stress-free, with access to occupational health whenever possible. They must ensure that the workload is manageable.
c. Governments must legislate standards for health care and support employers in creating stress-free working conditions, as well as facilitating return-to-work options for employees need them.

Appendix 9 presents an example of good practice for mental health in the workplace.

Employment and Mental Health

Tackling mental illness in the workplace is a global issue. Employment provides support to people with mental illness. However, the world over, rates of employment of people with mental illness are tragically low. If an employed person becomes mentally ill, they are more likely to lose their job. Thus, a vicious cycle of unemployment and mental illness continues.

Appropriate paid work is beneficial for individuals, and returning to suitable work can also improve mental health. Strategies for supporting people with mental illness in employment must include helping those without work to gain suitable employment, which may involve sheltered or supported employment if needed. Additionally, it important to help employed people with mental ill-health to remain in work or facilitate their gradual reintegration. Productivity can increase with enhanced support that reduces stress and addresses individuals according to their needs. By assisting and supporting people with mental health problems at work, employers can reduce sickness absences. Promoting well-being at work is an important preventive measure. Stronger links and a unified strategy between government departments of health and employment/labor can produce better outcomes.

Severe Mental Illness

People with severe mental illness (SMI) face significant barriers to employment, including workplace stigma, discrimination, and inadequate accommodations. Supported employment programs, particularly the individual placement and support (IPS) model, have been shown to improve job retention among individuals with severe mental illnesses, including schizophrenia and bipolar disorder. A comprehensive umbrella review synthesizing evidence from multiple studies found that combining supported employment with targeted interventions, such as neurocognitive therapy and job-related social skills training, has a positive impact on employment outcomes, including job retention, for people with severe mental illness (Suijkerbuijk et al., 2017) Furthermore, a systematic review and meta-analysis concluded that adults with schizophrenia and other psychoses receiving supported employment were more than twice as likely to obtain competitive employment compared to those receiving prejob training, sheltered employment, or standard psychiatric care. The study also noted that supported employment was most effective when augmented with additional interventions like social or cognitive skills training (National Institute for Health and Care Research [NIHR], 2018).

Managing Mental Health in the Workplace

Resilience in both the workplace and the home must be strengthened. It can be argued that any workplace-related stressors can be easily identified, therefore every effort should be made to reduce such stress in the environment. In the recruitment process, clear anti-stigma strategies should be put in place. Work-related stress factors can and must be identified and reduced. It is the common mental disorders such as anxiety, panic disorders, depression, and various phobias that affect a large number of people, especially adults of working age who are in jobs where the work environment may add extra stressors. Signs of mental ill-health in the workplace may reveal stress and poor functioning, such as underperformance and low productivity.

In the workplace, several steps can be taken to manage an employee's mental health. The first one is to identify and support those who are suffering from mental ill-health, whether it manifests as absenteeism or presenteeism (as discussed above). The next step is to support those who may have taken time off because of their mental ill-health; in this case, they need support in readjusting and settling into their job on their return, so due recognition of their needs is important. The employment practices that are effective in addressing risk factors, building resilience, and helping employees to overcome and manage life's stressors should be encouraged and welcomed. Having access to readily available occupational health services can be extremely helpful. A range of stepped-up services may be necessary, depending on the size of the workplace.

Global workplace mental health initiatives provide valuable insights into effective interventions across industries. For example, Japan's Workplace Mental Health Promotion Plan mandates stress checks for employees to reduce burnout (Kawakami & Tsutsumi, 2016). In Canada, the National Standard for Psychological Health and Safety in the Workplace provides guidelines for mental well-being at work (Canadian Standards Association & Bureau de normalization du Québec, 2013). Similar programs have been implemented in the European Union and Australia, focusing on early intervention and organizational mental health culture.

Examples of Good Workplace Mental Health Practice

The Deloitte report mentioned previously (Hampson & Siegel, 2017), details examples of good practice from different countries that are worth examining.

The German model works across employers, insurance companies, and the government to reduce mental health risk caused by stress. It focuses on information, sensitization, and motivation—that is, it informs employees and employers, motivates them, and shares information. Labor inspectors are trained to support and ensure that services are available, and they work closely with occupational medicine specialists. They are supported in a number of ways, from sharing examples of good practice to working out practicable ways of measuring stress and identifying those who are at a higher risk of developing mental ill-health. Clear targets (both achievable and aspirational) are set.

In Canada, although the practices set by the National Standard for Psychological Health and Safety are voluntary, the focus is on mental health promotion and the prevention of psychological harm at work, linking it to health and safety in the workplace in general. The standard addresses the identification of psychological hazards and the assessment of potential points of stress and their elimination or management; it also encourages implementation of better practices that support psychological health and safety with clear, regular reviews. The Deloitte report notes that 72 percent compliance with five elements of the standard has been achieved.

The Mentally Healthy Workplace Alliance in Australia provides strategy and resources divided into four areas—employers organizations, small businesses, the employees' role, and managers' responsibilities. Employers are encouraged to plan interventions after assessing needs and regularly monitor and review the plan. Similar action points are expected from employees. Small businesses are encouraged to introduce initiatives that help and support their staff. Managers are encouraged to protect the rights to privacy and confidentiality and to ascertain the impact of absences on the team and individual workloads.

The French strategy is to help improve work-life balance and flexible working conditions. The "right to disconnect" was enshrined in law so that individuals will not be required to check/reply to emails during their time off. The authorities expect regular assessment of psychosocial risk. Sweden has reduced daily working hours to six hours a day with a generous paternity allowance. Belgium has recognized burnout as a psychosocial risk, and employers are expected to carry out regular assessments and offer interventions such as counseling.

The UK example of BT is presented in appendix 9. British Telecom (BT) was at the forefront of addressing mental health in the workplace and developed a bespoke mental health plan within the overall framework. It was developed in partnership with the trade unions so that the ownership of the plan by both the unions and management would create a sense of co-ownership and lead to mutual respect and effective collaboration, which is exactly what happened. The basic aim was to normalize mental health problems and raise awareness of them, thereby ensuring that people who were stressed and needed help did not feel stigmatized. The key messages conveyed to the workforce were that individuals with mental illness are not unemployable and can contribute effectively to the organization and society at large. By using apps, BT created a culture of self-help while ensuring that those who needed help got it as soon as possible from trained staff as well as from experts. The company created a three-tier framework that focused on primary prevention, secondary intervention, and tertiary rehabilitation. Impressively, BT created a repository of resources to which individuals could gain access according to their needs. Furthermore, the resources were also organized into tiers and included access to developing resilience and mental health services within and outside the company. The company innovatively collects information on areas that are considered hot spots for producing stress and then creates suitable interventions accordingly. Employee satisfaction was rated to be very high. More importantly, employees felt that the company valued them by caring about their health. Another key aspect of feeling valued is when employees who take time off because of mental illnesses are made to feel welcome back into the workplace. Their gradual integration into the workplace without stigmatizing them makes them feel good about the company and, in turn, about themselves. It makes sense that returning to suitable work can itself improve mental health, well-being, self-image, and self-esteem.

Three years later, Deloitte (2020) published a follow-up report noting that there had been three positive changes in the workplace: greater support being provided to employees, especially in larger organizations; greater social awareness of mental health; and a reduction in stigma. At the same time, there were negative changes as well. A key observation was that the burden of poor mental health affected younger workers disproportionately, which is not surprising considering that they are in the vulnerable age group more likely to develop psychiatric disorders as discussed elsewhere in this book. Another interesting observation is a rise in "leavism," which is described as employees being unable to disconnect from use of technology, which contributes to burnout. This has other implications related to an increase in the use of social media and the post-COVID pandemic challenges of working from home. The third negative point raised by the report is an increase in short-term contracts that may not be accompanied by sufficient employer support. Furthermore, increase in zero hour contracts is likely to affect the mental health of individuals.

Recent trends in workplace mental health management include flexible work schedules and reduced-hour workweeks, both of which have been linked to improved mental well-being (Shifrin & Michael, 2021). Mental health monitoring tools that use artificial intelligence (AI), such as sentiment analysis in workplace communication, are also being used to detect stress levels and promote early intervention (Bendau et al., 2021). It is important to emphasize that middle-income and low-income countries may lack the resources to deliver these interventions. However, it is important for employers to maintain awareness of equity and social justice in ensuring that their employees have good mental health and well-being so that they can work better.

As discussed in chapter 3, the impact of commercial determinants needs to be taken into account, especially in low-income countries where multinational corporations may have production units. The impact of multinational corporations on the production environment and pollution, along with access to cheap labor, brings additional challenges to employee-employer relationships and responsibilities for employee mental health and well-being.

Conclusion

Interventions for a mentally healthy workforce are the responsibility of not only employers and the government but of civil society as a whole. These interventions include reducing work-related risk factors, providing education on well-being, promoting mental health by fostering the positive aspects of employment, helping to develop strength and resilience, and enhancing the atmosphere in the workplace. Employers, no matter how big or small, must have resources in place to address mental health problems among their employees, irrespective of the cause. Policymakers must make allowances for those with mental ill-health to find suitable sheltered employment, with a gradual increase in responsibilities accompanied by adequate support and assistance.

10 Tele-Mental Health and E-Mental Health

Introduction

Information technology has transformed mental health service delivery through digital platforms, telehealth, and AI-assisted diagnostics, improving diagnoses, aiding in the creation of better case summaries, and expanding communication and learning. Following the rapid growth of the internet and increased access to smartphones around the world, the possibilities related to service delivery using e-mental health and tele-mental health have expanded dramatically, especially during the COVID pandemic and since then. By using webcams and video applications, people who are suffering can be assessed from long distances and get treatment advice. Using apps or smartphones, psychological therapies and psychoeducational materials can be shared widely. Assessments conducted remotely also cut costs of travel for the patients while adding flexibility and contributing to a more diverse practice. Shore (2015a) points out that telepsychiatry can offer potential solutions to the challenges of restructuring health, and it can help improve quality and efficiency of care. Telepsychiatry has developed as a distinct field within psychiatry. The pandemic demonstrated that it is possible to carry out assessments at a distance, but the challenges of privacy and confidentiality need wider discussion within the profession and with key stakeholders.

Even before the pandemic, patients' use of apps and social media to research what might be wrong with them and what treatments are available was increasing, but this has now become even more dominant in many countries and clinical settings. In a changing world, it is important that professionalism keeps pace. In a World Psychiatric Association and Asian

Journal of Psychiatry (WPA-AJP) joint commission, Bhugra et al. (2023) recommend that knowledge about AI, newer apps, and social media be considered in psychiatric education and that adequate provisions be made so that all health care professionals are aware of ethical issues and are well prepared.

Another point worth bearing in mind that has been highlighted elsewhere in this book: the younger generation has different attitudes toward work-life balance and is more comfortable with modern technologies (Bernstein & Bhugra, 2011). However, in a survey of burnout among UK medical students (Bhugra et al., 2019), anecdotal evidence emerged that students find it difficult to learn with simulation and feel they are merely acting like technicians. As the students pointed out, they did not enter the field of medicine to become technicians, even if technical specialties do rely on technology. Furthermore, as medicine becomes more technical, training should integrate human aspects of medicine with technology. This makes it obvious that mental health care professionals need to ensure that the next generation of professionals is prepared for diagnostic and therapeutic challenges. In addition, as online supervision and telepsychiatry grow, clinicians and trainers must establish a suitable forum for mentoring and educational supervision.

Training in the use of telepsychiatry is of paramount importance, as there are key differences in carrying out assessments using telepsychiatry compared to face-to-face assessments and in talking to relatives or friends using online tools. Additional issues include gathering collateral information and working with off-site staff. Furthermore, issues related to confidentiality and privacy are important. The clinician also needs to be cognizant of the technical aspects of using equipment, making contemporaneous notes, and gathering relevant information while doing so. Training in the use of such procedures and their ethical implications is extremely patchy and needs closer observation. For those who use such methods, training must be made mandatory (Shore, 2015b).

Guidelines for the use of telemedicine and telepsychiatry are widely available (Seiferth et al., 2023) and provide clear indications for appropriate use of these approaches.

Definitions

The terms *telepsychiatry* and *tele-mental health* are often used interchangeably. They both describe two-way live interactive videoconferencing used to provide psychiatric care at a distance through telephone, email, and web-based systems and mobile applications. Telepsychiatry has been defined as the use of electronic communications and information technologies to provide or support clinical psychiatric care at a distance (Drago et al., 2016). Thus, telepsychiatry is the provision of psychiatric assessment and care using various forms of telecommunications.

Skills Needed

In order to use telepsychiatry successfully, clinicians need technical skills, assessment skills, communication and relational skills, interpersonal skills, medicolegal skills, and knowledge of the community and health care systems (Crawford et al., 2016). Among technical competencies, some are perhaps more focused on skills in using telepsychiatry, whereas others would be fairly similar to skills used in good clinical practice.

Teaching these skills needs to start at an undergraduate level in all countries and settings and across all disciplines. Health workers as well as community leaders need to be made aware of the potential advantages and disadvantages of the use of tele-mental health and e-mental health. It should be emphasized that these skills are crucial and no different from learning a new language. There are examples of good practice that should be made available widely (Sunderji et al., 2015). It might be possible to encourage undergraduates to learn about telepsychiatry during their elective periods or in internship programs.

Ethical Considerations

As technologies advance, it is likely that approaches to provide patients with detailed information and personalized assessments and interventions will become common place. Under these circumstances, ethical considerations need to be considered carefully. Data privacy and confidentiality will need to be understood and developed across regulatory and professional bodies. A careful balance between efficacy and privacy is needed, with safeguards in place to ensure that data is not accessed in an unauthorized manner. The interaction between human beings and machines and the risks related to mental illnesses need to be thought through carefully.

Range of Applications

Telepsychiatry was introduced in the US in 1959 (Brown, 1998); it has since grown in expertise as the field has advanced. It crosses national and international boundaries, linking clinicians and patients in terms of specialization, needs, and a common language. The American Telemedicine Association identifies other uses as part of telepsychiatry, such as the delivery of medical education, clinical supervision, patient education, and monitoring (American Telemedicine Association, 2018). Patients can be seen, assessed, monitored, and reviewed regularly using telecommunication. Videoconferencing is the oldest application observed within telepsychiatry. In many institutions, multisite conferencing facilities are available in different formats. Patients can use battery-operated systems and connect to the internet within the health care system. This increases both flexibility and access (Donley et al., 2017; Deslich et al., 2013). Patients can record their symptoms and queries and either email them or send them through an audio or video link to clinicians. Real-time approaches and assessments obviously do not require sophisticated telecommunication systems. Any machine that has secure access to the internet can prove to be useful (Hariman et al., 2019). In describing their own experiences, Yellowlees et al. (2015) suggest that patients and their doctors can have an empathic and powerful relationship using technology. It is possible for patients to have better control in videoconferencing, and patient satisfaction improves as videoconferencing reduces the power differential. These authors also point out that cultural consultations can be carried out using telepsychiatry through the use of apps that can provide live interpretation.

Portable equipment, such as smartphones or tablets, are extremely useful in this process (Cheng et al., 2018). Asynchronous telepsychiatry—otherwise known as the use of recorded, stored, and forwarded information—can be extremely helpful. This approach involves patients or their carers making a recording and sending it to the responsible clinician. The clinician can also review the results of investigations and advise the patient or their carers accordingly after reviewing the material. Such approaches have been shown to be extremely useful especially if patients speak a different language; they are also time efficient. Videos can be translated into appropriate languages and reviewed accordingly (Yellowlees et al., 2013). A very high inter-rater reliability has been reported using such approaches.

Apart from the use of videoconferencing and video recordings, other approaches within the field of telepsychiatry include providing accurate information and education. Butler and Yellowlees (2012) emphasize that a cost analysis of store-and-forward telepsychiatry as a consultation model for primary care indicates considerable savings, and such approaches can eliminate the need for simultaneous interpretation. Providing information through chatbot (computer programs designed to simulate human conversations) can facilitate early diagnosis of psychiatric and medical conditions, which may manifest as changes in voice modulation Chan et al., 2017; Fitzpatrick et al., 2017; Braun et al., 2016). Place et al. (2017) studied the level of activity on patients' smartphones to ascertain their physical and mental well-being. Interestingly, one approach that has been successfully tried is to dissuade alcohol dependent patients from going to pubs through the use of global positioning systems (Dulin et al., 2014). However, a patient's informed consent is of great importance in this context, and again cultural variations must be considered. Ready access to, and a degree of familiarity with, these tools and access to Wi-Fi are essential.

Text messaging can be used in many countries to remind individuals to attend their appointments or remind them to take medication at the right time. Using texts to provide adjunctive treatment in managing depression in Iran, authors found that use of bibliotherapy led to an improvement in the severity of depressive symptoms (Taleban et al., 2016). Real-time clinical assessments, although helpful, may well be prohibitively expensive and often impractical if the images are of poor quality (Bonnardot et al., 2014). Thus, asynchronous telepsychiatry may be helpful.

Social Media

Social media has become incredibly influential, but the full impact on population mental health is still not understood clearly. Social media includes a wide range of approaches from various apps and sites. (Negative mental health effects of social media are discussed in chapter 3 in section on digital platforms).

Algorithms have been developed to help social media providers identify vulnerable individuals (Hariman et al., 2019). Clinicians' presence on social media and interaction with their patients requires further detailed ethical discussion. Theoretically, it is possible that by keeping in contact with their patients on social media, clinicians may be in a position to monitor mood fluctuations. The challenge is whether this can lead to false positives or false negatives, causing unrealistic interventions and affecting both the patient-clinician relationship and broader issues of confidentiality. It is possible that on occasion, postings by patients may alert the clinician, who may then involve others to provide an appropriate intervention. Social media can be used for health promotion (Frankish et al., 2012). On the other hand, an online "relationship" between the patient and the clinician may compromise patient confidentiality and lead to social stigma, as Frankish et al. (2012) have emphasized.

Social media can provide rapid access to information, but this information may not always be accurate or up to date. Clinicians can use social media to share accurate information, but they need to be careful about what they should post on their personal accounts. Perhaps one solution is for clinicians to maintain a professional presence on social media and a separate personal one. Such a distinct division may create clear boundaries, although it is quite likely that some patients may deliberately or inadvertently choose to blur those boundaries.

Various social media sites and activities can be used for support. However, clinicians need to be aware that there are both positives and negatives in such approaches. Using machine learning techniques, it has been suggested that markers of depression are observed in the use of Instagram behavior, which may be recognized as a prodrome of depression (Reece & Danforth, 2017).

It is important to ensure that individuals, especially children and young people, use social media appropriately and wisely. They may need education, from their schools and families, to ensure that the extent and duration of their online usage are appropriate.

Mobile Applications

The reach of smartphones around the globe is truly impressive. The number of apps related to health were estimated to be around 15,000 in 2015, which included approximately 4,500 mental health–related mobile applications. By 2022, this number had risen to 54,546 (Statista, 2022). Inevitably, the range of services offered by these apps is wide-ranging, and the quality is variable, too. Some applications provide mental health information, whereas others provide therapies and interventions. These strategies include meditation, breathing exercises, and cognitive behavior therapies. Applications exist to keep a mood diary and engage in online counseling. There are applications to remind individuals or nudge them into various behaviors.

Turvey and Roberts (2015) highlight the use of mobile apps in a targeted manner for education, assessments, behavior logs, unobtrusive monitoring, web-based therapy, electronic personal health records, and patient portals for information exchange. In a meta-analysis, Firth et al. (2017a) reported that these applications can help reduce symptoms of depression, especially at mild levels. Firth et al. (2017b) noted that these apps are particularly helpful in managing anxiety. Mobile health (mHealth) apps, such as Moodpath and BetterHelp, have provided scalable self-help interventions and virtual counseling (Kruse et al., 2022).

There is no doubt that further developments of mental health apps will continue, but it is important that these are evaluated thoroughly. Another interesting development has been that of the Internet of Things (IoT), which connects various everyday objects through the internet, enabling the devices to record and transmit data to each other. These devices have been used to monitor blood pressure and blood glucose monitoring. These applications are rather limited in the field of mental health, although devices can record sleep patterns, and ingestible electronic sensors can be used to measure medication adherence (de la Torre Diez, 2019; Mason et al., 2022).

Artificial Intelligence (AI)

Advances in telepsychiatry, social media, and apps rely on the development of algorithms and AI—a term that has been applied to various domains, such as machine learning, natural language processing, and image processing. Artificial intelligence is already helping us to understand how mental disorders develop by using scans to assess the impact on the structures and functioning of the brain. This may lead to more personalized interventions. For example, understanding gene maps will enable clinicians to figure out whether the patient is a fast or slow metabolizer so that an appropriate and adequate dosage of medication can be given and titrated according to need. It is entirely possible that AI may change the way mental illness is classified. The use of big data can lead to identification of behavior patterns and possible relapsing behaviors. It is important that clinicians, in discussion with other key stakeholders—such as patients, carers, families, policymakers, and other professionals—develop ethics guidelines to ensure that the practice of digital psychiatry can provide not only appropriate investigation but also education and suitable interventions.

AI is increasingly being explored as a tool to proactively identify individuals at risk of suicide, allowing clinicians to intervene earlier. Machine learning algorithms that analyze electronic health records and social media data have shown potential in predicting suicidal behaviors (Pigoni et al., 2024). AI-powered risk assessments that integrate diverse data sources have been implemented to enhance suicide prediction in psychiatric patients (Parsapoor et al., 2023). AI-driven diagnostic tools for the early detection of mental health crises and depression show promise (Mao et al., 2023; Mansoor & Ansari, 2024).

AI-based mental health diagnostics raise critical ethical concerns about algorithmic bias, data privacy, and the role of human oversight. Bias in training data can result in misdiagnosis for marginalized populations, reinforcing existing health care disparities (Obermeyer et al., 2019). Furthermore, privacy concerns arise from the extensive data collection required for AI-driven mental health assessments, necessitating stringent regulatory frameworks (Leslie, 2019).

Benefits

As Hariman et al. (2019) note, with the increasing adoption of smartphones and advances in artificial intelligence, the use of telepsychiatry can change the way patients interact with their clinicians and receive and accept therapeutic interventions. Telepsychiatry utilization in rural areas has significant potential to transform both care delivery and clinician productivity (Paul et al., 2018). However, more research is needed, especially in the context of acceptability and the ethical issues related to confidentiality and privacy (discussed later in this chapter). There is some evidence that telepsychiatry is of equal value to face-to-face therapeutic encounters (Drago et al., 2016). Following their analysis of 26 randomized controlled trials, these authors cautioned that not enough data were available related to the use of psychotherapy in telepsychiatry. It can be argued that these are still early days, and further detailed observations and analysis are needed. Hubley et al. (2016) studied patients and clinician satisfaction following the use of telepsychiatry and reported that costs are low, satisfaction is high, and outcomes are on par with face-to-face consultations. These findings are evident particularly in high-income countries (Hilty et al., 2013). Salmoiraghi and Hussain (2015) have shown that the use of telepsychiatry can reduce the number of admissions to the wards, thereby leading to considerable financial savings.

Gloff et al. (2015) note that tele-mental health programs may be more beneficial for young people and children who are more familiar with technology, and such programs can be used in primary care, educational settings, correctional facilities, and at home. They may be used to provide psychotherapies and to assess suitability for medication. Similarly, Fortney et al. (2015) point out that telepsychiatry may be better suited to primary care settings, especially if there are workforce shortages. Its application in post-disaster assessments and management has been described by Augusterfer et al. (2015).

Hariman et al. (2019) emphasize that telepsychiatry can be of particular use and benefit in assessing and treating mentally ill offenders in prison. In the US, several states have partnered with universities and hospitals to provide assessments and interventions using telepsychiatry. This application has been welcomed by prison wardens and has reduced the risk of prisoners absconding. Prisoners themselves have felt that their health care needs are being addressed (Deslich et al., 2013; Cheng et al., 2018). Similar models can be used to assess and manage the health care needs of migrants, refugees, and asylum seekers who may be living in camps (Ye et al., 2012). Telepsychiatry can also be used in assessing and managing patients living in various institutions (Yeung et al., 2009) such as nursing homes and homes for the elderly and for immigrant groups (Yeung et al., 2016). Under these circumstances, collateral information gathered from care staff can be extremely helpful. Sunderji et al. (2015) emphasize that tele-psychiatry can be delivered at an institutional level, from academic centers and universities to community mental health settings and large multisite hospitals. Morland et al. (2015) suggest that clinical videoconferencing can be conducted at home and used successfully with underserved populations who may face issues related to mobility, transportation, scheduling, stigma, and privacy.

Challenges

Digital technology, particularly social media, has led to an increase in mental health awareness and access to information—although not all of the information found online is true. It has also contributed to cyberbullying and excessive screen exposure, which can negatively affect one's emotional well-being (Naslund et al., 2020). For policymakers, specific challenges in the development, delivery, and planning of telepsychiatry include ethical issues, as highlighted by Yellowlees et al. (2015) and Sabin and Skimming (2015). These authors point out various ethical dilemmas related to clinically competent and safe care, particularly concerning informed consent, privacy, and confidentiality. Morland et al. (2015) suggest that this approach may not be suitable for those who do not have access to a computer or camera, are unwilling to consent, or have severe psychosis, are actively suicidal, have impulse control issues, suffer from severe addiction or intoxication, or have cognitive or sensory impairments. It is therefore important for clinicians to have proper training in working with new technologies and methods. Hilty et al. (2015) have developed a framework using a competency-based curriculum and addressing how assessments can be carried out.

Personal, Privacy, and Confidentiality

Telepsychiatry raises specific challenges as far as privacy and confidentiality of the therapeutic encounter are concerned. How can a clinician be certain that the person being interviewed, assessed, and examined is the right person or that others around the person are not listening in? Some patients may see this as positive whereas others may feel stigmatized and depersonalized, so basic education for patients, caregivers, and families might be a good starting point.

Physical Distance Between the Clinician and the Patient

The physical distance between the clinician and the patient may be seen as a problem. The patient may not be confident about the confidentiality issues on the part of the clinician. Older, less educated individuals may find it more difficult to use technology, and many poor individuals may lack ease of access. If a proper therapeutic alliance is to be formed, then the clinician and the patient both need to feel comfortable with each other and the technology.

Physician Factors

Some clinicians may find it difficult to assess suicidal or homicidal risks using telepsychiatry. Hence, proper training is critical. Clinicians may find it difficult to form a working relationship and to assess verbal or nonverbal communication, thereby reducing the likelihood of developing a rapport with the patient.

Health Care System Factors

This challenge refers to the attributes within the health care system, such as whether it is public or private. Although telepsychiatry may be cost-effective, unless broader telecommunication systems are functioning adequately, the health care system will not work well. It has been argued that in some health care systems, clinicians may not be able to be reimbursed or collect their fees. These problems may be more complex if the patient and the clinician are communicating across geographical borders. This also may complicate the licensing and registration of doctors who may be registered in one country but not authorized to practice in another, thereby creating problems of accountability. These questions need global consideration and answers.

Technological Factors

Poor telecommunications infrastructure may create difficulties in implementation, particularly in developing countries and rural areas. Furthermore, the lack of encrypted communication systems may contribute to problems of confidentiality. Variables to consider include connectivity, hardware, clinic space, personnel, opportunity, and reimbursement. One development in China involves accessing booths where individuals can consult a virtual therapist for possible diagnosis and treatment (Yang, 2018). Hilty et al. (2015) propose that technology instruction, attitudes, expertise, evaluation, knowledge and skills, and learning styles all need to be taught and assessed.

Telepsychiatry in Low- and Middle-Income Countries

Telepsychiatry in low- and middle-income countries can be both helpful and problematic. The digital divide significantly affects access to tele-mental health services, with disparities observed in rural, low-income, and older populations (Ramsetty & Adams, 2020). Limited internet access, low digital literacy, and financial constraints prevent many individuals from benefiting from online mental health services (Hood, 2024). Digital inclusion schemes that provide loaned digital devices, internet connectivity, and personalized digital skills support to digitally excluded individuals could improve access to services, positively impact well-being, and empower individuals (Oliver et al., 2024).

In a systematic review of low- and middle-income countries, Acharibasam and Wynn (2018) noted that videoconferencing was the most commonly used tool. Telepsychiatry interventions were first deployed in 2004 after the Asian tsunami hit the coast of Tamil Nadu in South India. The Schizophrenia Research Foundation (SCARF), a nongovernmental organization in Chennai, used equipped vans to deliver consultation services, offering clinical assessments and treatments, with the medication subsequently dispensed by a pharmacist. In North India, services have been developed and delivered through a decision-support system using screening questions, functional and severity assessments, and a descriptive clinical diagnosis (Malhotra et al., 2014, 2015, 2017, 2019). These studies show that the online system is feasible, reasonably comprehensive, user-friendly, and associated with high levels of patient satisfaction, although diagnostic sensitivity varies across categories. The authors conclude that the digital model has the potential to serve as an effective alternative or adjunct for delivering comprehensive, high-quality mental health care in low- and middle-income countries.

Telepsychiatry bridges gaps in geography and services, making it possible for many more people to have better and easier access to care (Shore, 2015a) including in high-income countries with inequitable access (Sarvet et al, 2011). Although videoconferencing pilots in psychiatry started in the 1950s (Brown, 1998), the technological revolution has transformed approaches, and we are now looking at digital psychiatry and digital health/mental health. Shore (2015b) points out that with the increasing demand for videoconferencing, psychiatrists need to be trained and educated on various aspects of telepsychiatry. In many health care systems, telepsychiatry will influence emerging models of care and administrative issues such as funding and regulations. Yellowlees et al. (2015) suggest that the use of telepsychiatry puts the patient "in control," which may change the doctor-patient interaction and dynamic. In-person or dynamic online relationship may emerge. These authors argue that as cultures influence communication, telepsychiatry may provide much easier access to linguistic interpreters.

Yellowlees et al. (2015) emphasize that appropriate professional boundaries (ethical, physical, technical, and time-related) are maintained. Additional ethical issues include encouraging health equity and ensuring continuity of care (Sabin & Skimming, 2015). Clinical videoconferencing can be both home-based or institution-based. In addition to geographical access, teleconferencing can be used when the patient has a disability, mobility problems, or behavioral issues (Morland et al., 2015), although the authors caution that it may not be appropriate to assess suicidal patients, those with severe psychosis or poor mood regulation, severe substance misuse, or severe cognitive or sensory impairment. Teleconferencing can be used to assess children and young people, too, in primary care or in outpatient settings (Gloff et al., 2015).

Using online resources and mobile technologies is a part of digital health. It can be used for communication, diagnosis, and therapy. Increasingly, digital biomarkers—defined as physiological and behavioral measures collected through connected digital tools—are being used. They can be used to explain, influence, and protect against disease or certain health-related outcomes. It has been shown that patient behavior patterns can be monitored to assess a patient's mental state. For example, reduced use of mobile phone calls and texts may be related to the likelihood of relapse (Buck et al., 2019) and withdrawal. Changes in social behavior in the two weeks prior to relapse can be identified (Barnett et al., 2018). Patients can be monitored remotely, and their physical and mental health can be assessed (Turvey & Roberts, 2015). A patient's online activities, from filling prescriptions to seeking information about meditation and psychiatric disorders, can all be used effectively by clinicians.

Conclusion

With rapid advances in technology, the practice of not only medicine but also clinical psychiatry will change in the coming years. Telemedicine and e-health are likely to be adopted by different medical specialties at different rates. For example, online cameras can be easily applied to dermatology or pathology to examine photographs and lesions, but they may be harder to use in other specialties. In the past 50 years, clinical psychiatry has moved from asylums to community settings and now to care at home. The next logical step is the development and delivery of more targeted and individual-specific interventions. Using online videoconferencing for psychotherapy as well as for supervision and mentoring can be extremely helpful; however, issues related to confidentiality must be taken into account. E-mental health and regular use of electronic case records in patient care can make data-sharing much easier. There have been suggestions that patients should carry their medical case records on a USB drive for sharing with other professionals if necessary. However, these approaches require amendments in regulations, as well as assurances that ethical and confidential practices are being followed, in accordance with local privacy laws. The use of social media, videoconferencing, and smartphone apps will undoubtedly change not only clinician-patient interactions but also mutual expectations. Digital psychiatry is at an early stage, and future advancements bring both advantages and risks (Hariman, 2022). Clinicians need to start a dialogue with key stakeholders, including patients, their families and carers, policymakers, ethicists, and regulatory and training bodies. Ethical issues related to the use of telepsychiatry need to be addressed urgently. Its efficacy needs to be evaluated and developed further.

11 Mental Health for Nations in Pandemics

Introduction

Over the past millennia, human history has recorded hundreds of epidemics and pandemics. Different infectious agents have been responsible for deaths in large and small geographical areas. For the safety of their populations, governments of all hues have a moral and ethical responsibility to be prepared to deal with the spread of infections as well as manage their short-term and long-term sequelae along with their impact on people's mental health. They must invest in prevention through public health programs and find and fund research as well as suitable treatments and therapeutic interventions in the initial phases and in recovery and rehabilitation when needed. In the past, due to slow travel, the spread of infectious agents would have taken longer and information would have been shared more slowly. As globalization has shrunk the world, recent epidemics have spread rapidly across various nations. Equally important, though, the spread of information has been rapid.

In this chapter, we examine the impact of various epidemics in this century. Of these, the rapid spread of severe acute respiratory syndrome (SARS), Middle East respiratory syndrome (MERS), and Ebola, among others, has been truly remarkable. Due to climate change and other factors, it appears that the time period between epidemics is rapidly decreasing. The effect of epidemics on the mental health of individuals and populations can occur at different levels, from individual, familial, and neighborhood to community, regional, and national levels. The psychological effects of epidemics can result from stress that is related to the fear of infection, the actual loss of loved ones, survivor guilt, and the loss of employment, housing, and other basic needs. For those working particularly at the clinical front line, high rates of burnout and mental illness have been described. In anyone, fear and actual loss can contribute to depression, which may be further complicated by feelings of being trapped due to lockdown and self-isolation.

To begin with, we will briefly look at the history and lessons from some recent epidemics and their impact on mental health and well-being and what governments need to do. Social determinants of health will play an important role in the spread and management of epidemics.

Recent Pandemics

SARS CoV-1

In 2003, SARS CoV-1 virus was reported from China, although the first patient was seen in December 2002 (Christakis, 2020). The transmission of SARS CoV-1 virus initially was from animals to human beings and then human to human (Shereen et al., 2020). Wu et al. (2008) found that both individuals who had been infected and their carers showed high levels of anxiety and alcohol use during this epidemic. These researchers observed that younger individuals, those with limited education, and individuals who had been in quarantine were more likely to develop substance dependence. Understandably, symptoms of depression were frequently reported (Liu et al., 2012) and continued to persist even after three years, particularly among those who had experienced quarantine and trauma. These long-term effects are concerning, and health care providers need to be vigilant in identifying them and advocating for the implementation of appropriate policies and resources.

MERS

In 2015, the Middle East respiratory syndrome (MERS) virus appeared in Saudi Arabia and had a 20 percent mortality rate (Centers for Disease Control and Prevention [CDC], 2019). The virus appears to have transferred from bats to camels and then on to humans. Approximately 2,500 cases were reported, with 80 percent in Saudi Arabia and the remainder from 26 countries (Anonymous, 2019). A fear of contagion and anger was reported by 16 percent of those in isolation, but more worryingly, these emotions persisted in 25 percent of patients four to six months later (Jeong et al.,

2016). Anger can lead to aggression, and violence therefore is a crucial area of research for public mental health.

Ebola

There have been several outbreaks of Ebola virus on the African continent. The outbreak carries with it high rates of infection and mortality. O'Leary et al. (2018) observed that the Ebola epidemic in 2014 had 12 times more cases and 7 times more deaths than any of the previous 24 epidemics. During Ebola outbreaks, individuals from West Africa traveling to the US were received with panic and "a contagion of fear," which led to xenophobic racism and a climate of distrust of Africans, both travelers and residents. In a systematic review of mental health programs among populations affected by the Ebola virus, programs were implemented in hospitals, Ebola treatment centers, and communities, including in individuals exposed to Ebola. Evaluations of the programs showed improvements in the mental health of children and adults (Cénat et al., 2020).

SARS-2 (COVID-19)

With the SARS-2 (COVID-19) pandemic, countries responded in varying ways, from complete lockdowns to control through testing, tracking, and tracing to less restrictive approaches. Some countries initially denied that there was a problem. Tensions between various political factions in many countries contributed to confusing and contradictory messages. As tough leadership decisions were made, the tension between individual libertarian views and the common good led to conflicts about infection control. There is growing evidence that in many countries, the impact of the pandemic on people's mental health and well-being has been profound, adding to the existing burden of mental ill-health. Cases of long COVID are still being reported, causing further suspicion and panic.

Stages of an Epidemic

Epidemics unfold in distinct phases, each with its unique mental health challenges and responses. A comprehensive pandemic mental health strategy—including early intervention, crisis support, and long-term recovery programs—can help populations can recover and adapt in the aftermath of an epidemic (Litz et al., 2021; Watson, 2022). The CDC Preparedness and Response Framework for Influenza Pandemics identifies key epidemic stages (CDC, 2014) that are focused on public health prevention and response. For the purposes of this chapter, these have been mapped, adapted, and linked to mental health impacts and responses to mitigate distress and enhance resilience and recovery (table 11.1).

The effects of quarantine and isolation (discussed below) may apply to the emergence, acceleration, peak, and deceleration stages, depending on local contact restrictions in place.

Table 11.1
Stages of an epidemic, mental health impact, and key interventions

Epidemic stage	Mental health impact	Key mental health interventions
Preemergence (prodrome)	• Anxiety due to uncertainty and early warnings (Pfefferbaum & North, 2020) • Fear amplified by media and misinformation (Borges do Nascimento et al., 2022) • Psychological distress in vulnerable populations (Xiong et al., 2020)	• Risk communication and public awareness campaigns (Shultz et al., 2016) • Strengthening mental health system resilience (Moreno et al., 2020) • Training health care and community workers for crisis response (Greenberg et al., 2020)
Emergence (outbreak detection and early response)	• Heightened fear and distress due to unknown severity of the outbreak (Brooks et al., 2020) • Acute stress reactions in health care workers and the general public (WHO, 2020b) • Social and economic concerns beginning to emerge (Xiong et al., 2020)	• Clear, transparent communication to reduce panic (Pfefferbaum & North, 2020) • Psychological first aid (PFA) for those in distress (Shultz & Forbes, 2014) • Support systems for health care workers and at-risk populations (Greenberg et al., 2020)
Acceleration (rapid spread)	• Widespread distress due to rising cases and social isolation (Brooks et al., 2020) • Increased risk of depression, anxiety, and trauma-related disorders (Vindegaard & Benros, 2020) • Grief and loss affecting families and communities (Kontoangelos et al., 2020)	• Crisis counseling and mental health hotlines (Moreno et al., 2020) • Maintaining essential mental health services (Shultz et al., 2016) • Social support programs and virtual mental health care (WHO, 2020b)

Epidemic stage	Mental health impact	Key mental health interventions
Peak (health care systems overwhelmed)	• High psychological burden on health care workers (burnout, PTSD) (Greenberg et al., 2020) • Increased risk of suicide, moral injury, and severe distress (Sher, 2020) • Loss, grief, and trauma in affected communities (Brooks et al., 2020)	• Psychological crisis response teams for front-line workers (Shultz & Forbes, 2014) • Suicide prevention strategies (Gunnell et al., 2020) • Promoting coping mechanisms and stress management (Kontoangelos et al., 2020)
Deceleration (containment and declining cases)	• Lingering trauma, grief, and survivor's guilt (Greenberg et al., 2020) • Anxiety about returning to normal life and future uncertainties (Pfefferbaum & North, 2020) • Fatigue and mental exhaustion (WHO, 2020b)	• Continued psychological support and grief counseling (Kontoangelos et al., 2020) • Peer-support groups and therapy access (Moreno et al., 2020) • Workplace and community reintegration strategies (Shultz et al., 2016)
Recovery and rehabilitation (post-epidemic phase; preparation for the next one)	• Long-term mental health consequences ("Long COVID," PTSD, depression, anxiety) (Rogers et al., 2020) • Social stigma around mental illness and returning patients (Moreno et al., 2020) • Need for rebuilding mental health systems and resilience (Shultz et al., 2016)	• Long-term community-based mental health interventions including neuropsychiatric effects (Pfefferbaum & North, 2020) • Social prescribing and mental health policies (Moreno et al., 2020) • Public education campaigns to reduce stigma (Greenberg et al., 2020)

Mental Health Consequences of an Epidemic

Individual country responses to individual epidemics will vary based on cultural and socioeconomic factors. Epidemics carry with them several health (including mental health), social, and economic consequences (Morganstein & Ursano, 2020), which are discussed below. However, often mental health consequences of pandemics and epidemics are overlooked because the focus is on preventing further viral spread. Pandemics disproportionately affect vulnerable populations due to preexisting disparities in health care access, employment, and social support. For example, during the COVID-19 pandemic, individuals with disabilities faced greater social isolation and reduced health care services (Gleason et al., 2021). Low-income and ethnic minority communities also experienced higher rates of pandemic-related mental health distress resulting from financial insecurity and higher infection rates (Czeisler et al., 2020).

Prodrome

As soon as there was international recognition of the SARS-CoV-2 (COVID-19) epidemic, before it became a pandemic, populations around the world felt confused and threatened, resulting in both paranoid feelings and xenophobic attitudes. Some cultures, for political reasons, refrain from acknowledging health risks, focusing instead on economic factors, as has been observed in many parts of the US, which aligns with the political determinants of mental health. This debate between the common good and the economy is crucial in understanding and shaping the population's response. Policymakers have an ethical responsibility to provide clear and accurate information about the steps individuals need to take to protect themselves and their families.

The Impact of Quarantine

Chatterjee and Chanham (2020) remind us that historically, sailors who had sailed from infected ports had to wait for 40 (*quarenta*) days before being allowed to come ashore. Quarantine is differentiated from isolation, where those who are sick are separated from those who are not. Interestingly, while in quarantine, ships had to hoist the yellow flag. In the UK, in many streets and localities, people had been encouraged to have red or green signs in their windows so that neighbors could keep an eye on each other. Mass quarantine in many cities was particularly effective in containing the SARS epidemic in 2003 and Ebola outbreak in 2014 (Chatterjee & Chauhan, 2020). Such an approach can be seen as the first crucial step to enable asymptomatic carriers to avoid the spread of the infectious agents. Quarantine is defined as the process by which human beings or animals who are exposed to the pathogen are separated to prevent the spread of the disease. However, these periods can encourage spread of misinformation, rumors, and false news, thereby contributing to anxiety, panic, and a further sense of isolation. People may remain under direct or indirect observation for a period to ensure that they remain asymptomatic and are not carriers. From individuals being quarantined to communities and then cities or towns, quarantine has been used as a preventive technique for several centuries.

There is no doubt that the psychological impact of quarantine on individuals and communities but also on the family members quarantined or isolated together is significant (Brooks et al., 2020). Quarantine measures, while necessary for public health, have been linked to increased stress, depression, and anxiety resulting from loneliness and isolation. Strategies to mitigate these effects include maintaining structured daily routines, using digital platforms for social connectivity, and engaging in mindfulness exercises (Brooks et al., 2020). Evidence suggests that access to clear information and short quarantine durations help reduce psychological distress (Jeong et al., 2016).

In many settings after lockdown, the rates of domestic interpersonal violence went up dramatically (Porter et al, 2021). Being quarantined or isolated is not a pleasant experience. It can lead to frustration, loneliness, boredom, and uncertainty about the present and the future (Bai et al., 2004). The sense of feeling trapped in a pressure cooker setting can also lead to high levels of psychological morbidity. Individuals can experience panic, fear, anxiety, and post-traumatic stress disorder (Hawryluck et al., 2004). The duration of quarantine will contribute to the severity of these symptoms and responses. Furthermore, increased use of substances such as alcohol to ameliorate symptoms of anxiety and panic is well recognized. It is inevitable that being in quarantine or isolation will stop people from going outdoors, especially if access to green spaces is limited. Frustration and anger may be evident if those in power are seen not to be following the rules themselves; such feelings, if introjected, may lead to depression, while externalizing these feelings can lead to substance use, anger, frustration, or even violence.

It is possible that voluntary quarantine may work better, as the individual may feel that they have a degree of control. It is entirely possible that some individuals when asked to self-isolate after suspicion of infection may feel guilty, lonely, anxious, panicky, fearful, and depressed. Similarly, in vulnerable individuals, instructions on hand washing to prevent infections may well lead to compulsive behaviors.

Technology and Epidemics

Technology allows people to remain in contact but not in touch. However, there is a clear digital divide not only across countries but also within the same country influenced by levels of education, economic status, and across age groups. Individuals in quarantine should be encouraged to develop skills through activities such as learning, cognitive development, meditation, mindfulness, yoga, and relaxation. These approaches can help reduce anxiety and alleviate milder symptoms of other common mental disorders. Furthermore, individuals should be encouraged to follow news from reliable sources only and, if possible, to limit their daily consumption of news to specific time periods. Vulnerable groups and individuals (e.g., older adults who may not have access to technology or may be unfamiliar with it) along with children who may be missing school, friends, and education will require additional support.

Psychiatric Sequelae

As already noted, symptoms of anxiety may also lead to sleep disturbances that are likely to increase the risk for other difficulties (Zhen et al., 2018). Mellman et al. (1995) reported sleep difficulties in individuals without a history of psychiatric disorders in the previous six months after facing a hurricane. Morganstein and Ursano (2020) emphasize that psychological disorders following disasters lead to significant morbidity and mortality and therefore need appropriate interventions—an observation that is equally applicable to epidemics.

Psychiatric sequelae of epidemics may result from direct infection leading to changes in the brain and body, or it may arise from the indirect impacts of stress or social responses. The phases of epidemics can also shape individual and community reactions. Vulnerable and disadvantaged groups, such as children, older adults, migrants, and LGBTQ+ individuals, are more likely to experience infections and subsequent complications. Individuals in quarantine or isolation may increase their consumption of alcohol and substances such as tobacco. They might report feelings of separation anxiety, as well as challenges in managing anger, frustration, and a diminished sense of security and safety. The responses of individuals and communities will vary and may influence one another. Resilience at both levels—individual and community—will be essential to effectively manage responses to epidemics.

Psychiatric effects will be observed at the individual, community, and international levels (van Bortel et al., 2016), not ignoring the national or regional levels, and thus any interventions must be in place at all these levels. Not only may new cases appear even after the peak of the epidemic has subsided, but others may continue to experience distress and suffer in the medium to long term. Yao et al., (2020) note that patients with (pre-existing) mental disorders faced further barriers in seeking help during the pandemic due to factors such as poor awareness, discrimination, and a parallel epidemic of fear and anxiety. Equally important, pressures on health care facilities may deter people from seeking help in a timely fashion. Due to lockdowns and travel restrictions, they may not be able to make their appointments—hence, the importance of using technology for assessments and therapeutic interactions.

Stress Responses, Fear, and Anxiety

Stress responses are likely to be heightened in epidemics and disasters. These may emerge as a new episode of a disorder in vulnerable people or those predisposed to a psychiatric disorder. It may also exacerbate any pre-existing disorder. Some individuals may develop post-traumatic stress disorder (PTSD) or adjustment disorders, which are also more likely to be seen in frontline workers. Individuals may go on to develop a stress response that may or may not reach diagnostic levels (Esterwood & Saeed, 2020). These authors, after reviewing a number of top-cited papers, noted that alcohol use, anxiety, fear of contagion, perceived risk, uncertainty, and distrust can occur in the short term and, more worryingly, may persist in the long term. They highlight that not every individual with a genetic predisposition for a disease will go on to develop that disease, but early recognition of such predisposition may help some people if stressors are reduced. As they emphasize, a direct threat to one's life can result in psychological trauma, which can lead to intrusive thoughts, avoidance, and self-blame. While both the epidemics and pandemics contribute to traumatic thoughts, individuals will respond in different ways depending on a variety of internal and external factors, such as their personality traits, their support systems, and their access to physical, economic, social, and psychological resources in managing coping strategies.

O'Leary et al. (2018) observed a culture of fear during the Ebola epidemic, which adversely affected the economy and health care utilization. This phenomenon was described as the "fearonomic" effect (Shultz et al., 2016; Bali et al., 2016). Misinformation exacerbated fear and led to dangerous remedies. Stigma affected both survivors and those associated with Ebola transmission (Overholt et al., 2018; Thorson et al., 2016). Health workers caring for Ebola cases faced stigma, which affected their well-being (Sow et al., 2016). Frontline health care workers faced various risks, including infections as well as mental health issues stemming from stress and burnout. Ricci-Cabello et al. (2020) conducted a rapid review of 61 studies on the mental health effects of health emergencies, finding high rates of anxiety, depression, and PTSD among workers. Vulnerability factors included being female and of a younger age, a lack of support, stigma, isolation, occupational stress, and inadequate training. Bai et al. (2004) reported that quarantine negatively affected frontline workers, leading to burnout characterized by anxiety, irritability, and exhaustion.

A year after the Ebola outbreak in Sierra Leone, Jalloh et al. (2018) assessed anxiety, depression, and PTSD symptoms in the general population. They found that 48 percent in their sample reported anxiety symptoms, and 27 percent met the criteria for clinical PTSD. Knowing someone in quarantine was linked to increased anxiety, which has important implications for public health messaging. Rates of anxiety varied by country, with 22 percent of survivors in Sierra Leone reporting depression, compared to 13 percent in Guinea (Secor et al. 2020), suggesting that other influencing factors may be at play. Nyanfor and Xiao (2020) also reported high rates of anxiety, with one-third of their sample attempting suicide, emphasizing the need for effective mental health messaging. Mohammed et al. (2015) highlighted that health workers faced additional distress after the death of a colleague and the disruption of social support systems due to the epidemic (Shultz et al., 2014).

Long-Term Sequelae

At the time of writing, it is difficult to predict what the longer-term outcomes of the COVID-19 pandemic will be, but various neurological and neuropsychiatric sequelae have already been reported. It is worth recognizing that not every infected patient will develop psychiatric symptoms. "Long COVID' has already been described, where patients have long-term symptoms that may affect any body system. These have been divided into four syndromes (Mahase, 2020). A wide range of symptoms affecting virtually every organ of the body—the kidneys, respiratory system, brain, cardiovascular systems, heart, the gut, the liver, and the skin—have been identified. Undoubtedly, all these infections and related problems will have significant psychological impact on patients, their formal and informal carers, and their families.

A review from the National Institute for Health and Care Research (NIHR, 2020) highlights that while a lack of diagnostic consensus poses challenges for policymakers, these symptoms are likely to have significant psychological and social impacts, which in turn will result in long-term consequences both at the individual and societal levels. Disproportionate effects on ethnic minorities and other underprivileged populations are likely to add certain additional challenges (PHE, 2020; Sze et al., 2020) both in prevention and in management. In a systematic review and meta-analysis, Rogers et al. (2020) note that confusion, depressed mood, anxiety, impaired memory, and insomnia were common. In the post-illness stage, depressed mood, insomnia, irritability, poor memory, and fatigue were reported. Nearly one-third of individuals had symptoms of PTSD, around 15 percent had depression, and a similar number had anxiety. Long-term psychiatric consequences of pandemics include increased rates of PTSD, anxiety, and depression. Research on SARS survivors found that around a quarter developed PTSD within three years of recovery (Mak et al., 2009). Similar trends have been observed post-COVID-19, with prolonged stress and uncertainty exacerbating preexisting mental health conditions (Xiong et al., 2020).

The Management of Epidemics

Managing epidemics involves primary prevention and secondary and tertiary preventions. This is where planning at a national level and having clear policies with identified command structures can help deliver the interventions appropriately and promptly.

The responses in managing epidemics and pandemics must include managing mental health needs of those who are infected, those who look after them (both formal and informal carers), and the general population to avoid the spread of misinformation and provide educational materials in a commonsense manner. Misinformation during pandemics has significantly contributed to public anxiety and stress. During the COVID-19 pandemic, widespread misinformation on social media led to increased vaccine hesitancy and distrust in health authorities (Cinelli et al., 2020). Similarly, during the Ebola outbreak in West Africa, rumors about the virus being a government conspiracy heightened community resistance to health interventions (Allgaier & Svalastog, 2015).

International Management

Epidemics may start in one country but are highly unlikely to be confined to one. Given modern travel, viruses and other infectious agents spread very rapidly across the globe. Viruses do not respect national boundaries and do not require entry or exit visas. Hence, the first step must be sharing relevant information across the globe speedily so that data can be exchanged, treatment plans can be put in place, and if needed, protective equipment can be shared.

International collaboration is critical in pandemic mental health response. The WHO's Mental Health and Psychosocial Support (MHPSS) programs have been implemented globally to support mental well-being during crises (Tol et al., 2011). The United Nations also launched the COVID-19 Response and Recovery Fund to enhance mental health services in low-income countries, emphasizing cross-border cooperation (United Nations, 2020).

International collaboration can facilitate mutual learning, allowing the exchange of experiences in responses along with examples of good practices and lessons learned, which can be shared across communities. In addition, the development of new vaccines or the sharing of existing ones by increasing manufacturing capacity across national boundaries can be beneficial. It is worth remembering that smallpox was eradicated because of global cooperation and that polio is now being controlled and is confined to a small number of countries in a similar way. A non-blaming approach that involves working cooperatively and sharing data, research, and examples of good practice while collecting information on the psychological and psychiatric aspects of epidemics can be extremely helpful. Similarly, learning about the views of vaccine skeptics and objectors can be useful in developing and delivering strategies to vaccinate vulnerable populations.

National Management

Every country, irrespective of resources allocated to health, must have a clear and recognized disaster/emergency/epidemic management policy and plan. Planning exercises and dry runs can prove useful in controlling the spread of epidemics. There is no doubt that each country's response will depend on the resources allocated to health, especially public health.

Identifying the pattern of disease spread is the first step. In these days of social media, the use of test, trace, and track apps for identification and confirmation of cases is extremely important. Additionally, there needs to be clear messaging about the prevention of spread, and the public must be willing to follow the rules. Facilities to isolate those who may be infectious have to be easily accessible. Similarly, dealing with the bodies of those who may have succumbed to the infection must be done in a careful, culturally sensitive, and time-sensitive manner. Similar to the management of post-disaster situations, health care services must have the ability to ratchet up services depending on the immediate needs of the communities.

Managing epidemics does not mean that routine or emergency demands on health care for other conditions will disappear altogether; thus, managing the two in tandem can be a difficult task, but it needs to be carried out carefully. Using volunteers, community health workers or navigators to assist those in isolation or quarantine and those prone to infections can be an extremely useful first step. Resources for treatment must be adequate and easily accessible. Similarly, appropriate options for care—whether health, social, or material—must be made available to those who have recovered or are in the process of recovering. In many settings, the rehabilitative aspects may need to be delegated to nonmedical staff, volunteers, or others. The key is having a clear national plan and policy for managing disasters and epidemics, along with sufficient resources through international links and partnerships, to set in place primary, secondary, and tertiary prevention. Clear messaging and the sharing of information in a culturally sensitive manner can help engage populations and avoid alienating the public. Within each country, a degree of flexible variation will be needed to engage with local communities.

Community

National or federal policies can set national standards and expectations, but it is at the local or community level that true interventions have to take place. Appropriate and honest information is crucial, as misinformation shared through social media can prove to be damaging. There is no doubt that fear can affect engagement, stigma, and adherence to treatment. The information must be accessible and easily understandable. Using social media to share accurate information can be helpful. Trust in government policymakers, and leaders is crucial if people are going to follow relevant guidelines. Culturally appropriate information can help engage the population. During the COVID-19 pandemic, many streets set up local links and WhatsApp groups to share information, support each other, exchange goods and services, and assist those living alone. Using these methods in neighborhoods has brought communities closer together. However, it is important to recognize that heterogeneity within each community will continue to exist. Fake news, especially about the epidemic and pseudo treatments, needs to be identified early and debunked effectively. In some communities, religious leaders were helpful in establishing vaccination centers and hubs. Any intervention such as mass vaccinations can only be successful if communities are engaged properly through community or religious leaders, teachers, and other significant figures. The community can come together to deliver the national standards and policies.

Individual Management

Individuals have the right to good health, including mental health, but they also need to take responsibility for their own health, perhaps more so in the times of epidemics. They need to follow instructions on how to stay safe and, equally important, how to keep others safe around them. Furthermore, when required, they should follow the quarantine or self-isolation rules. These rules can be difficult to follow and can be perceived as impinging on an individual's freedom.

However, in order to stay safe and protect others, it is critical that rules are followed in isolation and quarantine to maintain everyone's physical and mental health and well-being. These quarantine recommendations are outline in box 11.1. They must be tailored according to individual needs

Health Workers

Frontline health care workers experience heightened stress during pandemics, making resilience-building strategies essential. Health care workers, whether they are on the frontline or working behind the scenes in the community, are more likely to show symptoms of burnout. Burnout is generally defined as an experience of physical, emotional, and mental exhaustion caused by a long-term involvement with emotionally demanding situations (Mateen & Dorji, 2009) and often because of stress stemming from a lack of control over working conditions. The symptoms of burnout include emotional exhaustion, depersonalization, and an absent sense of personal accomplishment (Tidy, 2015), which in itself can be traumatic for professionals who try to maintain professional standards and values but are unable to do so because of various stressors or resource limitations. Burnout

Box 11.1
Self-Care During Quarantine

- Prioritize self-care—Maintain a healthy lifestyle with balanced eating, regular exercise, and sufficient sleep. Incorporate mindfulness, meditation, and yoga to support mental well-being.
- Establish structure—Stick to a daily routine that balances work, breaks, and leisure. Take regular short breaks, and include a mix of stimulating and relaxing activities to maintain motivation.
- Set boundaries—Create space for oneself and loved ones, ensuring a balance between personal time and social interactions. Be mindful of work-life boundaries, especially when working from home.
- Stay connected—Maintain friendships and peer support, whether through virtual check-ins or workplace networks. Regular social interaction helps reduce feelings of isolation.
- Seek the right information—Control news intake by following reliable sources and limiting exposure to distressing content.
- Practice self-compassion—Be kind to yourself, acknowledge challenges, and develop resilience by embracing a sense of humor and focusing on what is within your control.
- Access support—Seek help early if struggling with mental ill-health. Engage in peer support, counseling, or professional resources as needed.

has key dimensions of disengagement, blunted emotion, and feelings of hopelessness and helplessness (i.e., feeling trapped) with low motivation and detachment. In contrast, stress is recognized by urgency, hyperactivity, overactive emotions, and over engagement. Institutions or organizations have a responsibility to look after their staff. To this end, they must offer relevant facilities for maintaining their staff's well-being, including occupational health. It is vital that such resources are publicized and that confidential private assistance is readily available.

Interventions such as resilience training have been shown to reduce burnout and improve coping mechanisms in nurses (Mealer et al., 2014). Mindfulness-based stress reduction (MBSR) interventions, which include mindfulness and relaxation techniques, have efficacy in reducing psychological distress among health care providers (Lamothe et al., 2016). Peer-support programs are also effective in reducing psychological distress as well as shifting organizational culture, equipping staff with skills to recognize and support distress, and supporting those already providing informal peer support. (Repper & Carter, 2011; Petera et al., 2021; Simms et al., 2023). Supervision and mentoring can help in managing distress (Milne & Reiser, 2017).

Leaders of institutions and organizations are responsible for ensuring that working conditions are safe and that staff are recognized and rewarded. Empowering the staff can help them manage their own stress more effectively and also better equips them to deal with stressors. Clear communication with an emphasis on the prevention of bullying and harassment, on the one hand, and coaching and mentoring, on the other, can be extremely beneficial. Encouraging health care workers to bring attention to issues when things are going awry can boost morale by addressing stressful situations appropriately at an early stage. Open listening and moral concerns need to be encouraged to help prevent burnout among health care workers (Moffic et al., 2020). National policies must address the stress experienced by health care staff, and adequate, appropriate, and additional resources must be allocated as needed to prevent burnout.

Resilience

Resilience was discussed in Chapter 2,but just to remind ourselves, it is defined as an individual's ability to adapt to and manage stress and adversity (Lown et al., 2015). At times of epidemics, both physical and psychological resilience are likely to be seriously tested. Resilience is needed to manage both psychological and physical stress and distress caused by epidemics. Furthermore, it must be recognized that resilience is a multidimensional and complex concept, likely to be affected by factors such as facing fear, moral compass, spirituality and religion, availability and access to social support, physical and brain fitness, cognitive and emotional flexibility, having meaning, purpose and growth in life, and realistic optimism (Southwick & Charney, 2012)

Conclusion

Epidemics and pandemics have occurred over millennia with varying rates of morbidity and mortality. New viruses as well as variations of existing viruses will continue to evolve and emerge. The spread of viruses and other infectious agents is rapid in a globally interconnected world, as demonstrated by the rapid spread of the COVID-19 virus, which enveloped the world within two to three months. In times of epidemics, the mental health needs of those at risk, those infected, those unaffected, and survivors are often ignored as the focus is on physical containment. This can lead to additional strain and stress on the population and resources. This situation especially affects those who may be developing mental illnesses unrelated to the epidemics, because delays in help-seeking will worsen their prognosis. At the same time, the mental health and well-being of the health care workers who look after affected individuals and those who provide essential services such as transport and catering, which put them at increased risk, are often ignored. The COVID-19 pandemic highlighted the critical need for integrating mental health considerations into public health responses across all epidemic phases. For instance, the rapid adoption of telepsychiatry ensured continuity of care during lockdowns, demonstrating the importance of adaptable mental health services. Additionally, proactive mental health strategies, such as resilience training and community support initiatives, have proved effective in mitigating psychological distress during health crises. It is crucial that governments, institutions, communities, and individuals take responsibility for ensuring that the population's mental health is looked after. In many settings, further evidence is needed to explore the long-term effects of epidemics on society and individuals. Furthermore, governments have a moral and ethical duty not only to look after their populations and those who care for them but also to be ready and prepared to do so. Lessons from the pandemic are still emerging, and societies need to be prepared not only for rehabilitation and recovery but also for similar future events.

12 Social Prescribing

Introduction

In this brief chapter, the concept of social prescribing will be described and its advantages and disadvantages discussed. It can be argued that its appeal has increased for clinicians because of increasing awareness of social factors within the biopsychosocial causation and intervention model of mental illnesses. Social prescribing has potential benefits but also risks for both patients and doctors who prescribe these activities. For countries where resources are limited, it offers a way to improve social connection and meaningful activities for people with mental illnesses, as well as increasing their engagement within the community. However, further research data are needed to evaluate its impact and outcomes in a variety of conditions and contexts.

As mentioned in chapter 12, the COVID-19 (SARS-2) pandemic highlighted the importance of social connection and meaningful activity. Reaching out through neighbors and volunteers to assist and support vulnerable groups who were shielding, in isolation, or in quarantine has illustrated the strength of many communities during the pandemic. Younan et al. (2020) concluded that the emergency situation induced by the pandemic made it feasible to offer social prescribing involving community health workers, a model used in Brazil to improve population health (Johnson et al., 2013; Macinko & Harris, 2015). Younan et al. (2020) proposed a realignment model of social prescribing with a household model based on the principles of universality, comprehensiveness, and integration. Various models of social prescribing can be used specifically for different vulnerable populations, including "community contractors" who facilitate access to services, increase community connections, and help improve knowledge and skills (NEF Consulting, 2019).

Background

Historically, in the UK and many other countries, psychiatric asylums provided patients with the experiences such as gardening, animal care, crafting, music, and exercise as part of therapeutic engagement and activities. As far back as 1847, lunacy commissioners observed that working in agriculture, gardening, and recreation in the open air were beneficial for patients, as these activities provided occupation and exercise (Hickman, 2014).

Components and Principles

Understanding that health and well-being are largely influenced by various social, economic, and environmental factors, social prescribing attempts to meet individuals' needs holistically while encouraging them to gain more control over their health (Buck & Ewbank, 2020). Social prescribing focuses on social interventions. It is defined as the process by which a clinician "prescribes" a variety of social and collaborative activities such as gardening, photography, sports, crafts, or hobbies. Individuals can be referred to nonclinical community services for these activities through social prescribing, which can help enhance mental, physical, and social well-being. (Younan et al., 2020). Social prescribing helps connect individuals—including those with long-term physical or psychiatric conditions and those who are lonely or isolated and may have complex social needs—with various community organizations, individuals or groups.

The reason is often to keep the individual occupied while awaiting further assessment or engagement, but there is also a focus on developing educational skills alongside learning new ones. Social prescribing supports individuals emotionally and also helps them in taking on more responsibility for developing and maintaining their health and well-being (Buck & Ewbank, 2020). Social prescribing can help overcome loneliness and isolation while fostering a sense of belonging and community. Such support can help reduce levels of distress in milder disorders such as anxiety or mild depression. It can also help reduce chronic stress (Bird et al., 2020).

Social prescribing can help people feel better without using medicine by focusing on what a person can do to be healthy and helping them build skills and confidence. Furthermore, because community activities are locally based, they can support the local community and economy (Jani and Gray 2019). As approximately one-fifth of consultations in primary care are said to be related to social needs (Primary Care Foundation & NHS Alliance, 2015), social prescribing and community activities can alleviate some of the pressures on primary care (Tønnesen, 2016). Jani and Gray (2019) argue that social prescribing activities can help strengthen communities and improve quality of life.

Social prescribing in both primary and secondary care can utilize the skills of community link workers, who are skilled practitioners with knowledge of existing community organizations and the ability to direct individuals according to their needs and accessibility. Link workers can also help create and develop new group activities. Social prescribing does not always require a medical prescription or decision and can therefore be provided by various sources, such as health visitors, community nurses, community link workers, or cultural brokers in the community. Since these individuals often live in the community, they know about local services and facilities, which can help build a sense of community and continuity.

Health care or social care professionals can make the referral to the community link worker. From the link worker, the individual is given trial access to engage in specific activities. Eventually, this may lead to full access to various community or third-sector organizations.

These activities can lead to community involvement and cohesion, with the secondary effect being a reduction in stigma. Younan et al. (2020) recommend that social prescribing be both comprehensive and go beyond the traditional biomedical model if it is to lead to improved population health, pointing out that social prescribing through community workers and community connectors can engage populations by identifying and supporting vulnerable individuals, especially in the post-COVID era. Social prescribing can also provide value in improving health education and monitoring chronic diseases, including stress.

Social prescribing can change behaviors related to lack of exercise, diet, and occupational skills that can affect mental health. Community link workers or navigators are the key in engagement since they can provide the right information about local activities and facilities and steer the individual to the right action or the correct community organization (PHE, 2019). Thus, community links and partnerships between health care professionals and community members and organizations will support communities and improve their knowledge about health habits. It is worth recognizing that many low- and middle-income countries where both human and financial resources may be limited have developed innovative strategies that combine social prescribing and task-shifting. For example, "Aunties" are trained in Cameroon to provide support to teenage mothers or those with substance abuse problems. In southern Thailand, villagers elect volunteers, with each volunteer taking responsibility for the health of ten households (see appendix 12 for more examples). These setups can be scaled up in times of emergency.

Social prescribing can function at light, medium, or high levels (Kimberlee, 2015), depending on the amount of time needed and available for activities. Carter et al. (2018) reported that most studies used individual navigators; however, in order to reach large numbers of people, systemic navigation was required. Care needs to be provided by individual navigators and community health workers with general skills or more specific skills such as health care, legal assistance, vocational rehabilitation, or financial advice.

The range of community activities available and accessible may include physical exercise, singing in choirs, playing music, reading, photography, gardening and working on allotments, visiting museums and galleries, or taking drawing classes. Local partnerships between health, housing, education, and employment programs are helpful and can operate through local community colleges, schools, libraries, theaters, or community centers where people can meet and participate in group activities on a regular basis. However, there must be a clear agenda and agreed-on outcomes before starting the activities. There is plenty of altruism and goodwill in communities; the challenge is to access it in a pragmatic manner.

Link Workers

The UK National Health Service (NHS) Long Term Plan has a clear focus on social prescribing as one of the targeted personalized interventions. The proposal is to have community link workers who become the central contact point or hub. The link worker devotes time and energy to informing and engaging both individuals and their families about what is suitable to meet their needs and available locally. Joint working with the care team, on the one hand, and the individual, on the other, can facilitate development and delivery of targeted personalized care.

As of 2023, more than 2.5 million people had been referred to more than 3,500 social prescribing link workers in England (NASP, 2023). Social prescribing is thus becoming a key part of primary care networks in the UK (NHS England, 2024). In a survey conducted by the Royal College of General Practitioners (RCGP, 2018), more than half (59 percent) of the GPs who responded felt that social prescribing could help their patients.

Community organizations and nongovernmental organizations (NGOs) are well positioned to employ link workers and may take on the responsibility for their selection, training, appraisal, and ethical practice as they are likely to be aware of local situations and resources. In some settings city councils are the employers. In any given geographical area and community, a single agency should be identified and recognized as the primary provider, thereby meeting the needs of the local people. Appropriate mapping of services and their functions can be helpful for those who need them. Creating a "metro map" (Carlile & Bhugra, 2014) that lets individuals know where to go for what they need can facilitate the appropriate use of link workers, who then can act as guides. Primary care, along with funders or commissioners, can take the lead. Professionals conducting needs assessments should be aware of the local support and activities available. Sharing health records can be beneficial for improving care and managing risk, but privacy and confidentiality must be managed carefully.

Finally, clear outcomes should be identified at the outset so that appropriate community organizations are engaged from the very beginning with funding that is well targeted.

Research Evidence

There is plenty of anecdotal evidence about social prescribing, although research evidence of its efficacy is varied. After evaluating 15 studies, Bickerdike et al. (2017) found a high risk of bias that they attributed to factors such as a lack of comparative controls, short follow-up durations, a lack of standardized and validated measuring tools, and missing data. Husk et al. (2019) point out that social prescribing has proliferated often without a concomitant evidence base and while ignoring community-based variations. Polley et al. (2017b) draw a distinction between evaluation and evidence, offering a checklist to ensure stronger evaluation of social prescribing activities. Dayson and Bashir (2014) analyzed data from Rotherham in the UK, which was one of the early sites to pioneer social prescribing. Their analysis included peer advocacy, group activity, advice, support, and activity coordination. Dayson et al. (2013) reported from the same dataset that almost a quarter of social prescribing participants (22 percent) requested community activity, 15 percent needed information only, 11 percent wanted befriending, and 9 percent required transport access. Among those accessing social prescribing, visits to emergency departments fell by almost a quarter (21 percent), and hospital admissions decreased by 9 percent. Interestingly, outpatient attendance also dropped by 29 percent compared to the six months prior to referral. Social outcomes also improved, with these authors observing that social prescribing had led to patients becoming more independent. Notably, the Rotherham sample was 80 percent female, which limits the generalizability of these findings.

In Somerset, England, a primary care service used an enhanced model to signpost community services, leading to a dramatic decrease in emergency hospital admissions (Abel et al., 2018). An evidence review from the Royal College of General Practitioners (RCGP, 2018) also reported an average drop of 28 percent in demand for primary care services following a referral to a social prescribing service. Cawston (2011), in a study of ten primary care services in Scotland, found that a key factor in patients' success was their strength in tackling their problems. General practitioners are part of the community and serve as key advisers to their patients; as such, they may facilitate greater acceptance of social prescribing (Brandling & House, 2009).

There is anecdotal evidence that some ethnic minority women may visit the doctor more frequently as a "genuine" reason to leave the house. Working with community organizations can thus help develop bonds, friendships, and both formal and informal support systems for those who need them. This can help improve their mental health and well-being as well as physical health. In some situations, the individual may need medication, which the primary care physician can supply. A study from New Zealand (Wilson & Read, 2001) noted that general practitioners tend to prescribe more medication because of the high cost of psychological therapies. However, it is possible to receive some psychological support through social prescribing. Moffat et al. (2017), in a qualitative survey of individuals with complex multi-morbidities, found that interventions by community link workers could generate feelings of control, self-confidence and well-being, leading to improved diet, increased physical activity, and reduced social isolation. In a randomized control trial, Grant et al. (2000) found that having access to a referrals-facilitator can reduce levels of anxiety while improving the ability to carry out daily activities and consequently quality of life. Surprisingly, they found that although the mean cost was greater, there were fewer referrals to mental health services, thereby saving referral costs. This reflects that collaboration is needed between primary care and secondary care. Carter et al. (2018) observed that social prescribing led to improved general wellness, reduced financial stress, increased employment, and improved knowledge and skills, all attributable to link workers. A review of the evidence assessing the impact of social prescribing on healthcare demand and costs found average reductions of 28 percent in GP (primary care) consultations, 24 percent in emergency room attendances, and statistically significant decreases in hospital referrals following participation in social prescribing schemes (Polley et al., 2017a).

Behavior change can result from improved self-care, increased physical activity, and improved motivation and can contribute to building voluntary capacity. Additionally, it helps to change some determinants of ill-health by reducing isolation and loneliness and increasing the likelihood of occupation and employment. Thus, individuals can coproduce with link workers locally and immediately and with health professionals at a distance.

Advantages

With increasing longevity, older individuals will require greater social and community interactions and support to avoid social isolation and subsequent loneliness. Abbasi (2019) suggests that, considering the pressures on health services and busy wards—as occurred during the COVID-19 pandemic—social prescribing could provide some interventions for individuals as well as the health care system as a whole, thereby offering relief to both, even if only in the short term.

Individuals are said to be happier in more scenic locations, but many residents especially in urban inner-city areas do not have access to green spaces, and many general or psychiatric hospitals do not offer outside space (Seresinhe et al., 2019). Thus, social prescribing can offer access to green spaces.

Disadvantages

There is a risk in that in some settings, social prescribing may be seen as an alternative to health care rather than as an adjunct. Policymakers may also see social prescribing as a means to deal with the social determinants of health (see chapter 3), which in reality need to be addressed at the national policy level. Social prescribing may be offered in deprived areas instead of more expensive services, thus creating a second-tier intervention, which may affect inner-city populations, including minority ethnic groups.

It is also important to know why some people are better at engaging with services whereas others are not. From their qualitative study, Pescheny et al. (2018b) reported that factors affecting uptake and adherence included the patient's trust in their health care provider—whether it was a primary care doctor, a community link worker, or a navigator. It is also worth recognizing that in many settings, doctors do have a certain status, which is what patients may prefer; thus link workers should be offered as a high-value choice so that the patient does not feel cheated. Furthermore, as South et al. (2008) point out, in many settings, the relationships between primary care physicians and voluntary sectors (non-governmental organizations also known as third sector in many countries) are often weak. These links can be strengthened by link workers, cultural brokers, and navigators (Dietze, 2018). The way the initial contact is established will play a major role in subsequent engagement. As these interventions are termed social *prescribing*, it is possible that they may be taken to be a medical recommendation as well as a forced one, thereby negating their potential advantages.

Conclusion

On balance, if appropriately offered and managed, social prescribing can in some cases help alleviate loneliness and social isolation and provide support; it can help people learn new skills and become more active, which can be beneficial for both physical and mental health. Even though research is mixed, social prescribing can facilitate better engagement with health care services and educate teams in a two-way process.

Through community link workers and mediators, individuals with complex needs can be introduced to a range of community activities that will help them feel like they belong and are part of a community. This engagement can reduce loneliness and isolation. Engaging in activities can also enhance health by promoting a better diet and exercise. Both aerobic and resistance exercise have demonstrated benefits for anxiety, depression, and PTSD (Smith & Merwin, 2021). Being healthy thus can be promoted at the community level.

Social prescribing should not be seen as a panacea but rather as one of many tools at the disposal of health care workers. In many countries, the economy has been strongly affected by the pandemic, and the closure of community institutions such as libraries, banks, and high street shops means that only a few places remain where people can gather, interact with one another, and share their experiences. People need access to publicly shared spaces and places where different generations can meet and share experiences. Older and younger generations can learn from each other, and community link workers or navigators may provide direction, saving time for statutory services to focus on other, perhaps more serious aspects of health care. Establishing community mental health teams offers a wonderful opportunity for them to engage with and be part of the community they serve. Social prescribing, done properly, can contribute to and indeed increase community engagement and help reduce stigma and discrimination. It can help engage individuals, improve their mental health and well-being, and reduce pressures on health care systems.

13 Conclusions

Over the past decades, medicine has changed dramatically with the rapid technological advances in diagnostic investigations, clinical interventions, and the use of AI (artificial intelligence) and algorithms. In many countries, the principle "No decision about me without me" has altered the therapeutic interaction and alliance. In this context, and with changing patient expectations, the doctor-patient relationship is also evolving. Simultaneously, the development and implementation of global health and mental health paradigms have resulted in increased authority being granted to the Western medical-industrial complex worldwide, where pharmaceutical companies wield considerable influence. This is not to say that global mental health or global health movements do little good, but neither are they without faults.

At the core of social justice, especially in the context of equity, is the ability to achieve good health. Social justice is about delivering equity by strengthening institutions (Bhugra et al. 2022; also see Tribe & Bhugra 2025). The difference between equity and equality is crucial. Health equality is about giving everyone a pair of glasses whether they need it or not, whereas health equity is to have the right kind of glasses for everyone, according to their need, while considering other variables, too.

The ability to be healthy depends on a many factors and can be strengthened at the individual, family, community, and national levels. At the national level, governments must provide support through education, employment, access to housing, and appropriate resources. Governments need strong public health and public mental health strategies. Public education about health, including mental health, happens at the community, family, and individual levels. Each level in turn has to be supported by federal, state, and local governments with sufficient resources and appropriate valid information. Geopolitical determinants, such as natural or human-caused disasters and climate change, affect the movement of people at intranational and international levels, thus affecting the social determinants within any nation-state. Charlson et al. (2021) underscore the mental health consequences of climate change, citing psychological distress, worsened mental health, higher mortality among people with pre-existing mental health conditions, increased psychiatric hospitalizations, and elevated suicide rates following extreme weather events. Furthermore, armed conflict and political instability exacerbate post-traumatic stress disorder and depression rates among displaced and undisplaced populations (Ahmed et al., 2024; Khadija et al., 2024).

Over 70 years ago, Hobson (1949) linked diseases with social environment and the Marmot-led WHO Commission on Social Determinants has shown that unemployment, poverty, overcrowding, lack of access to transport, and poor access to green spaces all contribute to poor health (WHO, 2008a). Geopolitical determinants influence social determinants in our much more globalized and interconnected world. However, there are differences across nations regarding relative and absolute poverty, and most if not all nations have experienced traumatic histories including colonialization, racism, war, and slavery, to different degrees. Cultures in transition from agrarian to urban economies and experiencing rapid industrialization and urbanization carry specific challenges in low- and middle-income countries. Economic factors that increase the discrepancy between high earners and poorer communities were a major factor in the rates of infection during the pandemic, such as ability to work from home with access to internet facilities or being in the frontline of running public services. Biopsychosocial models of mental illnesses emphasize social factors in the causation of psychiatric disorders in particular. Social factors through epigenetic factors also influence biology. Adverse childhood experiences influence brain structures and individual development, and this needs to be understood.

As a King's Fund (Williams et al., 2022) report highlights, health is strongly determined by a range of social, economic, and environmental factors, and thus all the factors need to be understood and taken into account when reaching a diagnosis. From a public mental health perspective, however, they need to included in the design and delivery of services.

Too often, the focus is on biomedical models, investigations, and interventions and the rest are ignored. Consequently, the patient may return to overcrowded conditions with little or no money, thus perpetuating the conditions. In recent proposals, the UK government is urging pharmacists to be first point of contact, which means that individual patients are more likely to be given medication.

Mental health and physical health services need to work together closely. The first step for any nation is to have a clear and inclusive mental health policy that focuses on local mental health needs and models of care. Policies must be interlinked with education, employment, housing, and so on so that various facets of everyone's functioning are taken into account. Policies must include resource allocation and models of good care in partnership with the community sector and nongovernmental organizations. Detention of patients and compulsory treatment may be necessary, but they should be exceptions rather than the rule.

Individuals with mental distress and mental illnesses often shy away from seeking professional help because they may perceive their experience as nonmedical, and in many settings, medical treatments can be expensive and physically inaccessible or limited. Stigma against mental illnesses may keep people from seeking professional help. Services may be seen as inappropriate or inadequate if models of care do not align with the expectations of informal carers, families, and individuals with mental illnesses themselves. Depending on their past experiences with health care systems and their explanatory models, individuals who go on to develop mental illnesses may seek help from nonmedical resources. In South Africa, for example, a country with well-developed government and private health care systems, an estimated 80 percent of people use traditional medicine (Mothibe & Sibanda, 2019).

A significant majority of individuals with mental illnesses in the UK are managed within primary care settings (RCGP, 2017). Specifically, around 90 percent of people with mental health problems receive their care entirely within primary care, including those with serious and enduring mental illnesses. However, less than 10 percent of the total expenditure on mental health is allocated to primary care services, highlighting a disproportionate funding emphasis on secondary care. This funding imbalance persists despite the high prevalence of mental health issues encountered in primary care. Approximately 30 percent of individuals consulting their general practitioner (GP) have a mental health component to their illness. Thus, individual nations may need to identify the pathways their populations choose and strengthen them according to need.

As mentioned earlier, stigma is a set of negative and rejecting attitudes and behaviors that result from a lack of knowledge and that lead to discrimination. It does play a role in confirming an individual's identity, so it may not be possible to eliminate it altogether. Although anti-stigma campaigns have proved to be partially successful in some countries and some settings, discrimination based on stigma can be challenged and abolished in law, making it even more important. By introducing antidiscrimination laws, the plight of individuals with mental illnesses can be changed by giving them equal rights. Rights to make decisions (to make a will, to marry, to vote) and rights to employment are all fundamental universal human rights. Urgent attention should be given to ensuring that the laws of each country are based on equal human rights and that they are compliant with international law especially in relation to mental health implications.

Psychiatric services must be geographically and emotionally accessible, affordable, and available to all who depend on them. A full range of services is required, from outpatients, primary care, inpatient services, intensive care, rehabilitation, day hospitals, and day centers, which ought to be based in local communities. Depending on specialist needs across the lifespan, services should be available for children, postnatal women, adults and older adults, and those with intellectual disabilities. For those in vulnerable groups—minority ethnic groups, LGBTQ+ individuals, prisoners, offenders with mental disorders, and those with intellectual disability—a specialized skill mix among the team members must be available.

A major lesson from wealthy countries is that when all these services are statutory, it is critical to have partnerships with policymakers, communities, and patients in order to develop not only services but also educational modules, peer support, and other relevant training. Specialized services, whether age-based or function-oriented, are to be encouraged. These must not exist within rigid boundaries so that patients and their carers and families suffer needlessly. Community teams must be outward looking and reach out to people who need help where they are, rather than always expecting people to come to get services. They should be working closely with the community as a whole, including community organizations.

A specific lesson from low- and middle-income countries is how to develop services in partnership with religious leaders, community members, teachers, and others, as the examples in appendix 12 describe. There is no doubt that despite increasing demand, resources for mental health care services will never be enough, even in high-income countries. Hence, service design must look outside the box and use community resources. With adequate availability of and access to social care and primary care services, suitable and appropriate interventions can be developed and delivered. More specialized services are important, but in many countries and cultures, these will remain aspirational because of a shortage of financial and human resources.

Protecting individuals with mental illness from exploitation needs to be enshrined in law, and that law must be given sufficient power. The legal framework must ensure that a human-rights-based approach is taken, that roles of formal carers who may be looking after people with mental illnesses are clearly agreed on and defined, and that suitable training is provided. It is critical that a range of resources are made available and funded in an equitable way with physical health services. Clear outcome measurers must be agreed on and followed. These targets need appropriate resourcing. Appropriate education at the right level for those with mental illness and for those who care for them (whether formal or informal carers) is also a must.

National standards for the delivery of mental health care must be established in each nation according to local cultural values and needs. However, the delivery of services must be localized with appropriate and suitable support. This book has been written largely from a psychiatric perspective, and it is not always possible to have enough psychiatrists. Yet as clinical leads, psychiatrists are well positioned to enable interagency collaboration and dialogue with policymakers and others, including patients and their carers. The training of psychiatrists and other mental health professionals is crucial, and nationally standards must be applied to it.

Morbidity and mortality because of psychiatric disorders are considerable, and the associated burden is second to none. Policymakers and professionals need to come together to make sure that there is equity of funding for research as well as clinical services so that those who develop mental illnesses are looked after in the most effective and best possible way.

Summary Challenges

1. Many of the social causes of mental ill-health are preventable. Social causes affect physical causes through epigenetics and other routes. Social causes include poverty, unemployment, discrimination, the built environment, and trauma; most of these are structural and require society-level change toward equity for all people (Furber et al., 2015).
2. There are significant variations in levels of mental health and rates of mental illnesses related to geography, socioeconomic status, culture, occupation, level of education, societal equity and safety, and a country's level of development (WHO, 2014c).
3. People with mental illness die prematurely, often 15 to 20 years younger than those who do not have mental illness (Walker et al., 2015). Deaths are not always due to medication or its side effects; other reasons include lifestyle factors (higher smoking, lower exercise rates), less engagement with health care services, and socioeconomic factors (Lawrence & Kisely, 2010; Thornicroft, 2011; Firth et al., 2020).

Summary Recommendations

By way of conclusion, a summary of recommended sets of basic principles, policy objectives, and targets is presented here. A program promoting mental health at the national level is also proposed.

Basic Principles for Mental Health for Nations

1. The mental health care needs of the whole population need to be assessed, with special attention given to vulnerable groups. This assessment is necessary to have an accurate idea of what the issues are and what is needed to ensure that the population is mentally healthy.
2. The goal is to provide the necessary services to ensure effective action is taken to maintain good mental health, prevent and treat mental ill-health, rehabilitate people to good mental health, and provide support and care for those with chronic mental illness.
3. It is crucial to ensure that all available services are appropriate, accessible, affordable, effective, efficacious, and of good quality—and that they are available to all.

4. A broader public mental health focus is needed and must be integrated with mental health care.
5. A broad coalition of partners is required to deliver these aims through strategic and coordinated action. These partners must include professionals but also patients, their carers and families, nongovernmental organizations, community and religious leaders when appropriate, and employers.
6. There must be better integration between health and social care and between physical and mental health care (which is already the case in countries where Cartesian mind-body dualism does not apply). Furthermore, a closer partnership between health and social care is essential in the delivery of mental health services.
7. The main theme is the prevention of mental ill-health and the promotion of positive mental health. This must be in combination with looking after those who have developed mental ill-health. Prevention, treatment, and rehabilitation must work together closely and in a cohesive manner.
8. Individuals, their families, and the societies in which they live must carry a degree of personal responsibility for developing and maintaining good mental health. A proper balance has to be struck between individual responsibility and governmental responsibility. In between the two are a range of organizations, such as local authorities, schools, and employers, who must be involved.
9. The capability to be healthy must be enshrined in law where national policies are set. Communities and families rely on these policies to build local mental health resources, and individuals must have easy access to information. This should be possible due to easy access to social media and the internet, even taking into account digital poverty in many parts of the world.
10. Each government must have and must own minimum targets, even if they are aspirational, in order to measure outcomes and also be accountable to its population for the results achieved. Local priorities with national support must be encouraged. Resources are finite, but health care demand is infinite, so examples of good clinical practice must be recognized and widely publicized and shared.

11. Mental health is determined by a number of factors, and it is critical to ascertain biological, social, and psychological vulnerabilities but also spiritual support. Any implementation will be at a local level, so involving people on the ground at an earlier level is essential. This will also help local populations to have ownership of ideas and practice.

Policy Objectives and Guiding Principles

Each nation must set key policy objectives and guiding principles in order to identify the mental health needs of its people.

i. To promote good mental health and to prevent mental ill-health through high-quality health services
ii. To recognize that health (including mental health) is influenced strongly by social determinants, such as housing, poverty, and overcrowding, as well as biological and genetic factors (which themselves are affected by social factors) and various psychological factors that are influenced by cultural and social factors and the way children are brought up
iii. To recognize that concerted action is needed across the lifespan and across national and local levels, as well as across biological, social. and psychological factors and boundaries
iv. To ensure the right balance between national governments, national plans and policies, and the local delivery of services
v. To ensure the best possible use of available resources in an efficient and efficacious manner, which requires making the best possible use of human as well as of financial resources
vi. To identify the main mental health problems by understanding the epidemiology of various types of mental illnesses (recognizing that rates of some illnesses may vary across nations, regions, and societies) and focusing on them
vii. To provide services that are geographically, culturally, and emotionally accessible, with policymakers working with service providers to ensure that services align with epidemiological, demographic, and cultural information and by gathering information on the use of services, treatment issues, take-up rates, and patient satisfaction
viii. To focus as much on the promotion of good mental health and the prevention of mental ill-health as on the treatment, care, and rehabilitation of those who fall ill and may need emotional and social support.

ix. To ensure that the responsibility for maintaining mental health is widely spread between the government and the individual, recognizing that mental health is determined by multiple genetic, psychological, social, and cultural factors

x. To foster concerted, ongoing action and collaboration across communities and across disciplines

xi. To aim for national standards and local delivery, with a strategy agreed to by central/federal governments, local authorities, and individuals

xii. To ensure the best possible use of available resources

xiii. To improve the ability to monitor the state of people's mental health through appropriate strategies and policies

xiv. To ensure that every child has the best start in life and every individual has the information they need to understand the influences on their mental health and well-being

xv. To involve people more directly and through local and voluntary organizations at strategic and operational levels

These objectives and principles are fundamental issues in enhancing the mental health of individuals across all nations. To achieve these objectives, targets are considered useful by this author.

Actions (Targets)

Targets provide an overall goal and give a sense of purpose. They should be SMART—specific, measurable, achievable, reasonable, and timed. They can be aspirational, but they should be achievable over a specified time period. If that does not happen, there must be adequate explanations. Targets need to be challenging if they are to help gain the maximum benefit from a strategic approach.

The following are examples of specific targets:

1. Make services accessible and local, with a range of services to provide the best care. Care should be equitable, according to need. Measuring the treatment gap (see chapter 2) is one metric.
2. Reduce suicide rates by a fixed percentage (say, 10 percent) over a specific period (say, 10 years), as was done in the UK (see chapter 6 and appendix 13 on mental health first aid).
3. Reduce alcohol consumption by 10 percent over 10 years through education and minimum unit pricing (see chapter 5).

4. Enhance understanding of mental health and mental illness by making them a part of school and university curricula. Metrics could be surveys of mental health literacy (see chapter 8).

In the context of mental health for nations, five of these targets (and their metrics) suggest themselves:

1. Increase understanding of the population's mental health needs (strategic needs assessments).
2. Reduce exposure to mental health risks from people's own behavior or the environment (violent crime, gambling, alcohol, tobacco consumption).
3. Inform people and give adequate, easy-to-understand, culturally sensitive information in order to educate them (patient surveys).
4. Expand access to universal health care as well as the efficiency and efficacy of services (treatment gaps, waiting times, treatment outcomes).
5. Eliminate or minimize the threats to individuals from the external world that they may not be able to control (crime rates, climate change, international cooperation, and factors impacting social connection and friendships—sometimes called friendship metrics)
6. Implement community-based mental health care models
7. Strengthen early intervention and prevention programs
8. Reduce structural inequalities in mental health access through targeted policies.

Constraints are twofold: knowledge and resources. There is thus a need to concentrate on what interventions are effective and efficacious and to make strategic investments in resources.

Strategic development is about establishing an ongoing process that provides an opportunity for decisions to be taken about what matters most for the population's mental health, with a focus on securing improvement in these areas.

A Six-Point Program Promoting Mental Health at National Level

A program promoting mental health at the national level must include the following six components:

1. Mental health promotion and prevention of mental illnesses
2. The urgent addressing of discrimination, resource mobilization, and equity

3. The provision of a range of services, from partnerships in the community to inpatient care
4. The delivery of evidence-based treatments, with minimum acceptable standards
5. The adoption of a life course approach, in policy, planning, and service delivery
6. The empowerment of patients, carers, and their families and their inclusion as key stakeholders

In the past few decades, the rates of psychiatric disorders have increased. In many countries, newer diagnostic categories have emerged, and patients and their informal carers have become more aware of these conditions. In some ways, this has helped reduce stigma, which means that demand for services has increased. However, failing to meet these needs efficiently and promptly may produce further stigma. Medicalization and psychiatrization of normal human emotions must be eliminated. Working in teams across disciplines is a must. Partnerships with community organizations and religious and community leaders can provide increased dividends, especially in cultures that rely on community support. With the increasing use of the internet, patients and their carers may attend their clinical appointments with either correct or incorrect information from the web. This also means that the previous models of patriarchal care must give way to a partnership model. This may not be easy in many countries, but it is the way forward.

Appendices

Appendix 1 Minimum Standards for Services

1. Promote an information revolution around mental health and well-being.
2. Tackle inequalities related to access to mental health services.
3. Expand access to psychological therapies for children and young people.
4. Uphold the right of adults to make choices about their care.
5. Minimize, to the extent possible, restrictive practices and high-risk restraints.
6. Involve friends and family when gathering feedback
7. Identify poor quality services and act on them
8. Strengthen support for carers and establish better partnerships with them.
9. Improve integration between physical and mental health care.
10. Improve the response to self-harm.
11. Ensure that no one needing services is turned away.
12. Deliver targeted support for new mothers.
13. Equip schools to identify mental health problems sooner.
14. Facilitate better transitions for adolescents moving to adult services if needed.
15. Implement suitable measures to help people with mental ill-health live longer and healthier lives.
16. Ensure more people with mental health problems have homes that support recovery.
17. Help identify liaison and diversion services for offenders.

18. Enhance support for those with mental illness who are victims of crime.
19. Provide support to employers so that they keep employees with mental illness in employment longer.
20. Assist people with mental illness in gaining suitable employment if needed.
21. Work against discrimination.

Appendix 2 Core Competencies for Mental Health Workers

Mental health workers have specialist skills when managing individuals with severe mental illness and require certain competencies and training. Health workers also must have some training in managing individuals with mental illness.

Four areas of competencies for all health workers (including mental health workers) include knowledge of the subject, attitudes, attributes, and skills that include managing others as well as themselves.

Competencies:

1. Health workers must be aware of and provide practical skills for daily living—accommodation, education, employment, and social support.
2. Health workers must be sensitive to the cultural, religious, social, racial, and lifestyle variations and differences among patients, their carers and families, and the workers.
3. Health workers must be aware of the physical, mental, and spiritual health needs of individuals as well as their emotional and psychological needs.
4. Health workers must be trained in trauma-informed care (TIC) to reduce re-traumatization and increase treatment adherence.
5. Health workers must be trained in proper risk assessment and risk management in vulnerable individuals.
6. Health workers must be trained to follow evidence-based interventions insofar as it is possible.
7. Health workers must be trained in building and sustaining effective working relationships with individuals with mental illness and their carers and families.

8. Health workers should be aware of other resources available in the community that can be called on for support, help, and assistance.
9. Mental health workers should be competent, empathetic, flexible, and able to deal with the ambiguity and anxiety embedded in individuals with mental illness and their carers.
10. Health workers require appropriate training and continuing professional development to keep up to date with developments in managing patients and educating families and communities.
11. Staff must be recruited according to their qualities as well as their academic abilities.
12. Patients and their carers must be involved in education and training of staff.
13. More emphasis should be placed on primary prevention, relapse prevention, and early intervention. Staff and communities need to be educated accordingly.
14. Nongovernmental organizations (NGOs) should be involved in training and ongoing education.
15. Community liaison workers may be needed.

Appendix 3 WPA Position Statement: Roles and Responsibilities of the Psychiatrist of the Twenty-First Century

Introduction

In the past few decades, progress in research and clinical practice of psychiatry has continued apace. However, the resources for mental health services around the globe have not kept pace with the increasing burden of mental illness (WHO, 2008b) and certainly do not bear equity with physical illness. The reasons for this variation include stigma in funding as well as often limited training in psychiatry in undergraduate curricula. In addition, in many countries, places for training are limited and not adequate for local needs. Consequently, in most countries around the globe, recruitment into psychiatry remains problematic.

Psychiatrists are physicians who manage mental illness. They are the only mental health professionals trained to combine physical (organic or medical), psychological and social factors in understanding aetiology and recommending management of psychiatric disorders. Spiritual models and matters as well as anthropological factors are of importance in understanding aetiology and also in planning interventions. They are therefore, well placed to develop collaborative care which places the patient at the heart of intervention and thus can use their knowledge and skills in managing mental illness and in alleviating mental distress. Equally importantly, they should be able to recognize physical and mental illness. This places a unique responsibility upon psychiatrists to utilize their medical skills, knowledge and experience to provide integrated collaborative care.

In a series of articles in *World Psychiatry* in 2010, there was a fierce debate about psychiatry as a profession under siege. In an editorial, Professor Mario Maj (2010), Past President of the WPA, challenged the notion that psychiatrists were an endangered species. He argued passionately that if psychiatry was in crisis, it was a developmental one. In the same issue, Katschnig (2010) highlighted three challenges (from inside) to psychiatry, which included decreasing faith in the knowledge base of psychiatry (in diagnosis and in management) and a lack of coherent theoretical base and, from outside, challenges included client discontent, competition from other professions, and a negative image. However, these challenges should be seen as straw men. In the same issue, a number of authors take the Katschnig position to task, recommending various strategies.

We believe that the issue about confidence among psychiatrists and in psychiatry is a red herring, and this position has been discussed in the past. We do consider that the confidence in our position and role has to emanate from a balanced view. Just because there is stigma does not mean that our role is less relevant but that our role must include challenges to stigma and discrimination on the basis of equity and advocacy for our patients. Psychiatrists have the expertise, skills and knowledge to deliver services to some of the most vulnerable and neglected individuals, and we must take pride in what we do.

The WPA recognizes that many national organizations already have documents relating to the psychiatrists' roles and responsibilities. The present document is not meant to replace them but sets the scene for the twenty-first century.

In this position statement, the WPA describes the role and responsibilities for psychiatrists, no matter where in the world they practice.

Background: Changes in social expectations, patient-doctor relationships, social media, and factors such as globalization, urbanization, rapid industrialization in many countries, biological factors (such as psychopharmacogenomics), neuroscience of emotions, therapies without therapists and other factors, mean that as a profession we need to look at the role of psychiatrists in the future and their changing responsibilities.

The WPA-Lancet Psychiatry commission on psychiatry (2017) has highlighted that psychiatry in the twenty-first century will be affected by human and financial resources and demographic and societal factors. Aging of the population, an increase in urban sprawl, migration, and the digital world will all influence psychiatric services and pathways into care. Under these changing circumstances, the role of the psychiatrist is also due to change in a number of arenas.

The British Medical Association (BMA, 2017) in its Presidential Project noted that the doctor-patient relationship is changing, and the medical practice needs to reflect these changes. The report notes that doctors have to walk a fine line between being realistic with their patients and destroying all their hope. Patients require both reassurance and empathy.

The definition of roles and responsibilities is important for a number of reasons. Foremost is that, once roles and responsibilities are clearly identified, the profession is able to set standards for training, competencies, and skills that then can be used to develop competencies and subsequently recruit suitable individuals. Our patients need good psychiatrists and deserve excellent care; and as a profession, we need to train and support best practice.

CanMEDS model: The CanMEDS physician competency network, adopted in 1996 (revised subsequently) by the Royal College of Physicians and Surgeons of Canada (2015), places competency of being a medical expert at its core. Rapid technological advancements bring with them changes in expectations, competencies, and perhaps more precision too, but they also put a strain on resources.

Medical expert: The core role of a clinician is providing medical care by delivering clinical skills, leading to improvement and better outcomes for patients through the application of medical knowledge and professional attitudes. The patient is at the heart of health care delivery.

Communicator: In clinical practice, doctors must communicate with patients, their families, and their carers, as well as with the team and the community and society at large. Teaching communication to doctors should start at the undergraduate level and continue throughout their careers.

Collaborator (team player): Doctors, especially psychiatrists, need to work in teams; hence, they need to be fully aware of the role that team members play and work in a collaborative fashion in order to deliver optimal patient care.

Manager (of resources)/leader: Doctors need to know how to manage teams and human and financial resources, as well as how to allocate responsibilities and resources. In managing resources, they must be aware of the efficacy and efficiency of therapeutic interventions and sustainable practices.

Health advocate: Doctors are uniquely positioned, both as clinicians and as respected members of society, to advocate for their patients, especially in reducing stigma and discrimination and in advancing the health and well-being of patients, communities, and society.

Scholar: Doctors have an obligation to their patients to stay up to date and engage in reflective learning as well as in the creation, dissemination, and clinical translation of medical research and knowledge.

Professional: Being professional means adhering to professional standards and regulations, keeping up to date, and demonstrating the highest personal standards of behavior and ethical practice (see also Bhugra and Malik, 2011a). The psychiatrist has additional competencies that include the ability to hold hope for patients and contain the anxiety experienced by patients, their families, and their carers, teams, and society at large.

As a profession, we need to demonstrate excellence in all these domains, which are at the heart of clinical practice. This allows us to illustrate the unique nature of clinical psychiatry. These roles are listed in box A3.1 but described in detail below. Psychiatrists need to be clinical leaders who are both responsible and accountable to society and to the profession as represented by the regulator. As psychiatrists and clinicians, we must demonstrate a continual drive for better service and quality in the services we provide, whether in the private or the public sector.

Role of the psychiatrist: The roles and responsibilities for the psychiatrist are multifaceted and significantly interrelated and should be seen in that context.

a. *Caring for the patient:* Providing efficient and efficacious care in the best possible manner is the core role of the psychiatrist. Services, whether in the public or the private sector, have to be accessible and affordable, and the clinical practice must be nondiscriminatory. Patients must be treated with dignity and respect, irrespective of the patient's gender, religion, age, socioeconomic status, and sexual orientation. A psychiatrist is a medically qualified doctor who deals with mental illness but also with the interaction between physical and mental illness. Understanding psychological and social factors, along with integrating the biopsychosocial model, is crucial for comprehending etiology and delivering effective therapeutic interventions.

b. *Managing complexity and comorbidity:* The psychiatrist's medical expertise in identifying the complex and comorbid nature of mental illness (be it between personality disorder and mental illness, substance abuse and mental illness, or physical and mental illness) is critical in managing these situations. Managing complexities within the system also affects clinical care. A good manager can enable the team and the patients to traverse these complex settings. As clinical scientists, psychiatrists are able to sift and manage the information and provide the best possible interventions according to the needs of the patient.
c. *Managing risk:* In many countries, psychiatrists are expected to identify and manage risk, whether it is in the patient's best interest or that of society. Psychiatrists therefore need to work within the statutory framework. The psychiatrists should be aware of the bill of rights for the patients with mental illness (Bhugra, 2016b).
d. *Identifying and managing patient support systems:* In order for patients to get back to their best level of functioning, clinicians—directly or through their teams—are best placed to identify and manage support systems through the families, kinships, nongovernmental or statutory organizations, or communities. Identifying positive resources is an important clinical skill and, indeed, a responsibility.
e. *Enabling the patient:* Identifying positive support systems can help the patient reach their full potential in social functioning. By focusing on a patient's strengths and capabilities, the clinician can identify the best options for housing, employment, and education. The team, directly or through specialists such as social workers, can help the psychiatrist. A key responsibility lies with the psychiatrist in supporting the patient and educating them about their strengths.
f. *Facilitating recovery:* Patients can learn to live with their symptoms if they can achieve a social potential that is compliant with their abilities. The recovery model for severe mental illness is an important approach.
g. *Containing anxiety:* Psychiatrists, like other doctors, must learn to combat and contain their own anxiety as well as that of the team, the patients,

their families, and their carers. Individual and group skills may help the psychiatrist in this regard.

Responsibilities of psychiatrists are related to their roles and have to be considered together.

h. *Holding hope:* In addition to containing anxiety, psychiatrists also need to hold hope for their patients, their families, and their carers. This responsibility is at the heart of medical care but, for various reasons, is often ignored. For patients, however, it is one of the major roles they look for in their clinician. Training to acquire this skill (irrespective of how difficult it may seem) is important.
i. *Teaching and training:* Not all psychiatrists need to teach or train, but they require sharing skills with their teams. With personal and lifelong commitment to reflective learning, they still have a responsibility to educate patients and their carers. Suitable resources are essential to carry out this teaching and training role. Psychiatrists also have a responsibility to better inform the public and policymakers about the roles and responsibilities of psychiatrists as medically trained leaders and experts in treating mental illness. There is also an important role in helping patients, their carers, and families to recognize the strengths of patients in dealing with their illness.
j. *Research and innovation:* Again, not all psychiatrists are researchers or innovators, but they must have the scientific approach and skills to interpret new research and data and use these to improve services and their clinical practice. The research evidence, if applied appropriately, may help clinicians to seek appropriate equitable resources to provide better services. In many countries, the resources for research and research training will be limited, but it is important that psychiatrists are trained to recognize research findings and their application in clinical matters.
k. *Public mental health and advocacy:* By challenging stigma and discrimination, psychiatrists are well placed to advocate for our patients. Psychiatrists also need to continue advocating for the profession. Furthermore, we need to put evidence that public mental health works into practice and educate the public, communities, and policymakers.
l. *Clinical leadership:* Psychiatrists are best positioned to provide clinical leadership and accountability (an undertaking to ensure that something is done) as well as responsibility (a personal undertaking to do something). These skills are outlined in box A3.2.

m. *Drive for quality:* Psychiatrists have the responsibility to ensure that services continue to improve according to the new research that can be translated into clinical care. Providing affordable and effective services and care is a major challenge in such a context.

Values embedded within the clinical practice of psychiatry are defined as positive or negative factors weighted as a guide to decision and action (Royal College of Psychiatrists, 2017). The four dimensions that describe the values in psychiatry include their role as a doctor, their role as a leader, being transparent, and their role as a co-producer (working with patients and their carers and families with a range of characteristics and qualities). Working with patients in a collaborative manner and joint decision-making is preferred, although this approach may vary across cultures. These core values present the role of the psychiatrist in a slightly different manner but contain all the characteristics already described. Co-production (or team-working) is an important role and responsibility of the psychiatrist. Ethical values and conforming to local ethics-based practice is a significant aspect of an individual's functioning. However, it needs to be recognized that co-production can also be with others, such as physicians, surgeons, primary care practitioners, and other professionals across disciplines and specialties. All medicine, including psychiatry, is value based, and these values must be inculcated among undergraduates from an early stage.

Next steps: The major challenges to psychiatry and psychiatrists is from within, where we feel stigmatized and let down. We believe that psychiatry as a profession indeed has a bright future. With our understanding of brain structures and the functioning of the brain improving on a daily basis, and with better knowledge of interactions between biological vulnerabilities and social factors through the development of the field of epigenetics, we are becoming more focused on targeted interventions. Psycho-pharmacogenomics has shown us the way in identifying drug responses in individuals according to their genes so that we can titrate the dosage of medications more specifically. Using social media and web-based apps, we are in a position to take on public mental health and education agendas in a more focused and constructive way. The future of psychiatry is bright, and we need to use new inventions in delivering the best for our patients according to their needs.

Box A3.1
Roles of the Psychiatrist

- Caring for patients: through appropriate knowledge and management
- Managing complexity and comorbidity
- Dealing with ambiguity and anxiety of patients, their families and carers, and teams
- Identifying and managing support systems
- Enabling the patient and dealing with ambiguity
- Facilitating patient recovery
- Containing the anxiety of their patients and their teams
- Holding hope for the patient and the team
- Teaching and training
- Applying research and innovation to clinical practice
- Advocating for public mental health
- Providing clinical leadership
- Driving for equality

Box A3.2
Roles and Responsibilities as Clinical Leaders

- Clinical decision-making in the multidisciplinary context if available
- Management of team dynamics
- Support for colleagues' development
- Service improvement
- Drive for quality improvement
- Equity of access to services
- Affordable accessible services
- Ambassadorial role of the profession
- Awareness of legal frameworks
- Horizon scanning

Appendix 4 WPA Position Statement: Good Psychiatric Practice

Several national organizations already have papers highlighting the components of good psychiatric practice. The present statement (WPA, 2017) is not meant to replace them. This should be read in conjunction with the WPA position statement on roles and responsibilities of psychiatrists (WPA, 2019b). The WPA urges its member societies (which do not have a similar document) to use this and modify it according to local and national needs.

Role of the Psychiatrist

A. Caring for the Patient

1. Carry out a thorough accurate assessment.
    a Take a full history and collateral history.
    b Take developmental history.
    c Conduct comprehensive mental state examinations.
    d Carry out necessary physical examination and investigations.
2. Adopt a consultation style directed toward therapeutic alliance.
    a. Depending on cultural values and expectations, engage the patient, their carers, and families.
    b. Demonstrate good communication skills.
3. Be fully cognizant of at least one of the major diagnostic systems and of the latest developments in therapeutic intervention.
4. Ensure that appropriate therapeutic interventions are available and offered using evidence-based and appropriate guidelines.
5. Work with detained patients and their carers and families as indicated.
6. Be aware of when and who to refer to between agencies and across specialties.

7. Maintain good quality case notes and consent access by patients if local regulations allow that.
8. Keep up to date with and provide services that are nondiscriminatory related to gender, age, sexual orientation, religion, or disability.

B. Managing Complexity and Comorbidity

1. Whenever psychiatric patients have complex and comorbid conditions, take due care in assessing, investigating, managing, and recording these details.
2. Communicate any changes in treatment or treatment decisions appropriately, taking into account local confidentiality arrangements.
3. Keep up to date with clinical advances relevant to clinical practice, and seek help wherever appropriate.
4. Throughout one's practicing career, work with teams and colleagues to improve clinical care.

C. Managing Risk

1. Carry out a thorough and proper assessment of risk to self and others through examination, collateral history, and developmental history.
2. Work with patients, their carers and families, and the team wherever available and possible to assess and manage risk.
3. Be readily accessible.
4. Carry out regular review of risk assessment.

Relationships with patients depend on mutual respect, openness, trust, and good communication. These relationships can be sometimes difficult and strained, especially if patients are detained against their will. Relationships with patients and their families and carers have to be open and mutually respectful.

D. Identifying and Managing Patient Support Systems

1. It is important to identify a patient's support systems, which may include carers, families, friends, peers, or others in the community, even possibly nongovernmental organizations.
2. The psychiatrist must listen to the patient and ask for and respect their views while engaging them.

3. The patient's support system needs information about the illness, treatment options, and possible outcomes. The psychiatrist must share appropriate risk and benefits of recommended therapeutic interventions.
4. The psychiatrist must share adequate information regarding the patient's diagnosis, treatment, and outcome in simple-to-understand language.
5. Psychiatrists should recognize and respect patients' lifestyles and personal goals and take their gender, sexual orientation, religion, and disability into account. They should be able to deal with the patient's and team's anxiety, hold hope for the patient and their carers and manage ambiguity in diagnoses and outcomes.
6. When the patient lacks the capacity to consent, the psychiatrist should share appropriate information and explanations with the person who is responsible for the care of the patient.

Appendix 5 Minimum Standards for Inpatient Services

This material is modified from Scizophrenia Research Foundation Chennai (SCARF) India Standard Procedures with permission.

Introduction

Inpatient admission is a valuable component in the management of certain aspects of psychiatric disorders like suicidal risk, acute exacerbation of symptoms, and catatonia. If used appropriately and the processes and resources are adequate, inpatient care can make a significant difference to a patient's journey through psychiatric care.

To ensure that inpatient care is delivered effectively, it is important to standardize the process of inpatient journey by defining who will benefit from such care, identifying the problems for which it will be useful, describing the roles and responsibilities of different staff involved in the care, and having a clear procedure in place for the different elements of inpatient journey.

Centers should be able to offer placements to the following:

1. Patients requiring acute care
2. Patients requiring short respite admissions at times of crises
3. Patients requiring long-term inpatient psychosocial rehabilitation

Which conditions will benefit from inpatient admission?

1. Acute and severe symptom presentation/relapse that is unmanageable at home by the family with outpatient supervision
2. Suicidal risk

3. Verbal aggression
4. Catatonia
5. Medication change/initiation that cannot be undertaken in the community (e.g., clozapine trial) for reasons such as risks of side effects, distance from the center impeding close monitoring, or compliance issues
6. Electroconvulsive treatment
7. Negative symptoms requiring psychosocial rehabilitation
8. Patients with only alcohol dependence or drug dependence requiring inpatient detoxification (which may need expert intervention)
9. Patients with suspected delirium/delirium tremens (which may need medical support and care)
10. Patients acutely unwell and currently physically violent or with a history of significant physical violence to self, others. or property (will need proper a comprehensive risk assessment)
11. Acute medical/surgical comorbidities requiring immediate medical care, especially patients requiring intense physical nursing care, physically frail elderly, or those with an intellectual disability

In outpatient departments, the following tasks are indicative and not comprehensive; local protocols and guidance should be followed:

1. Patient should be assessed by the medical staff, and a recommendation for admission should be made following discussion with the patient and their family, with consent obtained.
2. The decision for admission, along with the reasons for the same and an inpatient treatment plan, should be clearly documented.
3. A detailed physical examination should be carried out.
4. Appropriate chaperones (female for a female patient and a male for a male patient) should be present. Physical examination findings should be documented in the medical records contemporaneously.
5. If the female patient is in the reproductive age group and has amenorrhea, pregnancy should be ruled out before administering psychotropic medications.
6. Ideally, a suitable case manager should be allocated to the patient wherever possible.

7. If a patient has not had investigations within the last month or if previous reports indicate abnormalities, the patient should have lab investigations and an ECG at admission.
8. The patient should be accompanied by family members until the admission process has been completed.

Admission procedures on the ward should be followed:

1. Inpatient case notes should be made if needed.
2. The ward should have a checklist according to local procedures.
3. The details about the ward, roles, and expectations should be explained to the patient and their family, including visiting times.
4. Allergy to medications should be explored and noted.
5. The patient should be shown to their bed area, and induction to the ward should be carried out.
6. The admitting doctor should document clinical management plans.
7. All medications, including those for physical health problems should be recorded in the drug treatment order.
8. Patient should hand over any medication that they have been taking to the nurses and have it recorded.
9. Only medications (for both physical and mental health problems) written in the drug treatment order can be administered to the patient.

Inpatient stays on the ward should follow these procedures:

1. All patients should have a named Consultant Psychiatrist and recognized trained staff, insofar as possible, responsible for their care.
2. Patients should have an identified bed space and a secure storage space for their belongings.
3. Patients should receive their medications from nursing staff at the correct time.
4. Patients should receive regular nutritious meals on the ward.
5. Meals should take into consideration any medical recommendations (e.g., salt restriction, diabetic diet). Any medically recommended diet should be documented in the medical notes.

6. Patients should know who their care worker on the ward is.
7. Families should be kept informed of progress by the treating team regularly, and any meetings with the family should be documented in the patient's notes with details of who from the treating team and the family were present for the meeting.

Nursing responsibilities for patient care on the ward are as follows:

1. Check daily blood pressure, pulse, temperature.
2. Check weight weekly.
3. Record height at admission.
4. Carry out any other physical monitoring as instructed by the medical staff (monitoring input/output, noting consciousness using standard scales).
5. For female patients, ask and record the date of their monthly menstrual periods regularly.
6. Check the patient's self-care and hygiene (e.g., brushing teeth, taking bath with soap and water, combing hair, wearing clean clothes) and eating and sleep patterns daily.
7. Observe the patient's behavior (e.g., hallucinatory behavior, irritability, suicidal gestures, interactions with staff and other patients).
8. Carry out any special instructions for patient care as advised by the doctors.
9. Arrange for investigations to be completed as soon as they are requested.
10. If the patient is recommended to leave the hospital premises for any reason, record the absence.
11. When the patient returns to the ward, document the time and date of arrival on the ward and take feedback about the visit from the patient and the accompanying person, and document the same in the notes.
12. If a patient leaves the ward alone with permission of the treating doctor documented in the medical notes, document the same information, except for the accompanying person details.
13. If a patient who leaves the ward does not return at the time expected, follow the procedure documented for this situation.
14. If a patient absconds from the ward, immediately follow the absconding patient protocol.

Appendix 6 Minimum Standards of Care for Individuals with Schizophrenia

This material is modified from Schizophrenia Research Foundation (SCARF) Chennai, India guidelines, courtesy Dr. R. Thara. This is an example. The standards cover the following:

- Initial assessment on an urgent basis, review, and follow-up
- Pharmacological management: basic, evidence-based affordable medication accessible by all
- Psychosocial interventions
- Physical health assessments on a regular basis
- Special vulnerable groups such as pregnant women, the elderly, and children, and their special requirements

Initial Assessment

1. All persons with psychoses are to be seen, preferably, along with an informant who is familiar with the history of the patient's illness and is reliable.
2. After an in-depth interview and mental state examination, the diagnosis of schizophrenia should be confirmed, using standard criteria.
3. A physical examination and measurement of pulse and blood pressure are desirable.
4. A management plan should be drawn up in consultation with the patient and a family member. If the patient is violent, aggressive, or lacks insight, this discussion may have to happen at a later date.
5. It is desirable to review persons with a first episode once a week for the first month and then once a month.

Pharmacological Interventions

1. Treatment is started with any of the second-generation antipsychotics, such as risperidone, olanzapine, or quetiapine, if cost is not a constraint.
2. When these drugs are not available or there are cost constraints, treatment can be started with first-generation antipsychotics (haloperidol or chlorpromazine).
3. It is preferable to start with adequate dosage of one antipsychotic for a minimum period of four weeks.
4. For those who do not respond to adequate dose and duration of one antipsychotic medicine, adding another may be considered. Polypharmacy should be avoided insofar as possible.
5. For those who do not respond to adequate dose and duration of other antipsychotic medicines alone or in combination, clozapine may be considered; blood counts and an EKG need to be done before starting clozapine.
6. Ethnic differences contribute to adverse effects, so dosages should be modified accordingly.
7. For women who are planning a pregnancy or are pregnant or breastfeeding, low-dose oral haloperidol or chlorpromazine or olanzapine may be considered.
8. Those who had their first episode of psychosis will need medication for at least 12 months after the beginning of remission. Any further continuation of antipsychotic drug treatment should be based on a clinical review, preferably by a mental health specialist, and taking into account the preferences of the individuals, in consultation with the family.
9. Those with multiple relapses will require medication for several years and possibly even a lifetime.
10. Stopping antipsychotic medication should be gradual, keeping in mind the increased risk of relapse, possible adverse effects of medicines, and individual preferences, in consultation with the family.
11. When medicines are withdrawn, individuals and family members need to be educated to detect early symptoms of relapse, and close clinical monitoring should be done.
12. For those whose adherence to medication is not satisfactory, consider switching over to depot medication.

Psychosocial Interventions

1. Education and information—written, oral, and increasingly video information—may be offered to persons with schizophrenia and their family members/caregivers on a one-to-one basis or in groups.
2. Supportive psychotherapy and cognitive therapies may be considered if there are persistent cognitive deficits and may be needed on a long-term basis.
3. Recovery-oriented psychosocial interventions (e.g., life skills training, social skills training) to enhance independent living skills must be offered to individuals as well as their carers and families.
4. Some individuals may require assisted living and supported housing.
5. Every effort must be made to place patients in supported employment programs or even in open employment with good professional support.
6. Active family intervention may be required in some cases.
7. Recovery orientation must involve patient empowerment and patient rights.

Physical Health

Individuals with schizophrenia sometimes develop problems with their physical health. This could be due to unhealthy lifestyles, lack of exercise, smoking, and abuse of other drugs. Some of the medicines used can also lead to metabolic disturbances like obesity, diabetes, and lipid-related disorders. It is essential to monitor their physical health regularly and conduct all basic blood and urine investigations and an EKG at least once a year.

Elderly:

1. In elderly patients, first rule out organicity (e.g., delirium, dementia, substance induced mental illnesses, Parkinson's disease in cases of late or very late onset schizophrenia).
2. Check hearing and vision in elderly patients because symptoms can be attributed to deficits in these areas.
3. "Start low and go slow" should be the principle of pharmacotherapy.
4. Keeping in mind safety and tolerability, administer the drugs of choice, which are risperidone (1–2 mg), olanzapine (2.5–5 mg) or quetiapine (25–100 mg). Avoid depot medication.

5. Watch for drug-induced side effects (Parkinsonism, drug-induced movement disorders,) especially tardive dyskinesia in women.
6. Watch for complications, such as hyponatremia due to antipsychotics.
7. Consider comorbid medical conditions and possible drug interactions while initiating the antipsychotics.
8. Lastly, as psychosis remits, watch for any decline in cognitive functioning and activities of daily living in the future because symptoms could be a precursor to underlying dementia.

Children:

1. In children with schizophrenia, screen for all possible causes—substance-induced causes (e.g., cannabis, alcohol, polysubstance) or psychoses that may be related to epilepsy. Neuroimaging, EEG, and urine drug screening may be necessary.
2. Schizophrenia prodrome (comprising of sudden or gradual academic decline, odd behavior, anxiety sleep disturbances, anger, paranoia, fleeting hallucinations) should not be ignored. Treatment with antipsychotics or benzodiazepines can be decided on an individual basis, depending on the severity of symptoms and dysfunction. However, treating prodrome conclusively as schizophrenia should be avoided.
3. High-risk groups—children of patients with schizophrenia—may present with frank psychotic symptoms or prodrome and should be treated with a low dose of antipsychotics. Commonly used drugs are risperidone (1–2 mg), aripiprazole (5–10 mg), or olanzapine (5–10 mg).
4. Delays in seeking treatment or nonadherence are commonly encountered in this population.
5. Psychoeducation of family members and group intervention for affected children are necessary.

Pregnant Women:

1. Pregnancy results in the abrupt discontinuation of antipsychotics. Intrapartum and postpartum exacerbations should be treated preferably with a low dose of antipsychotics.
2. Stable pregnant schizophrenia patients are advised to continue the antipsychotics. Change the drugs in the case of diabetes. Noncompliant

patients on depot should be continued on their depot medication and monitored regularly.

3. Breast feeding can be continued, with drugs dispensed as once-daily doses; mothers should be advised to express foremilk in the morning prior to feeding.
4. Antiparkinsonian medications must be avoided.
5. In the case of high blood sugar, change from atypical antipsychotics to typical antipsychotics during pregnancy.
6. Unwell mothers need close monitoring. Those with negative symptoms may be apathetic and those with positive symptoms may pose potential harm to the infant. Families will need support.

Appendix 7 Minimum Standards of Care for Individuals with Dementia

This material is modified from Schizophrenia Research Foundation (SCARF), Chennai, India, courtesy Dr. R. Thara. This is an example.

Aim:

The main aim is to provide comprehensive care and support for persons with dementia and their families and caregivers.

Process:

1. Conduct an assessment to develop a patient- and caregiver-centered care plan.
2. Support the individual with dementia and their families with the care plan.
3. Periodically review the care plan.

The Care Plan:

The patient- and caregiver-centered care plan aims to deliver tailored care and support for the individuals with dementia and their families, taking into account the needs of persons with dementia and their caregivers.

Caregiver Burden:

Caregiver burden in dementia care is a significant issue, requiring targeted support strategies. Interventions such as psychoeducation, respite care, and caregiver support groups have been shown to reduce stress and improve well-being by also improving education and awareness of relapses (Brodaty & Donkin, 2009). Physical activities, exercises, tai chi, yoga, mindfulness-based interventions, structured exercise programs, and social prescribing also enhance resilience among all carers (also see Oken et al., 2010).

Assessments:

Assessments will be made from the point of first contact with the persons with dementia and their families. They can be achieved either in the clinic or during home visits or at any other place convenient to both the assessor and the patient (e.g., community hub). The aim will be to complete all appropriate and applicable assessments within the first three months of initial contact. The assessments will include the following broad areas:

1. Person with dementia
   a. The nature and severity of cognitive impairment
   b. The nature and severity of functional impairment
   c. Presence and severity of associated behavioral and psychological symptoms in dementia (BPSD)
   d. Comorbid medical and mental illnesses
   e. Psychosocial circumstances
   f. Environment
   g. Quality of life
2. Caregiver
   a. Knowledge and awareness about dementia
   b. Practical coping and problem-solving skills
   c. Mood changes
   d. Physical health
   e. Confidence in dealing with challenges
   f. Financial and psychosocial support
   g. Knowledge of caregiver burden and burnout and how to cope

Interventions:

Following the assessment, a comprehensive intervention and support strategy will be developed in collaboration with the multidisciplinary team, the person with dementia, and the caregivers. The interventions will be delivered individually or in groups as appropriate and acceptable. The person- and family-centered care plan will include the following interventions as appropriate:

1. Person with dementia
    a. Post-diagnostic information about the condition and support available
    b. Medication
        i. Cognitive enhancers as appropriate
        ii. Antipsychotics (with a clear treatment goal and review plan)
        iii. Other psychotropic drugs as appropriate (e.g., antidepressants)
    c. Non-pharmacological interventions
        i. Reminiscence
        ii. Cognitive stimulation
        iii. Environmental changes, as appropriate
        iv. Practical and emotional support
2. Caregiver
    a. Post-diagnostic information about the condition and support available
    b. Practical and emotional support
        i. Individual
        ii. Support groups (for the individual and their caregivers)
    c. Knowledge, skills, and problem-solving
        i. Individual caregiver training
        ii. Group caregiver training

Review of Person- and Family-Centered Care Plan

The care plan should be reviewed regularly, at least every six months or sooner, depending on the clinical need.

Table A7.1
Assessments for person with dementia—tools used

No.	Assessment	Tool(s) used
1	The nature and severity of cognitive impairment	1. History pro-forma 2. Dementia diagnosis checklist 3. One of the following instruments as appropriate: a) Montreal Cognitive Assessment (MoCA) b) Mini-mental state examination (MMSE) c) Vellore Screening Instrument for Dementia
2	The nature and severity of functional impairment	1. Dementia diagnosis checklist 2. Instrumental Activities of Daily Living Scale 3. Global Deterioration Scale (GDS)
3	Presence and severity of associated behavioral and psychological symptoms in dementia (BPSD)	1. Neuropsychiatric Inventory (NPI) 2. Biopsychosocial assessment for potential causes and intervention
4	Comorbid medical and mental illnesses	1. Physical assessment 2. Mental state examination 3. Drug review
5	Psychosocial circumstances	Home visits
6	Environment	Environment audit
7	Quality of life	Quality of life tools

Table A7.2
Assessments for caregivers—tools used

No.	Assessment	Tool(s) used
1	Knowledge and awareness about dementia	1. Caregiver assessment pro forma 2. DEMCARES Dementia Awareness Questionnaire
2	Practical coping and problem-solving skills	Caregiver assessment pro forma
3	Mood changes	1. Caregiver assessment pro forma 2. Patient Health Questionnaire (PHQ-9)
4	Physical health	Caregiver assessment pro forma
5	Confidence in dealing with challenges	Caregiver assessment pro forma
6	Financial and psychosocial support	1. Caregiver assessment pro forma 2. Home visit assessment
7	Knowledge of caregiver burden and burnout and how to cope	1. Caregiver assessment pro forma 2. Zarit Burden Interview

Appendix 8 Minimum Standards for Child and Adolescent Psychiatric Disorders

This material was developed at Schizophrenia Research Foundation (SCARF), Chennai, India, courtesy Dr. R. Thara. This should be seen as an example.

Background:
Child and psychiatric disorders are often under-recognized and inappropriately treated conditions in many low- and middle-income countries. Reasons include inadequate training and exposure to the subject during the course of training in psychiatry.

Minimum standards include ease of access to services and working with schools to train and educate teachers and families.

Assessment:
The assessment of a child differs from that of adults with mental health problems in a number of ways. First, the clinical phenomenology of certain adult-type disorders may be modified in presentation according to developmental factors, even though the same criteria are used. Next, children's abnormalities may consist of deficiencies in positive adaptive behaviors and a failure to progress in the expected fashion along one or more dimensions of behaviors rather than a specific psychopathology. Further, a child's ability to conceptualize and discuss their experiences and feelings is influenced by maturational and developmental factors.

Child interviews and mental status examinations must account for the characteristic lability of children and their tendency to revert to more immature forms of communication when tired, sick, apprehensive, or in unfamiliar situations. The child's functioning and psychological well-being are dependent on the family and school situations; therefore, to obtain a full picture, obtaining information from multiple sources is essential. These two reasons may necessitate multiple interviews.

Purposes of the diagnostic assessment are

1. to determine whether psychopathology exists,
2. to determine whether treatment is indicated,
3. when treatment is indicated, to determine the best treatment and recommendations and plans, and
4. to facilitate the family and child's cooperative engagement in the development and implementation of the treatment plan.

Specific aims of the diagnostic assessment are to

1. identify the stated reasons and factors leading to the referral,
2. obtain an accurate picture of the child's developmental functioning and the nature and extent of the child's behavioral difficulties, functional impairment, and subjective distress, and
3. identify potential individual family or environmental factors that may account for, influence, or ameliorate these difficulties.

The sources of information are as follows:

The *full diagnostic assessment* usually requires gathering data from the child, the family, the school, and other health providers, including the pediatrician and any prior mental health providers (e.g., psychiatrist, psychologist, occupational and speech therapist).

The styles and techniques of interviewing children vary according to the age, gender, and developmental status of the child and thus will not be detailed in this document.

The child interview contributes to the clinician understanding of the child's perception of the presenting problems and the degree of personal suffering. The interview also collects information concerning affects and mental phenomena that the child may choose not to share with others.

Assessment of preverbal infants and toddlers requires careful developmental assessment and direct observation of the child-parent interactions.

Content of the history is documented in the record under specific headings:

- Information obtained from relevant sources.
- Diagnostic formulation and treatment planning.
- Standardized assessments.
- Standardized instruments, including tests to assess psychological functioning. Development will be administered based on the need of the specific child. As much as possible, the use of validated scales and instruments in the cultural context will be used.

Appendix 9 Example of Good Practice

Mental Health in the Workplace—BT Story

This example is adapted from BT Public Affairs Briefing, January 18, 2016. British Telecom (BT) has set up a tailored mental health plan within the overall framework developed with the trade unions. Normalizing mental health problems and raising awareness of mental health issues has led to ensuring that individuals with mental illness are not unemployable or unproductive members of society. BT has a culture of self-help among the workforce and manages with added support from experts. The three-tier framework focuses on primary prevention, secondary intervention, and tertiary rehabilitation. The mental health toolkit developed by BT contains a range of resources of escalating sophistication, including mental health service and resilience training. BT collects and reports on a number of metrics, thereby identifying "hot spots" and intervening accordingly. Among employees, 81 percent acknowledged that opportunities to participate in health promotion campaigns made them feel that the company cared about their health, and more than half of employees felt valued.

Resources include managing pressure, work-fit, managing mental health, dealing with distress, a mental health dashboard, a health and well-being passport, employee assistance programs, mental health and resilience toolkits, and training.

Appendix 10 Minimum Standards of Information for Carers

This checklist aims to provide clinicians (psychiatrists) with guidelines for informing patients and their carers. The checklist is a framework and does not have to be followed strictly. Not every carer or family member needs all of the information. The medical information to be provided will depend on the level of medical confidentiality present in the culture and country. This checklist may help reduce anxiety and can be supplemented by providing extra written information.

The checklists should be used in conjunction with other information. Patients and carers may not be receptive to detailed information.

A. About the Illness

- What is the diagnosis? Differential diagnosis?
- What are the reasons for diagnosis?
- What would be the causes for the illness?
- What is the likely treatment?
- What is the likely outcome?

B. About the Assessment

- What are the investigations needed, if any?
- What other assessments may be needed?
- What physical examinations are needed?
- Are any physical conditions diagnosed?
- What are the cultural aspects of the assessment?

C. About Care and Treatment

- What is needed?
- Who will provide what?

- When is follow-up needed?
- How long is treatment needed?
- What will happen if the person stops the treatment?
- What will happen if they refuse treatment?
- Are other treatments available? Who will provide them? How can they be accessed?

D. The Carer and Treatment

- What is the role of the carer?
- How does the patient feel about it?
- How does the carer contact you?
- How will the carer deal with emergencies?
- Have confidentiality issues been discussed?

E. Medication

- What medication is provided?
- Why this medication?
- What will it do?
- What is the right dose? Can they start at a low dose?
- Are there any dietary taboos?
- When is the medication to be reviewed? Who will review it?
- Does any additional information need to be made available? Written or otherwise?
- What are the likely effects and side effects?

F. Hospitalization

- Is hospitalization needed? Why? For how long?

G. If Admission Is Not Required

- Who will look after the patient?
- Who will monitor their medication?
- Are daytime activities allowed?

H. Carers' Needs

- Are there any specific needs for carers?
- How carers should look after their health?
- What support do they need, and who will provide it?

I. Information

- How much information do the patient and the patient's carers need? Who will provide it? Is it needed on an ongoing basis or one-time only?
- Is any information about the illness confidential?

Appendix 11 Minimum Standards of Information for Individuals with Mental Illnesses

The following checklist provides a framework that can be used by individuals with mental illness to explore information about their illness.

A. About the Diagnosis

- If a diagnosis has been made, what is it?
- What are the reasons for the diagnosis?
- What tests are needed, if any?
- Are there any accompanying physical illnesses?
- What is the long-term outcome?
- Is any written information available about this particular illness?
- If the diagnosis is not yet made, what are the possible alternative diagnoses?

B. Treatment

- What are the aims of treatment?
- What treatment is needed? For how long?
- What medication do I need? What will it do? What are its side effects? What do I take it with? What food should I avoid, if any?
- What other treatment options are available?
- How often do I need to be seen?

C. Getting Help

- Who do I contact if I become unwell?
- Who do I contact in an emergency?

D. About My Carer

- What do they need to know?

- How do they contact the doctor or any other member of treating team?
- What details are to be given to the carer?

E. Medication

- Why is this (particular) medication recommended?
- How long will it take to work?
- What happens if it does not work?
- What side effects should I look out for?
- What will happen if I stop the medication suddenly?
- Where can I get additional information?

F. Hospitalization

- Do I need to be admitted? If so, why?
- For how long?
- What will happen in the hospital?

G. If Not Admitted

- If my carer cannot look after me, who will?
- What can I do to help myself?
- Are there any support groups I can approach?

Appendix 12 Examples of Good Practice: Task-Shifting

Problem Management Plus—PM+ (WHO, Global Implementation)

Developed by the World Health Organization (WHO), PM+ is a low-intensity psychological intervention delivered by trained non- specialists to individuals experiencing distress. Trials in Kenya, Pakistan, and Nepal have demonstrated its effectiveness in reducing symptoms of depression and anxiety (Bryant et al., 2017; Rahman et al., 2016; Sangraula et al., 2021; also see WHO, 2022g).

Friendship Bench (Zimbabwe)

The Friendship Bench initiative is a globally recognized task-shifting mental health intervention that originated in Zimbabwe in 2006 to address the mental health treatment gap in low-resource settings. The initiative trains lay health workers (grandmothers) to provide problem-solving therapy (PST) to individuals experiencing common mental disorders (CMDs) such as depression and anxiety using a structured approach on a wooden bench in a primary care setting (Chibanda et al., 2016). The Friendship Bench has since expanded to other African nations (e.g., Malawi, Kenya) as well as global cities like New York and London. The program's success lies in its simplicity, cultural adaptation, and cost-effectiveness, making mental health care accessible and acceptable to underserved populations.

A randomized controlled trial (RCT) in Zimbabwe found that Friendship Bench participants had significantly lower depression scores, higher remission rates, and reduced suicidal ideation (2 percent versus 12 percent) at six-month follow-up (Chibanda et al., 2016). The Friendship Bench continues to demonstrate that low-cost, lay-delivered therapy can be highly effective, particularly when integrated within community and primary care settings.

Cooperation with Traditional Healers—The Dava-Dua Program (India)

In Gujarat State in Western India, an innovative collaborative program has been introduced at a dargah (a Muslim holy site where people with mental illness go to pray). Collaboration between faith-based healers and allopathic practitioners, although fraught with initial mistrust, has been achieved following a long dialogue that allows the belief systems on both sides to play a shared role in care and recovery. Despite differing practices, a close collaboration between faith-based and allopathic mental health practitioners is feasible and indeed should be encouraged (see Shields et al, 2016).

In countries where multiple health care systems coexist, pluralistic health care means that individuals who develop mental illness are likely to seek help from several sources. Such examples show what can be achieved by engaging different stakeholders. Building trust and rapport takes time, but this investment is critical. Mutual respect is the key here. Extensive sensitization and training are needed with an open frame of mind. Health improvement, employment, and integration into society are desired outcomes.

Thinking Healthy Program (Pakistan)

This intervention, which is based on cognitive behavioral therapy (CBT), trains community health workers—known as Lady Health Workers—to provide structured psychosocial support to perinatal women experiencing depression. A randomized controlled trial demonstrated significant reductions in perinatal depression, with recovery rates up to 75 percent and effects lasting up to seven years postpartum (Rahman et al., 2008)

STRONG (Canada/USA)

STRONG—Supporting Transition Resilience of Newcomer Groups—is a school-based intervention codeveloped by Dr. Sharon Hoover and School Mental Health Ontario (SMHO) to support refugee and immigrant youth in managing stress and trauma. Studies indicate that it improves coping skills and enhances resilience among participants (Santiago et al., 2025).

War Trauma Foundation's Peer Support (Various Countries)

This model, implemented in conflict-affected regions, trains laypeople in psychological first aid (see appendix 14) and structured peer counseling. It has been applied in settings such as Bosnia, South Sudan, and Syria, showing positive effects on post-trauma resilience (WHO, War Trauma Foundation & World Vision International, 2011).

Aunties in Cameroon

Teenage girls learn about sexual health through their peers—a role that aunties used to play. Aunties are now often neighbors who have been trained to support those with substance abuse disorders and teenage mothers; they also monitor the mental health and well-being of these individuals (Goergen & Ndonko, 2025). This network of women in Cameroon is helping survivors of sexual abuse. It is estimated that around half a million of the country's women and girls have experienced rape and other forms of sexual violence.

Volunteers in Thailand

Over one million village health volunteers help with the delivery of health care in rural areas (WHO, n.d.). They have been active for several decades, upgrading their interventions during times of crisis, as they did during the Asian tsunami and more recently during the COVID pandemic.

Exercise and Training Gym Instructors

There have been attempts to train gym teachers to help people with mental illnesses. Exercise can help in managing anxiety and depression (Smith & Merwin, 2021), and it also promotes weight loss. During exercise sessions, the gym instructor can also assess a person's mental state and bring in health care professionals if necessary.

Appendix 13 Mental Health First Aid

Mental health first aid (MHFA) originated in Australia in 2001 to enhance public mental health literacy. Initial courses aimed to improve understanding and attitudes toward mental ill-health while equipping individuals to identify those at risk or in the early stages of mental health issues. Kitchener and Jorm (2008) highlight that the aim of MHFA is to identify early signs and risk factors for various conditions, such as anxiety, depression, substance abuse disorders, suicidal ideation, panic attacks, and responses to trauma.

The five steps of MHFA are abbreviated into the acronym ALGEE:

- Assess—risk of suicide and harm (to self or others)
- Listen—nonjudgmentally
- Give—reassurance and information
- Encourage—professional help
- Encourage—self-help strategies (Morgan et al., 2018)

MHFA training has been successfully implemented among a diverse range of groups including social workers (Rose et al., 2017), military personnel (Mohatt et al., 2017), family members of military veterans with a mental health condition (Evans et al., 2021), firefighters (Moffitt et al., 2014), university staff (Richardson et al., 2017), nursing students (Crawford et al., 2015; Fessey et al., 2016), administrative staff (Hashimoto et al., 2016), financial counselors (Bond et al., 2015), refugee communities (Subedi et al., 2015), student welfare staff (Massey et al., 2014), pharmacists (Chowdhary et al., 2019), pharmacy students (O'Reilly et al., 2011), high school students Hart et al., 2016), teachers (Jorm et al., 2010), football coaches (Pierce et al., 2010), and extension agents supporting farmers (Hossain et al., 2010. Cultural modifications of these programs have demonstrated effectiveness (Crooks et al., 2018), suggesting relevance for community-based public mental health interventions in most countries.

A summary of research evidence was published by MHFA International (2022) and Morgan et al. (2018). In brief, MHFA increases participants' knowledge about mental health, decreases their negative attitudes, and increases supportive behaviors toward individuals with mental health problems.

Appendix 14 Psychological First Aid

Psychological first aid (PFA) is an evidence-informed, early intervention approach designed to reduce initial distress and foster resilience in individuals exposed to trauma, disasters, or crises (Bisson et al., 2021). Studies indicate that PFA is effective in promoting emotional stabilization, reducing acute stress reactions, and enhancing long-term coping strategies (Shultz & Forbes, 2014). Unlike debriefing interventions, which have been linked to potential harm, PFA is nonintrusive, adaptable to diverse cultural contexts, and aligned with trauma-informed care principles (WHO, War Trauma Foundation, & World Vision International, 2011). Meta-analyses suggest that PFA contributes to improved psychological outcomes by reinforcing social support networks and encouraging adaptive coping behaviors (Fox et al., 2012). Research in disaster settings, including humanitarian crises and pandemics, has demonstrated that PFA helps mitigate post-traumatic stress symptoms, particularly when provided by trained responders in community-based or health care settings (Hermosilla et al., 2023). While more randomized controlled trials (RCTs) are needed, existing studies support PFA as a scalable, low-cost, and evidence-aligned intervention for psychological crisis response.

PFA is widely endorsed but criticized for limited empirical validation, inconsistent implementation, and a lack of standardized outcomes (McCabe et al., 2014). Most evidence for PFA relies on expert consensus rather than robust RCTs, which complicates assessments of its true efficacy compared to other interventions (Fox et al., 2012). Critics note that PFA lacks long-term follow-up studies for its impact on post-traumatic stress, depression, and recovery (Dieltjens et al., 2014). There is also inconsistency in training, as

PFA is often delivered by non-specialists, raising concerns about recognizing high-risk cases (Shultz & Forbes, 2014). Some studies indicate PFA may be insufficient for severe trauma, necessitating structured interventions like trauma-focused cognitive behavioral therapy (TF-CBT) or Eye Movement Desensitization Reprograming (Bisson et al., 2010; 2015). Despite these issues, PFA remains a pragmatic approach, though further research is essential to refine its protocols and assess the long-term outcomes.

References

Abba Hassan, A. u., Ibrahim, A. M., & Nadkarni, A. (2024). A systematic review of task-sharing interventions for substance use and substance use disorder in low- and middle-income countries. *Drug and Alcohol Dependence*, 256, 111093. https://doi.org/https://doi.org/10.1016/j.drugalcdep.2024.111093

Abbasi, K. (2019). There's something about social prescribing. *Journal of the Royal Society of Medicine, 112*(11), 451. https://doi.org/10.1177/0141076819887837

Abdullah, T., & Brown, T. L. (2011). Mental illness stigma and ethnocultural beliefs, values, and norms: an integrative review. *Clinical Psychology Review, 31*(6), 934–948. https://doi.org/10.1016/j.cpr.2011.05.003

Abebe, D. S., Lien, L., & Elstad, J. I. (2014). Immigrants' utilization of specialist mental healthcare according to age, country of origin, and migration history: A nationwide register study in Norway. *Social Psychiatry and Psychiatric Epidemiology, 49*(11), 1779–1789. https://doi.org/10.1007/s00127-017-1381-1

Abel, J., Kingston, H., Scally, A., Hartnoll, J., Hannam, G., & Thomson-Moore, A. (2018). Reducing emergency hospital admissions: A population health complex intervention of an enhanced model of primary care and compassionate communities. *British Journal of General Practice, 68*(676), e803–e810. https://doi.org/10.3399/bjgp18X699437

Abrams, E. M., & Szefler, S. J. (2020). COVID-19 and the impact of social determinants of health. *The Lancet Respiratory Medicine, 8*(7), 659–661. https://doi.org/10.1016/S2213-2600(20)30234-4

Acharibasam, J. W., & Wynn, R. (2018). Telemental health in low- and middle-income countries: A systematic review. *International Journal of Telemedicine and Applications, 2018*, 9602821. https://doi.org/10.1155/2018/9602821

Adler, N. E., & Rehkopf, D. H. (2008). US disparities in health: Descriptions, causes, and mechanisms. *Annual Review of Public Health, 29*, 235–252. https://doi.org/10.1146/annurev.publhealth.29.020907.090852

Ahad, A. A., Sanchez-Gonzalez, M., & Junquera, P. (2023). Understanding and addressing mental health stigma across cultures for improving psychiatric care: A narrative review. *Cureus, 15*(5), e39549. https://doi.org/10.7759/cureus.39549

Ahmed, S. H., Zakai, A., Zahid, M., Jawad, M. Y., Fu, R., & Chaiton, M. (2024). Prevalence of post-traumatic stress disorder and depressive symptoms among civilians residing in armed conflict-affected regions: A systematic review and meta-analysis. *General Psychiatry, 37*(3), e101438. https://doi.org/10.1136/gpsych-2023-101438

Akbulut, N., & Razum, O. (2022). Why othering should be considered in research on health inequalities: Theoretical perspectives and research needs. *SSM—Population Health, 20*, 101286. https://doi.org/10.1016/j.ssmph.2022.101286

Alaimo, K., Olson, C. M., & Frongillo, E. A. (2002). Family food insufficiency, but not low family income, is positively associated with dysthymia and suicide symptoms in adolescents. *Journal of Nutrition, 132*(4), 719–725. https://doi.org/10.1093/jn/132.4.719

Albrecht, G. (2011). Chronic environmental change: Emerging "psychoterratic" syndromes. In I. Weissbecker (Ed.), *Climate change and human well-being* (pp. 43–56). Springer. https://doi.org/10.1007/978-1-4419-9742-5_3

Allgaier, J., & Svalastog, A. L. (2015). The communication aspects of the Ebola virus disease outbreak in Western Africa—Do we need to counter one, two, or many epidemics? *Croatian Medical Journal, 56*(5), 496–499. https://doi.org/10.3325/cmj.2015.56.496

Alonso-Rodríguez, I., Pérez-Jorge, D., Pérez-Pérez, I., & Olmos-Raya, E. (2025). Restorative practices in reducing school violence: A systematic review of positive impacts on emotional wellbeing. *Frontiers in Education, 10*. https://doi.org/10.3389/feduc.2025.1520137

American Association of Medical Colleges. (2016). *Advancing health equity: A guide to language, narrative and concepts*. Retrieved February 5, 2025, from https://www.aamc.org

American Psychiatric Association (APA). (2013). *Diagnostic and statistical manual of mental disorders* (5th ed.). American Psychiatric Publishing.

American Psychological Association. (2017). *Stress in America: The state of our nation*. https://www.apa.org/news/press/releases/stress/2017/state-nation.pdf

American Telemedicine Association. (2018). *Services provided by telemedicine*. Retrieved February 10, 2023, from https://www.americantelemed.org/resource/why-telemedicine/

Anaf, J., Baum, F., & Fisher, M. (2023). Global health and equity burden of commercial determinants of health. In N. Maani, M. Petticrew, & S. Galea (Eds.), *The commercial determinants of health* (pp. 17–26). Oxford University Press.

Anda, R. F., Croft, J., Felitti, V., Nordenberg, D., Giles, W. H., & Williamson, W. F. (1999). Adverse childhood experiences and smoking during adolescence and adulthood. *JAMA, 282*, 1652–1658. https://doi.org/10.1001/jama.282.17.1652

Anda, R. F., Felitti, V., Bremner, J. D., Walker, J. D., Whitfield, C., Perry, B., Dube, S. R., & Giles, W. H. (2006). The enduring effects of abuse and related adverse experiences in childhood: A convergence of evidence from neurobiology and epidemiology. *European Archives of Psychiatry and Clinical Neuroscience, 256,* 174–186. https://doi.org/10.1007/s00406-005-0624-4

Anda, R. F., Whitfield, C., Felitti, V., Chapman, D., Edwards, V. J., Dube, S. R., & Williamson, D. F. (2002). Adverse childhood experiences, alcoholic parents, and later risk of alcoholism and depression. *Psychiatric Services, 53,* 1001–1009. https://doi.org/10.1176/appi.ps.53.8.1001

Anonymous. (2019). *Middle East respiratory syndrome coronavirus (MERS-CoV).* World Health Organization.

Appelbaum, P. S. (2007). Assessment of patients' competence to consent to treatment. *New England Journal of Medicine, 357*(18), 1834–1840. https://doi.org/10.1056/NEJMcp074045

Arango, C., Díaz-Caneja, C. M., McGorry, P. D., Rapoport, J., Sommer, I. E., Vorstman, J. A., McDaid, D., Marín, O., Serrano-Drozdowskyj, E., Freedman, R., & Carpenter, W. (2018). Preventive strategies for mental health. *The Lancet Psychiatry, 5*(7), 591–604. https://doi.org/10.1016/s2215-0366(18)30057-9

Arias, D., Saxena, S., & Verguet, S. (2022). Quantifying the global burden of mental disorders and their economic value. *eClinicalMedicine, 54,* 101675. https://doi.org/10.1016/j.eclinm.2022.101675

Armstrong, T. (2015). The myth of the normal brain: Embracing neurodiversity. *AMA Journal of Ethics, 17*(4), 348–352. https://doi.org/10.1001/journalofethics.2015.17.4.msoc1-1504

Arseneault, L. (2018). Annual research review: The persistent and pervasive impact of being bullied in childhood and adolescence: Implications for policy and practice. *Journal of Child Psychology and Psychiatry, 59*(4), 405–421.https://doi.org/10.1111/jcpp.12841

Arseneault, L., Walsh, E., Trzesniewski, K., Newcombe, R., Caspi, A., & Moffitt, T. E. (2006). Bullying victimisation uniquely contributes to adjustment problems in young children: A nationally representative cohort study. *Pediatrics, 118,* 130–138. https://doi.org/10.1542/peds.2005-2388

Augusterfer, E. F., Mollica, R. F., & Lavelle, J. (2015). A review of telemental health in international and post-disaster settings. *International Review of Psychiatry, 27*(6), 540–546. https://doi.org/10.3109/09540261.2015.1082985

Babor, T. F., Caetano, R., Casswell, S., Edwards, G., Giesbrecht, N., Graham, K., Grube, J., Hill, L., Holder, H., Homel, R., Livingston, M., Österberg, E., Rehm, J., Room, R., & Rossow, I. (2010). *Alcohol: No ordinary commodity—Research and public policy* (2nd ed.). Oxford University Press.

Badano, V. (2024). The Basaglia Law. Returning dignity to psychiatric patients: The historical, political and social factors that led to the closure of psychiatric hospitals in Italy in 1978. *History of Psychiatry, 35*(2), 226–233. https://doi.org/10.1177/0957154X231224650

Bai, Y., Lin, C.-C., Lin, C.-Y., Chen, J.-Y., Chue, C.-M., & Chou, P. (2004). Survey of stress reactions among health workers involved with the SARS outbreak. *Psychiatric Services, 55*(9), 1055–1057. https://doi.org/10.1176/appi.ps.55.9.1055

Bailey, Z. D., Krieger, N., Agénor, M., Graves, J., Linos, N., & Bassett, M. T. (2017). Structural racism and health inequities in the USA: Evidence and interventions. *The Lancet, 389*(10077), 1453–1463. https://doi.org/10.1016/S0140-6736(17)30569-X

Baker, D. A., Krieger, H., & LeRoy, A. (2016). Fear of missing out: Relationships with depression, anxiety, and social media engagement. *Computers in Human Behavior, 64*, 280–286. https://doi.org/10.1016/j.chb.2016.06.020

Baker-Henningham, H., Scott, S., Jones, K., & Walker, S. (2012). Reducing child conduct problems and promoting social skills in a middle-income country: Cluster randomised controlled trial. *British Journal of Psychiatry, 201*(2), 101–108. https://doi.org/10.1192/bjp.bp.111.096834

Bakst, S. S., Braun, T., Zucker, I., Amitai, Y. & Shohat, T. (2016). The accuracy of suicide statistics: Are true suicide deaths misclassified? *Social Psychiatry and Psychiatric Epidemiology, 51*, 115–123. https://doi.org/10.1007/s00127-015-1119-x

Bali, S., Stewart, K., & Pate, M. (2016). Long shadow of fear in an epidemic: Fearonomic effects of Ebola on the private sector in Nigeria. *BMJ Global Health, 1*(3), e000111. https://doi.org/10.1136/bmjgh-2016-000111

Bardol, O., Grot, S., Oh, H., Poulet, E., Zeroug-Vial, H., Brunelin, J., & Leaune, E. (2020). Perceived ethnic discrimination as a risk factor for psychotic symptoms: A systematic review and meta-analysis. *Psychological Medicine, 50*(7), 1077–1089. doi:10.1017/S003329172000094X.

Barnett, I., Torous, J., Staples, P., Sandoval, L., Keshavan, M., & Onnela, J.-P. (2018). Relapse prediction in schizophrenia through digital phenotyping: A pilot study. *Neuropsychopharmacology, 43*(8), 1660–1666. https://doi.org/10.1038/s41386-018-0030-z

Baron-Cohen, S. (2000). Theory of mind and autism: A fifteen year review. In S. Baron-Cohen, H. Tager-Flusberg, & D. J. Cohen (Eds.), *Understanding other minds: Perspectives from developmental cognitive neuroscience* (2nd ed., pp. 3–20). Oxford University Press.

Bauman, Z. (1991). *Modernity and ambivalence*. Polity Press.

Baumann, M., Spitz, E., Guillemin, F., Ravaud, J. F., Choquet, M., Falissard, B., Chau, N., & Lorhandicap group (2007). Associations of social and material deprivation with tobacco, alcohol, and psychotropic drug use, and gender: A population-based study. *International Journal of Health Geographics, 6,* 50. https://doi.org/10.1186/1476-072X-6-50

BBC News. (2023, April 20). KitKat maker Nestle urged to cut unhealthy food sales. https://www.bbc.co.uk/news/business-65328763

Beauchamp, T. L., & Childress, J. F. (2013). *Principles of biomedical ethics* (7th ed.). Oxford University Press.

Beckfield, J., & Krieger, N. (2009). Epi+demos+cracy: Linking political systems and priorities to the magnitude of health inequities—evidence, gaps, and a research agenda. *Epidemiologic Reviews, 31*(1), 152–177. https://doi.org/10.1093/epirev/mxp002

Beeston, C., McCartney, G., Wimbush, E., Beck, S., MacDonald, W., & Fraser, A. (2013). *Health inequalities: Policy review for the Scottish Ministerial Task Force on Health Inequalities.* NHS Health Scotland. https://publichealthscotland.scot/publications/health-inequalities-policy-review/

Bellis, M. A., Hughes, K., Leckenby, N., Hardcastle, K., Perkins, C., & Lowey, H. (2015). Measuring mortality and the burden of adult disease associated with adverse childhood experiences in England: A national survey. *Journal of Public Health (Oxford, England), 37*(3), 445–454. https://doi.org/10.1093/pubmed/fdu065

Bellis, M. A., Hughes, K., Leckenby, N., Jones, L., Baban, A., Kachaeva, M., Povilaitis, R., Pudule, I., Qirjako, G., Ulukol, B., Raleva, M., & Terzic, N. (2014a). Adverse childhood experiences and associations with health-harming behaviours in young adults: Surveys in eight eastern European countries. *Bulletin of the World Health Organization, 92*(9), 641–655. https://doi.org/10.2471/BLT.13.129247

Bellis, M. A., Hughes, K., Leckenby, N., Perkins, C., & Lowey, H. (2014b). National household survey of adverse childhood experiences and their relationship with resilience to health-harming behaviors in England. *BMC Med 12*, 72 (2014). https://doi.org/10.1186/1741-7015-12-72

Bendau, A., Petzold, M. B., Pyrkosch, L., Mascarell Maricic, L., Betzler, F., Rogoll, J., Große, J., Ströhle, A., & Plag, J. (2021). Associations between COVID-19 related media consumption and symptoms of anxiety, depression and COVID-19 related fear in the general population in Germany. *European Archives of Psychiatry and Clinical Neuroscience, 271*(2), 283–291. https://doi.org/10.1007/s00406-020-01171-6

Benedict, R. E., & Farel, A. M. (2003). Identifying children in need of ancillary and enabling services: A population approach. *Social Science & Medicine, 57*(11), 2035–2047. https://doi.org/10.1016/S0277-9536(03)00080-7

Berg, A. O., Melle, I., Rossberg, J. I., Romm, K. L., & Larsson, S. (2011). Perceived discrimination is associated with severity of positive and depression/anxiety symptoms in immigrants with psychosis: A cross-sectional study. *BMC Psychiatry, 11*, Article 77. https://doi.org/10.1186/1471-244X-11-77

Bernstein, C. A., & Bhugra, D. (2011). The next generation of psychiatrists: What is needed in training. *Asian Journal of Psychiatry, 4*(2), 88–91. https://doi.org/10.1016/j.ajp.2011.04.004

Bhugra, D. (2011). Introduction. In D. Bhugra, A. Malik, & G. Ikkos (Eds.), *Psychiatry's contract with society: Concepts, controversies, and consequences* (pp. 1–7). Oxford University Press.

Bhugra, D. (2014). Medicine's contract with society. *Journal of the Royal Society of Medicine, 107*(4), 144–147. https://doi.org/10.1177/0141076814525068

Bhugra, D. (2016a). Mental health for nations. *International Review of Psychiatry, 28*, 342–374. https://doi.org/10.1080/09540261.2016.1211095

Bhugra, D. (2016b). Bill of rights for persons with mental illness. *International Review of Psychiatry, 28*, 335. https://doi.org/10.1080/09540261.2016.1210580

Bhugra, D. (2024). Medicine's social contract. *Journal of the Royal Society of Medicine, 117*(3),102--103. doi: 10.1177/01410768241230772

Bhugra, D., Molodynski, A., & Ventriglio, A. (2021). Well-being and burnout in medical students. *Industrial Psychiatry Journal, 30*(2), 193–197. https://doi.org/10.4103/ipj.ipj_224_21

Bhugra, D. (Ed.). (2021). *Oxford textbook of migrant psychiatry*. Oxford University Press.

Bhugra, D., & Becker, M. A. (2005). Migration, cultural bereavement, and cultural identity. *World Psychiatry, 4*(1), 18–24. https://pmc.ncbi.nlm.nih.gov/articles/PMC1414713/

Bhugra, D., & Bhui, K. (2020). *Textbook of cultural psychiatry* (2nd ed.). Cambridge University Press.

Bhugra, D., Craig, T., & Bhui, K. (2010). *Mental health of refugees and asylum seekers*. Oxford University Press.

Bhugra, D., Gupta, K. R., & Wright, B. (1997). Depression in North India: Comparison of symptoms and life events with other patient groups. *International Journal of Psychiatry in Clinical Practice, 1*, 83–87.

Bhugra, D., & Gupta, S. (2010). *Migration and mental health*. Cambridge University Press.

Bhugra, D., Killaspy, H., Kar, A., Levin, S., Chumakov, E., Rogoza, D., Harvey, C., Bagga, H., Owino-Wamari, Y., Everall, I., Bishop, A., Javate, K. R., Westmore, I., Ahuja, A., Torales, J., Rubin, H., Castaldelli-Maia, J., Ng, R., Nakajima, G. A., . . . & Ventriglio A. (2022). IRP commission: Sexual minorities and mental health: Global perspectives. *International Review of Psychiatry, 34*(3–4):171–199. https://doi.org/10.1080/09540261.2022.2045912.

Bhugra, D., & Malik, A. (Eds.). (2011a). *Professionalism in mental healthcare*. Cambridge University Press.

Bhugra, D., & Malik, A. (2011b). Psychiatry's contract: Where next? In D. Bhugra, A. Malik, & G. Ikkos (Eds.), *Psychiatry's contract with society: Concepts, controversies, and consequences* (pp. 241–243). Oxford University Press.

Bhugra, D., Mallet, R., & Leff, J. (1999). Schizophrenia and African Caribbeans: A conceptual model of aetiology. *International Review of Psychiatry, 11*, 145–152. https://doi.org/10.1080/09540269974311

Bhugra, D., Pathare, S., Gosavi, C., Ventriglio, A., Torales, J., Castaldelli-Maia, J., Tolentino, E. J. L., & Ng, R. (2016a). Mental illness and the right to vote. *International Review of Psychiatry, 28*, 395–399. https://doi.org/10.1080/09540261.2016.1211096

Bhugra, D., Pathare, S., Joshi, R., Nardodkar, R., Torales, J., Tolentino, E. J. L., Dantas, R., & Ventriglio, A. (2016b). Right to property, inheritance, and contract with persons with mental illness. *International Review of Psychiatry, 28*, 402–408. https://doi.org/10.1080/09540261.2016.1210576

Bhugra, D., Pathare, S., Nardodkar, R., Gosavi, C., Ng, R., Torales, J., & Ventriglio, A. (2016c). Legislative provisions related to marriage and divorce of persons with mental illness. *International Review of Psychiatry, 28*, 386–392. https://doi.org/10.1080/09540261.2016.1210577

Bhugra, D., Smith, A., Ventriglio, A., Hermans, M. H. M., Ng, R., Javed, A., Chumakov, E., Kar, A., Ruiz, R., Oquendo, M., Chisolm, M. S., Werneke, U., Suryadevara, U., Jibson, M., Hobbs, J., Castaldelli-Maia, J., Nair, M., Seshadri, S., Subramanyam, A., . . . & Liebrenz, M. (2023). World Psychiatric Association-Asian Journal of Psychiatry Commission on psychiatric education in the 21st century. *Asian Journal of Psychiatry, 88*, 103739. https://doi.org/10.1016/j.ajp.2023.103739

Bhugra, D., Tasman, A., Pathare, S., Priebe, S., Smith, S., Torous, J., Arbuckle, M. R., Langford, A., Alarcón, R. D., Chiu, H. F. K., First, M. B., Kay, J., Sunkel, C., Thapar, A., Udomratn, P., Baingana, F. K., Kestel, D., Ng, R. M. K., Patel A., . . . & Ventriglio A. (2017). The WPA-Lancet Psychiatry Commission on the future of psychiatry. *The Lancet Psychiatry, 4*(10), 775–818. https://doi.org/10.1016/S2215-0366(17)30333-4

Bhugra, D., Till, A., & Sartorius, N. (2013). What is mental health? *International Journal of Social Psychiatry, 59*(1), 3–4. https://doi.org/10.1177/0020764012463315

Bhugra, D., & Ventriglio, A. (2023a). Commercial determinants of mental health. *International Journal of Social Psychiatry, 69*, 1065–1067. https://doi.org/10.1177/00207640231175047

Bhugra, D., & Ventriglio, A. (2023b). Geographical determinants of mental health. *International Journal of Social Psychiatry, 69*(7), 1702–1706. https://doi.org/10.1177/00207640231169816

Bhugra, D., & Ventriglio, A. (2023c). Political determinants of mental health. *International Journal of Social Psychiatry, 69*(3), 521–522. https://doi.org/10.1177/00207640231168544

Bhugra, D., Ventriglio, A., Castaldelli-Maia, J., & McCay, L. (2019). *Urban mental health*. Oxford University Press.

Bhugra, D., Ventriglio, A., & Bhui, K. (2021). Cultural competence in mental health care: Practice and policy. *European Psychiatry, 64*(1), e7. https://doi.org/10.1192/j.eurpsy.2020.106

Bhugra, D., Wijesuriya, R., Gnanapragasam, S., & Persaud, A. (2020). Black and minority mental health in the UK: Challenges and solutions. *Forensic Science International: Mind and Law, 1*, 100036. https://doi.org/10.1016/j.fsiml.2020.100036

Bickerdike, L., Booth, A., Wilson, P. M., Farley, K., & Wright, K. (2017). Social prescribing: Less rhetoric and more reality. A systematic review of the evidence. *BMJ Open, 7*(4), Article e013384. https://doi.org/10.1136/bmjopen-2016-013384

Bird, W., Adamo, G., Pirin, E., Gray, M., & Jani, A. (2020). Reducing chronic stress to promote health in adults: The role of social prescriptions and social movements. *Journal of the Royal Society of Medicine, 113*(3), 105–109. https://doi.org/10.1177/0141076819890547

Bisson, J. I., Roberts, N. P., Andrew, M., Cooper, R., & Lewis, C. (2010). Psychological therapies for chronic post-traumatic stress disorder (PTSD) in adults. The Cochrane Database of Systematic Reviews, 2010(11), CD003388. https://doi.org/10.1002/14651858.CD003388.pub3

Bisson, J. I., Cosgrove, S., Lewis, C., & Roberts, N. P. (2021). Post-traumatic stress disorder. *BMJ, 372*, Article n94. https://doi.org/10.1136/bmj.h6161.

Black, J. A., Cunningham, G., Fluckiger-Hawker, E, Robson, E., and Zólyomi, G. (1998–2025). The Electronic Text Corpus of Sumerian Literature (https://etcsl.orinst.ox.ac.uk/index1.htm), University of Oxford.

Bleidorn, W., Schönbrodt, F., Gebauer, J. E., Rentfrow, P. J., Potter, J., & Gosling, S. D. (2016). To live among like-minded others: Exploring the links between person-city personality fit and self-esteem. *Psychological Science, 27*(3), 419–427. https://doi.org/10.1177/0956797615627133

Bolton, P., West, J., Whitney, C., Jordans, M. J. D., Bass, J., Thornicroft, G., Murray, L., Snider, L., Eaton, J., Collins, P. Y., Ventevogel, P., Smith, S., Stein, D. J., Petersen, I., Silove, D., Ugo, V., Mahoney, J., El Chammay, R., Contreras, C., . . . Raviola, G. (2023). Expanding mental health services in low- and middle-income countries: A task-shifting framework for delivery of comprehensive, collaborative, and community-based care. *Global Mental Health, 10*, e16. https://doi.org/10.1017/gmh.2023.5

Bond, K., Chalmers, K., Jorm, A., Kitchener, B., & Reavley, N. (2015). Assisting Australians with mental health problems and financial difficulties: A Delphi study to develop guidelines for financial counsellors, financial institution staff, mental health professionals, and carers. *BMC Health Services Research, 15*, 218. https://doi.org/10.1186/s12913-015-0868-2

Bond, G. R., & Drake, R. E. (2015). The critical ingredients of assertive community treatment. *World Psychiatry, 14*(2), 240–242. https://doi.org/10.1002/wps.20234.

Bonell, C., Allen, E., Warren, E., McGowan, J., Bevilacqua, L., Jamal, F., Legood, R., Wiggins, M., Opondo, C., Mathiot, A., Sturgess, J., Fletcher, A., Sadique, Z., Elbourne, D., Christie, D., Bond, L., Scott, S., & Viner, R. M. (2018). Effects of the Learning Together intervention on bullying and aggression in English secondary schools (INCLUSIVE): A cluster randomised controlled trial. *The Lancet, 392*(10163), 2452–2464. https://doi.org/10.1016/S0140-6736(18)31782-3

Bonnardot, L., Liu, J., Wootton, E., Amoros, I., Olson, D., Wong, S., & Santi, L. (2014). The development of a multilingual tool for facilitating the primary-specialty care interface in low-resource settings: The MSF Tele-Expertise system. *Frontiers in Public Health, 2*, 126. https://doi.org/10.3389/fpubh.2014.00126

Borges do Nascimento, I. J., Pizarro, A. B., Almeida, J. M., Azzopardi-Muscat, N., Gonçalves, M. A., Björklund, M., & Novillo-Ortiz, D. (2022). Infodemics and health misinformation: A systematic review of reviews. *Bulletin of the World Health Organization, 100*(9), 544–561. https://doi.org/10.2471/BLT.21.287654

Bowleg, L. (2012). The problem with the phrase women and minorities: Intersectionality-an important theoretical framework for public health. *American Journal of Public Health, 102*(7), 1267–1273. https://doi.org/10.2105/AJPH.2012.300750

Boysen, G. A., & Doonan, A. (2014). Expansion of the concept of mental disorder in the DSM-5. *Journal of Mind and Behavior, 35*(3–4), 225–244. https://www.jstor.org/stable/43854371

Brandling, J., & House, W. (2009). Social prescribing in general practice: Adding meaning to medicine. *British Journal of General Practice, 59*(563), 454–456. https://doi.org/10.3399/bjgp09X421085

Brandt, L., Henssler, J., Müller, M., Wall, S., Gabel, D., & Heinz, A. (2019). Risk of psychosis in refugees: A systematic review and meta-analysis. *JAMA Psychiatry, 76*(11), 1133–1140. https://doi.org/10.1001/jamapsychiatry.2019.1937

Braubach, M., Jacobs, D. E., & Ormandy, D. (2011). Environmental burden of disease associated with inadequate housing: A method guide to the quantification of health impacts of housing risks in the WHO European Region. World Health Organization Regional Office for Europe. https://www.euro.who.int/__data/assets/pdf_file/0003/142077/e95004.pdf.

Braun, S., Annovazzi, C., Botella, C., Bridler, R., Camussi, E., Delfino, J. P.,Mohr, C., Moragrega, I., Papagno, C., Pisoni, A., Soler, C., Seifritz, E., & Stassen, H. H. (2016). Assessing chronic stress, coping skills, and mood disorders through speech analysis: A self-assessment "voice app" for laptops, tablets, and smartphones. *Psychopathology, 49*(6), 406–419. https://doi.org/10.1159/000450959

Braveman, P., & Gottlieb, L. (2014). The social determinants of health: It's time to consider the causes of the causes. *Public Health Reports, 129*(Suppl. 2), 19–31. https://doi.org/10.1177/00333549141291S206

British Broadcasting Corporation (BBC). (2016, November 29). Hate crime "surge" after Trump win. BBC News. https://www.bbc.co.uk/news/world-us-canada-38149406.

British Medical Association. (2019). *Medicine's social contract.* https://www.bma.org.uk/media/1840/bma-medicines-social-contract-2019.pdf

Brodaty, H., & Donkin, M. (2009). Family caregivers of people with dementia. *Dialogues in Clinical Neuroscience,* 11(2), 217–228. https://doi.org/10.31887/DCNS.2009.11.2/hbrodaty

Brooks, S. K., Webster, R. K., Smith, L. E., Woodland, L., Wessely, S., Greenberg, N., & Rubin, G. J. (2020). The psychological impact of quarantine and how to reduce it: Rapid review of the evidence. *The Lancet, 395*(10227), 912–920. https://doi.org/10.1016/S0140-6736(20)30460-8

Brown, D. W., Anda, R. F., Tiemeier, H., Felitti, V. J., Edwards, V. J., Croft, J. B., & Giles, W. H. (2009). Adverse childhood experiences and the risk of premature mortality. *American Journal of Preventive Medicine, 37*(5), 389–396. https://doi.org/10.1016/j.amepre.2009.06.021

Brown, F. W. (1998). Rural telepsychiatry. *Psychiatric Services, 49*(8), 963–964. https://doi.org/10.1176/ps.49.7.963

Brown, S., Learmonth, A., & Mackereth, G. (2015). *Promoting public mental health and wellbeing: Principles into practice.* Jessica Kingsley Publishers.

Brunstein Klomek, A., Sourander, A., & Gould, M. S. (2010). The association of suicide and bullying in childhood to young adulthood: A review of cross-sectional and longitudinal research findings. *Canadian Journal of Psychiatry, 55*(5), 282–288. https://doi.org/10.1177/070674371005500503

Brunwasser, S. M., Gillham, J. E., & Kim, E. S. (2009). A meta-analytic review of the Penn Resiliency Program's effect on depressive symptoms. *Journal of Consulting and Clinical Psychology, 77*(6), 1042–1054. doi:10.1037/a0017671.

Bryant, R. A., Schafer, A., Dawson, K. S., Anjuri, D., Mulili, C., Ndogoni, L., Koyiet, P., Sijbrandij, M., Ulate, J., Harper Shehadeh, M., Hadzi-Pavlovic, D., & van Ommeren, M. (2017). Effectiveness of a brief behavioural intervention on psychological distress among women with a history of gender-based violence in urban Kenya: A randomised clinical trial. *PLoS Medicine, 14*(8), e1002371. https://doi.org/10.1371/journal.pmed.1002371

Buck, B., Scherer, E., Brian, R., Wang, R., Wang, W., Campbell, A. T., Choudhury, T., Hauser, M., Kane, J. M., & Ben-Zeev, D. (2019). Relationships between smartphone social behavior and relapse in schizophrenia: A preliminary report. *Schizophrenia Research, 208*, 167–172. https://doi.org/10.1016/j.schres.2019.03.014

Buck, D., & Ewbank, L. (2020, November 4). *What is social prescribing?* The King's Fund. https://www.kingsfund.org.uk/insight-and-analysis/long-reads/social-prescribing

Bullough, V. L. (1976). *Sexual variance in society and history*. University of Chicago Press.

Buss, C., Entringer, S., & Wadhwa, P. D. (2012). Fetal programming of brain development: Intrauterine stress and susceptibility to psychopathology. *Science Signaling, 5*(245), pt7. https://doi.org/10.1126/scisignal.2003406

Butler, T. N., & Yellowlees, P. (2012). Cost analysis of store-and-forward telepsychiatry as a consultation model for primary care. *Telemedicine and e-Health, 18*(1), 74–77. https://pubmed.ncbi.nlm.nih.gov/22085113/

Butterworth, P., Rodgers, B., & Windsor, T. D. (2009). Financial hardship, socio-economic position and depression: Results from the PATH Through Life Survey. *Social Science & Medicine, 74*(5), 732–740. https://doi.org/10.1016/j.socscimed.2009.05.008

Byambasuren, S., & Tsetsegdary, G. (2005). Mental health in Mongolia. *International Psychiatry, 2*(8), 9–12. https://www.ncbi.nlm.nih.gov/pmc/articles/PMC6733123/

Cacioppo, J. T., Cacioppo, S., Capitanio, J. P., & Cole, S. W. (2015). The neuroendocrinology of social isolation. *Annual Review of Psychology, 66*, 733–767. https://doi.org/10.1146/annurev-psych-010814-015240

Calati, R., Ferrari, C., Brittner, M., Oasi, O., Olié, E., Carvalho, A. F., & Courtet, P. (2019). Suicidal thoughts and behaviors and social isolation: A narrative review of the literature. *Journal of Affective Disorders, 245*, 653–667. https://doi.org/10.1016/j.jad.2018.11.022

Campion, J., Bhui, K. S., & Bhugra, D. (2012). European Psychiatric Association (EPA) guidance on prevention of mental illness. *European Psychiatry, 27*(2), 68–80. https://doi.org/10.1016/j.eurpsy.2011.10.004

Canadian Mental Health Association. (2014). Cross-cultural mental health. https://bc.cmha.ca/documents/cross-cultural-mental-health-and-substance-use-2/

Canadian Standards Association & Bureau de normalisation du Québec. (2013). *Psychological health and safety in the workplace—Prevention, promotion, and guidance to staged implementation* (CAN/CSA-Z1003-13/BNQ 9700-803/2013).

Canetto, S. S. (2015). Suicidal behaviour among Muslim women: Patterns, pathways, meanings and prevention. *Crisis, 33*, 447–458. https://doi.org/10.1027/0227-5910/a000347

Cannon, M., Jones, P. B., & Murray, R. M. (2002). Obstetric complications and schizophrenia: Historical and meta-analytic findings. *American Journal of Psychiatry, 159*(7), 1080–1092. https://doi.org/10.1176/appi.ajp.159.7.1080

Cantor-Graae, E., & Selten, J. P. (2005). Schizophrenia and migration: A meta-analysis and review. *American Journal of Psychiatry, 162*(1), 12–24. https://doi.org/10.1176/appi.ajp.162.1.12

Carlile, A., & Bhugra, D. (2014). *Future of mental health services*. Mental Health Foundation.

Carter, N., Valaitis, R., Lam, A., Feather, J., Nicholl, J., & Gleghorn, L. (2018). Navigation delivery models and roles of navigators in primary care: A scoping literature review. *BMC Health Services Research, 18*, 896. https://doi.org/10.1186/s12913-018-2889-0

Casswell, S. (2023). A policy agenda for the commercial determinants of health. In N. Maani, M. Petticrew, & S. Galea (Eds.), *The commercial determinants of health* (pp. 341–352). Oxford University Press.

Castaldelli-Maia, J. M., & Bhugra, D. (2022). Analysis of global prevalence of mental and substance use disorders within countries: Focus on sociodemographic characteristics and income levels. *International Review of Psychiatry, 34*(1), 6–15. https://doi.org/10.1186/s12888-025-07041-6

Cattan, M., White, M., Bond, J., & Learmouth, A. (2005). Preventing social isolation and loneliness among older people: A systematic review of health promotion interventions. *Ageing and Society, 25*(1), 41–67. doi:10.1017/S0144686X04002594

Cawston, P. (2011). Social prescribing in very deprived area. *British Journal of General Practice, 61*(586), 350. https://doi.org/10.3399/bjgp11X572517

Centers for Disease Control and Prevention (CDC). (2014). *Updated preparedness and response framework for influenza pandemics*. https://www.cdc.gov/mmwr/preview/mmwrhtml/rr6306a1.htm

Centers for Disease Control and Prevention (CDC). (2019). *Middle East respiratory syndrome*. https://www.cdc.gov/coronavirus/mers/index.html

Centers for Disease Control and Prevention (CDC). (2024a). *About adverse childhood experiences*. https://www.cdc.gov/aces/about/index.html

Centers for Disease Control and Prevention (CDC). (2024b). *Understanding the opioid overdose epidemic*. https://www.cdc.gov/overdose-prevention/about/understanding-the-opioid-overdose-epidemic.html

Cénat, J., Mukunzi, J., Noorishad, P.-G., Rousseau, C., Derivois, D., & Bukaka, J. (2020). A systematic review of mental health programs among populations affected by the Ebola virus disease. *Journal of Psychosomatic Research, 131*, 109966. https://doi.org/10.1016/j.jpsychores.2020.109966

Centre for Mental Health. (2007). *Mental health at work: Developing the business case*. Centre for Mental Health. https://www.centreformentalhealth.org.uk/wp-content/uploads/2018/09/mental_health_at_work.pdf

Chae, D. H., Clouston, S., Hatzenbuehler, M. L., Kramer, M. R., Cooper, H. L. F., Wilson, S. M., Stephens-Davidowitz, S., & Link, B. G. (2015). Association between an Internet-based measure of area racism and Black mortality. *PLoS ONE*, 10(4), e0122963 . https://doi.org/10.1371/journal.pone.0122963

Chan, S., Godwin, H., Gonzalez, A., Yellowlees, P. M., & Hilty, D. M. (2017). Review of use and integration of mobile apps into psychiatric treatments. *Current Psychiatry Reports, 19*, 96. https://doi.org/10.1007/s11920-017-0848-9

Chandra, V., Pandav, R., Laxminarayan, R., Tanner, C., Manyam, B., Rajkumar, S., Silberberg, D., Brayne, C., Chow, J., Herman, S., Hourihan, F., Kasner, S., Morillo, L., Ogunniyi, A., Theodore, W., & Zhang, Z.-X. (2006). Neurological disorders. In D. T. Jamison, J. G. Breman, A. R. Measham, G. Alleyne, M. Claeson, D. B. Evans, P. Jha, A. Mills, & P. Musgrove (Eds.), *Disease control priorities in developing countries* (2nd ed., pp. 627–646). World Health Organization. https://doi.org/10.1596/978-0-821-36179-5

Chandra, P. S., & Stewart, D. E. (2017). WPA International Competency-Based Curriculum for Mental Health Providers on Intimate Partner Violence and Sexual Violence Against Women. *World Psychiatry, 16*(2), 223–224. https://doi.org/10.1002/wps.20432.

Charlson, F., Ali, S., Benmarhnia, T., Pearl, M., Massazza, A., Augustinavicius, J., & Scott, J. G. (2021). Climate Change and Mental Health: A Scoping Review. *International Journal of Environmental Research and Public Health, 18*(9), 4486. https://doi.org/10.3390/ijerph18094486

Chatterjee, K., & Chauhan, V. S. (2020). Epidemics, quarantine and mental health. *Medical Journal Armed Forces India, 76*(2), 125–127. https://doi.org/10.1016/j.mjafi.2020.03.017

Chen, H., Lai, K., He, L., & Yu, R. (2020). Where you are is who you are? The geographical account of psychological phenomena. *Frontiers in Psychology, 11*, 536. https://doi.org/10.3389/fpsyg.2020.00536

Chen, Y., Su, J., Zhang, Y., & Yan, W. (2021). Optimism, social identity, mental health: Findings from Tibetan college students in China. *Frontiers in Psychology, 12*, 747515. https://doi.org/10.3389/fpsyg.2021.747515

Cheng, K. M., Siu, B. W. M., Yeung, C. C. Y. A., Chiang, T. P., So, M. H., & Yeung, M. C. W. (2018). Telepsychiatry for stable Chinese psychiatric out-patients in custody in Hong Kong: A case-control pilot study. *Hong Kong Medical Journal, 24*, 378–383. https://doi.org/10.12809/hkmj187217

Chiao, J. Y., & Blizinsky, K. D. (2010). Culture–gene coevolution of individualism–collectivism and the serotonin transporter gene. *Proceedings of the Royal Society B: Biological Sciences, 277*(1681), 529–537. https://doi.org/10.1098/rspb.2009.1650

Chibanda, D., Weiss, H. A., Verhey, R., Simms, V., Munjoma, R., Rusakaniko, S., Chingono, A., Munetsi, E., Bere, T., Manda, E., Abas, M., & Araya, R. (2016). Effect of a primary care–based psychological intervention on symptoms of common mental disorders in Zimbabwe: A randomized clinical trial. *JAMA, 316*(24), 2618–2626. https://doi.org/10.1001/jama.2016.19102

Chicote-Beato, M., González-Víllora, S., Bodoque-Osma, A. R., & Olivas, R. N. (2024). Cyberbullying intervention and prevention programmes in primary education (6 to 12 years): A systematic review. *Aggression and Violent Behavior, 77*, 101938. https://doi.org/10.1016/j.avb.2024.101938

Chida, Y., & Steptoe, A. (2008). Positive psychological well-being and mortality: a quantitative review of prospective observational studies. *Psychosomatic medicine, 70*(7), 741–756. https://doi.org/10.1097/PSY.0b013e31818105ba

Chowdhary, A., Zlotnikova, V., Lucas, C., & Lonie, J. (2019). How do Mental Health First Aid interventions influence patient help-seeking behaviours? A dilemma for pharmacist Mental Health First Aid responders. *Research in Social and Administrative Pharmacy, 15*(1), 106–108. https://doi.org/10.1016/j.sapharm.2018.02.010

Christakis, N. A. (2020). *Apollo's arrow*. Little, Brown Spark.

Chua, R. Y., Huang, K. G., & Jin, M. (2019). Mapping cultural tightness and its links to innovation, urbanization, and happiness across 31 provinces in China. *Proceedings of the National Academy of Sciences, 116*(14), 6720–6725. https://doi.org/10.1073/pnas.1815723116

Cinelli, M., Quattrociocchi, W., Galeazzi, A., Valensise, C. M., Brugnoli, E., Schmidt, A. L., Zola, P., Zollo, F., & Scala, A. (2020). The COVID-19 social media infodemic. *Scientific Reports, 10*(1), 16598. https://doi.org/10.1038/s41598-020-73510-5

Clarke, A., & Barry, M. (2015). Supporting a whole school approach to mental health promotion and wellbeing in post-primary schools in Ireland. In S. Kutcher, Y. Wei, & M. D. Weist (Eds.), *School mental health: Global challenges and opportunities* (pp. 112–124). Cambridge University Press.

Classen, T., & Dunn, R. (2012). The effect of job loss and unemployment duration on suicidal risk in the United States: A new look using mass-layoffs and unemployment duration. *Health Economics, 21*(3), 338–350. https://doi.org/10.1002/hec.1719

Colantone, I., Crinò, R., & Ogliari, L. (2019). Globalization and mental distress. *Journal of International Economics, 119*, 181–207. https://doi.org/10.1016/j.jinteco.2019.04.008

Collins, P. H. (2000). *Black feminist thought: Knowledge, consciousness, and the politics of empowerment* (2nd ed.). Routledge.

Committee on the Rights of Persons with Disabilities (CRPD). (2014). *General comment No. 1 (2014) on Article 12: Equal recognition before the law*. United Nations. https://www.ohchr.org/en/treaty-bodies/crpd/general-comments

Compton, M. T. (2015). Food insecurity. In M. T. Compton & R. Shim (Eds.), *The social determinants of mental health* (pp. 145–160). American Psychiatric Publishing.

Connolly, S. M., Vanchu-Orosco, M., Warner, J., Seidi, P. A., Edwards, J., Boath, E., & Irgens, A. C. (2021). Mental health interventions by lay counsellors: A systematic review and meta-analysis. *Bulletin of the World Health Organization, 99*(8), 572–582. https://doi.org/10.2471/BLT.20.269050

Cooper, J. E., Kendall, R., Gurland, B. J., Sharpe, L., & Copeland, J. E. M. (1972). *Psychiatric diagnosis in New York and London.* Oxford University Press.

Cooper, R., Goldenberg, R., Das, A., Norman, G., Cliver, S. P., & Andrews, W. W. (1996). The preterm prediction study: Maternal stress is associated with spontaneous preterm birth at less than thirty-five weeks gestation. *American Journal of Obstetrics and Gynecology, 175*(5), 1286–1292. https://doi.org/10.1016/s0002-9378(96)70042-x

Cooper, S. A., Smiley, E., Morrison, J., Williamson, A., & Allan, L. (2007). Mental ill-health in adults with intellectual disabilities: Prevalence and associated factors. *British Journal of Psychiatry, 190*(1), 27–35. doi:10.1192/bjp.bp.106.022483

Corrigan, P., Watson, A. L., Heyrman, M., Warpinski, A., Gracia, C., Slopen, N., & Hall, L. (2005). Structural stigma in state legislation. *Psychiatric Services, 56*(5), 557–563. https://doi.org/10.1176/appi.ps.56.5.557

Cossu, G., Preti, A., & Carta, M. C. (2018). Treatment of mental health problems in refugees and asylum seekers. In D. Bhugra, K. Bhui, S. Y. S. Wong, & S. E. Gilman (Eds.), *Oxford textbook of public mental health* (pp. 289–304). Oxford University Press.

Council of Europe. (2023). *Improving well-being at school.* https://www.coe.int/en/web/campaign-free-to-speak-safe-to-learn/improving-well-being-at-school

Cowie, H. (2022). Pastoral care in education today: Its continuing role in promoting mental health in children and young people. *Pastoral Care in Education, 40*(3), 321–327. https://doi.org/10.1080/02643944.2022.2093955

Community Partners in Care (CPIC). (2016). *Policy brief by Wells K. & Miranda J.* CPIC, UCLA Center for Health Services and Society.

Crawford, A., Sunderji, N., López, J., & Soklaridis, S. (2016). Defining competencies for the practice of telepsychiatry through an assessment of resident learning needs: Approaches to teaching and learning. *BMC Medical Education, 16*(1), 28. https://doi.org/10.1186/s12909-016-0529-0

Crawford, G., Burns, S. K., Chih, H. J., Hunt, K., Tilley, P. J. M., Hallett, J., Coleman, K., & Smith, S. (2015). Mental health first aid training for nursing students: A protocol for a pragmatic randomised controlled trial in a large university. *BMC Psychiatry, 15*(1), 26. https://doi.org/10.1186/s12888-015-0403-3

Crenshaw, K. (1989). Demarginalizing the intersection of race and sex: A Black feminist critique of antidiscrimination doctrine, feminist theory and antiracist politics. *University of Chicago Legal Forum, 1989*(1), 139–167.

Crooks, C., Lapp, A., Auger, M., van der Woerd, K., Snowshoe, A., Rogers, B. J., Tsuruda, S., & Caron, C. (2018). A feasibility trial of Mental Health First Aid First Nations: Acceptability, cultural adaptation, and preliminary outcomes. *American Journal of Community Psychology, 61*(3–4), 459–471. https://doi.org/10.1002/ajcp.12241

Cruess, S. R. (2006). Professionalism and medicine's contract with society. *Clinical Orthopaedics and Related Research, 449*, 170–176. https://doi.org/10.1097/01.blo.0000229275.66570.97

Cunsolo, A., & Ellis, N. R. (2018). Ecological grief as a mental health response to climate change-related loss. *Nature Climate Change, 8*(4), 275–281. https://doi.org/10.1038/s41558-018-0092-2

Czeisler, M. É., Lane, R. I., Petrosky, E., Wiley, J. F., Christensen, A., Njai, R., Weaver, M. D., Robbins, R., Facer-Childs, E. R., Barger, L. K., Czeisler, C. A., Howard, M. E., & Rajaratnam, S. M. W. (2020). Mental health, substance use, and suicidal ideation during the COVID-19 pandemic—United States, June 24–30, 2020. *Morbidity and Mortality Weekly Report, 69*(32), 1049–1057. https://doi.org/10.15585/mmwr.mm6932a1

Dawes, D. (2020). *The political determinants of health*. Johns Hopkins University Press.

Dayson, C., & Bashir, N. (2014). *The social and economic impact of the Rotherham social prescribing pilot: Main evaluation report*. Sheffield Hallam University. https://shura.shu.ac.uk/18961/1/Dayson-SocialAndEconomicImpact-Rotherham(VoR).pdf

Dayson, C., Bashir, N., & Pearson, S. (2013). *From dependence to independence: Emerging lessons from the Rotherham social prescribing pilot* (CESR Report). Sheffield Hallam University.

Dekker, J., Sears, S. F., Åsenlöf, P., & Berry, K. (2023). Psychologically informed health care. *Translational Behavioral Medicine, 13*(5). https://doi.org/10.1093/tbm/ibac105

de Jonge, P., Roest, A. M., Lim, C. W., Levinson, D., & Scott, K. M. (2018). Panic disorder and panic attacks. In K. M. Scott, P. de Jonge, D. J. Stein, & R. C. Kessler (Eds.), *Mental disorders around the world* (pp. 93–105). Cambridge University Press.

de la Torre Díez, I., Alonso, S. G., Hamrioui, S., Cruz, E. M., Nozaleda, L. M., & Franco, M. A. (2019). IoT-based services and applications for mental health in the literature. *Journal of Medical Systems, 43*, Article 4. https://doi.org/10.1007/s10916-018-1130-3

de Lacy-Vawdon, C., & Livingstone, C. (2020). Defining the commercial determinants of health: A systematic review. *BMC Public Health, 20*(1), 1022. https://doi.org/10.1186/s12889-020-09126-1

de Mooij, L. D., Kikkert, M., Theunissen, J., Beekman, A. T. F., de Haan, L., Duurkoop, P. W. R. A., Van, 'H. L., & Dekker, J. J. M. (2019). Dying too soon: Excess mortality in severe mental illness. *Frontiers in Psychiatry, 10*, 855. https://doi.org/10.3389/fpsyt.2019.00855

De Witte, H., Pienaar, J., & De Cuyper, N. (2016). Review of 30 years of longitudinal studies on the association between job insecurity and health and well-being: Is there causal evidence? *Australian Psychologist, 51*(1), 18–31. https://doi.org/10.1111/ap.12176.

Degenhardt, L., Charlson, F., Ferrari, A., Santomauro, D., Erskine, H., Mantilla-Herrara, A., Whiteford, H., Leung, J., Naghavi, M., Griswold, M., Rehm, J., Hall, W., Sartorius, B., Scott, J., Vollset, S. E., Knudsen, A. K., Haro, J. M., Patton, G., Kopec, J., . . . Vos, T. (2018). The global burden of disease attributable to alcohol and drug use in 195 countries and territories, 1990–2016. *The Lancet Psychiatry, 5*(12), 987–1012. https://doi.org/10.1016/S2215-0366(18)30337-7

Degenhardt, L., Grebely, J., Stone, J., Hickman, M., Vickerman, P., Marshall, B. D. L., Bruneau, J., Altice, F. L., Henderson, G., Rahimi-Movaghar, A., & Larney, S. (2019). Global patterns of opioid use and dependence: Harms to populations, interventions, and future action. *The Lancet, 394* (10208), 1560–1579. https://doi.org/10.1016/S0140-6736(19)32229-9

Degenhardt, L., Torres, Y., Hinkov, H., ten Have, M., & Glantz, M. D. (2018). Drug use disorders. In K. M. Scott, P. de Jonge, D. J. Stein, & R. C. Kessler (Eds.), *Mental disorders around the world* (pp. 243–262). Cambridge University Press.

Deloitte. (2020). *Mental health and employers: Refreshing the case for investment.* Deloitte. https://www2.deloitte.com/content/dam/Deloitte/uk/Documents/consultancy/deloitte-uk-mental-health-and-employers.pdf

Deng, L., & Fang, X. (2015). Mental health education for children and adolescents in China. In S. Kutcher, Y. Wei, & M. D. Weist (Eds.), *School mental health: Global challenges and opportunities* (pp. 80–94). Cambridge University Press.

Desai, G., & Chaturvedi, S. K. (2018). Neurotic disorders. In D. Bhugra & K. Bhui (Eds.), *Textbook of cultural psychiatry* (pp. 205–214). Cambridge University Press.

Deslich, S., Stec, B., Tomblin, S., & Coustasse, A. (2013). Telepsychiatry in the 21st century: Transforming healthcare with technology. *Perspectives in Health Information Management, 10,* 1–17. https://pmc.ncbi.nlm.nih.gov/articles/PMC3709879/

Department of Health and Social Care (DHSC). (2020). *Tackling obesity: Empowering adults and children to live healthier lives.* https://www.gov.uk/government/publications/tackling-obesity-government-strategy/tackling-obesity-empowering-adults-and-children-to-live-healthier-lives

Di Forti, M., Quattrone, D., Freeman, T. P., Tripoli, G., Gayer-Anderson, C., Quigley, H., Rodriguez, V., Jongsma, H. E., Ferraro, L., La Cascia, C., La Barbera, D., Tarricone, I., Berardi, D., Szöke, A., Arango, C., Tortelli, A., Velthorst, E., Bernardo, M., Del-Ben, C. M., . . . van der Ven, E. (2019). The contribution of cannabis use to variation in incidence of psychotic disorder across Europe (EU-GEI). *The Lancet Psychiatry, 6*(5), 427–436. https://doi.org/10.1016/S2215-0366(19)30048-3

Dickinson, P., & Peterson, R. (2015). Flourishing schools in Aotearoa, New Zealand and wellbeing in school model. In S. Kutcher, Y. Wei, & M. D. Weist (Eds.), *School mental health: Global challenges and opportunities* (pp. 170–185). Cambridge University Press.

Dieltjens, T., Moonens, I., Van Praet, K., De Buck, E., & Vandekerckhove, P. (2014). A systematic literature search on psychological first aid: Lack of evidence to develop guidelines. *PLoS ONE, 9(12)*. https://doi.org/10.1371/journal.pone.0114714

Diener, E., Oishi, S., & Lucas, R. E. (2003). Personality, culture, and subjective wellbeing: Emotional and cognitive evaluations of life. *Annual Review of Psychology, 54*, 403–425.

Dietze, A. (2018). Cultural brokers and mediators. In M. Middell (Ed.), *Routledge handbook of transregional studies*. Routledge.

Dingle, G. A., Cruwys, T., & Frings, D. (2015). Social identities as pathways into and out of addiction. *Frontiers in Psychology, 6*, 1795. https://doi.org/10.3389/fpsyg.2015.01795

Department of Health (DoH). (2011). *No health without mental health*. Department of Health.

Donabedian, A. (1980). *The definition of quality and approaches to its assessment*. Health Administration Press.

Donkin, A., Goldblatt, P., Allan, J., Nathanson, V., & Marmot, M. (2018). Global action on the social determinants of health. *BMJ Global Health, 3*, e000603. https://doi.org/10.1136/bmjgh-2017-000603

Donley, E., McClaren, A., Jones, R., Katz, P., & Goh, J. (2017). Evaluation and implementation of a telepsychiatry trial in the emergency department of a metropolitan public hospital. *Journal of Technology in Human Services, 35*(4), 292–313. https://doi.org/10.1080/15228835.2017.1367351

Doshmangir, L., Sanadghol, A., Kakemam, E., & Majdzadeh, R. (2025). The involvement of non-governmental organisations in achieving health system goals based on the WHO six building blocks: A scoping review on global evidence. *PloS one*, 20(1), e0315592. https://doi.org/10.1371/journal.pone.0315592.

Downing, J. (2016). The health effects of the foreclosure crisis and unaffordable housing: A systematic review and explanation of evidence. *Social Science & Medicine, 162*, 88–96. https://doi.org/10.1016/j.socscimed.2016.06.014

Drago, A., Winding, T. N., & Antypa, N. (2016). Videoconferencing in psychiatry: A meta-analysis of assessment and treatment. *European Psychiatry, 36*, 29–37. https://doi.org/10.1016/j.eurpsy.2016.03.007

Dulin, P. L., Gonzalez, V. M., & Campbell, K. (2014). Results of a pilot test of a self-administered smartphone-based treatment system for alcohol use disorders: Usability and early outcomes. *Substance Abuse, 35*(2), 168–175. https://doi.org/10.1080/08897077.2013.821437

Durkin, M. S., Schneider, H., Pthania, V., Nelson, K. B., Solarsh, G. C., Bellows, N., Scheffler, R. N., & Hofman, K. J. (2006). Learning and developmental disabilities. In World Health Organization & Disease Control Priorities Project (Eds.) *Disease control priorities related to mental, neurological, developmental and substance abuse disorders* (pp. 39–56). World Health Organization.

Durlak, J. A., Weissberg, R. P., Dymnicki, A. B., Taylor, R. D., & Schellinger, K. B. (2011). The impact of enhancing students' social and emotional learning: A meta-analysis of school-based universal interventions. *Child Development, 82*(1), 405–432. https://doi.org/10.1111/j.1467-8624.2010.01564.x

Eisenberg-Guyot, J., & Prins, S. (2022). The impact of capitalism on mental health: An epidemiological perspective. In D. Bhugra, D. Moussaoui, & T. Craig (Eds.), *Oxford textbook of social psychiatry* (pp. 195–204). Oxford University Press.

El-Guebaly, N., Carrà, G., & Galanter, M. (Eds.). (2015). *Textbook of addiction treatment: International perspectives*. Springer.

Elliott, S. (2014). Health geography. In A. C. Michalos (Ed.), *Encyclopedia of quality of life and well-being research* (pp. 2750–2754). Springer.

Estanislau, G. M., Vieira, M. A., Moriyama, T. S., Neto, A. G. A., Bordini, I., & Bressan, R. (2015). The "Cool Mind" programme: Mental health literacy for middle and high school teachers in Brazil. In S. Kutcher, Y. Wei, & M. D. Weist (Eds.), *School Mental Health: Global challenges and opportunities* (pp. 21–29). Cambridge University Press.

Esterwood, E., & Saeed, S. A. (2020). Past epidemics, natural disasters, COVID-19, and mental health: Learning from history as we deal with the present and prepare for the future. *Psychiatric Quarterly,* 91(4), 1121–1133. 10.1007/s11126-020-09808-4

European Convention on Human Rights. (1950). *The convention in 1950.* Council of Europe. https://www.coe.int/en/web/human-rights-convention/the-convention-in-1950

Eurostat. (2018, December 5). *Number of psychiatrists: How do countries compare?* https://ec.europa.eu/eurostat/web/products-eurostat-news/-/ddn-20181205-1

Evans, C. (2006). Child development and the physical environment. *Annual Review of Psychology, 57*, 423–445. https://doi.org/10.1146/annurev.psych.57.102904.190057

Evans, G. W., & Kim, P. (2013). Childhood poverty, chronic stress, self-regulation, and coping. *Child Development Perspectives, 7*(1), 43–48. https://doi.org/10.1111/cdep.12013

Evans, J., Romaniuk, M., & Theal, R. (2021). Evaluation of mental health first aid training for family members of military veterans with a mental health condition. *BMC psychiatry, 21*(1), 128. https://doi.org/10.1186/s12888-021-03139-9

Every-Palmer, S. (2011). Synthetic cannabinoid JWH-018 and psychosis: An explorative study. *Drug and Alcohol Dependence, 117*(2–3), 152–157. https://doi.org/10.1016/j.drugalcdep.2011.01.012

Eyberg, S. M., Nelson, M. M., & Boggs, S. R. (2008). Evidence-based psychosocial treatments for children and adolescents with disruptive behavior. *Journal of Clinical Child & Adolescent Psychology, 37*(1), 215–237. https://doi.org/10.1080/15374410701820117

Faculty of Public Health & Mental Health Foundation. (2016). Better mental health for all: A public health approach to mental health improvement. London: Faculty of Public Health and Mental Health Foundation. https://www.fph.org.uk/media/1644/better-mental-health-for-all-final-low-res.pdf.

Fanon, F. (1952). *Black skin, white masks*. Éditions du Seuil.

Fantegrossi, W. E., Wilson, C. D., & Berquist, M. D. (2018). Pro-psychotic effects of synthetic cannabinoids: Interactions with central dopamine, serotonin, and glutamate systems. *Drug Metabolism Reviews, 50*(1), 65–73. https://doi.org/10.1080/03602532.2018.1428343

Fardouly, J., & Vartanian, L. R. (2016). Social media and body image concerns: Current research and future directions. *Current Opinion in Psychology, 9*, 1–5. https://doi.org/10.1016/j.copsyc.2015.09.005

Faris, R. E. L., & Dunham, H. W. (1939). *Mental disorders in urban areas: An ecological study of schizophrenia and other psychoses*. University of Chicago Press.

Fazel, M., Hoagwood, K., Stephan, S., & Ford, T. (2014). Mental health interventions in schools in high-income countries. *The Lancet Psychiatry, 1*(5), 377–387. https://doi.org/10.1016/S2215-0366(14)70312-8[1]

Fazel, M., Reed, R. V., Panter-Brick, C., & Stein, A. (2012). Mental health of displaced and refugee children resettled in high-income countries: Risk and protective factors. *The Lancet, 379*(9812), 266–282. https://doi.org/10.1016/S0140-6736(11)60051-2

Felitti, V. J., Anda, R. F., Nordenberg, D., Williamson, D. F., Spitz, A. M., Edwards, V., Koss, M. P., & Marks, J. S. (1998). Relationship of childhood abuse and household dysfunction to many of the leading causes of death in adults: The Adverse Childhood Experiences (ACE) Study. *American Journal of Preventive Medicine, 14*(4), 245–258. https://doi.org/10.1016/S0749-3797(98)00017-8

Fernando, S. (2010). *Mental health, race and culture*. Palgrave Macmillan.

Fernando, S., Brown, T., Datta, K., Chidhanguro, D., Tavengwa, N. V., Chandna, J., Munetsi, E., Dzapasi, L., Nyachowe, C., Mutasa, B., Chasekwa, B., Ntozini, R., Chibanda, D., & Prendergast, A. J. (2021). The Friendship Bench as a brief psychological intervention with peer support in rural Zimbabwean women: a mixed methods pilot evaluation. *Global mental health, 8,* e31. https://doi.org/10.1017/gmh.2021.32

Ferrari, A. J., Charlson, F. J., Norman, R. E., Patten, S. B., Freedman, G., Murray, C. J. L., Vos, T., & Whiteford, H. A. (2013). Burden of depressive disorders by country, sex, age, and year: Findings from the Global Burden of Disease Study 2010. *PLoS Medicine, 10*(11), e1001547. https://doi.org/10.1371/journal.pmed.1001547

Fessey, V., James, G., & Pengelly, T. (2016). Mental health first aid: Equipping the nurses of the future. *British Journal of Nursing, 25*(15), 858–859. https://doi.org/10.12968/bjon.2016.25.15.858

Figgis, J. N. (1914). *The divine right of kings*. Cambridge University Press.

Figueiredo, A. R., & Abreu, T. (2020). Suicide among LGBT individuals. *European Psychiatry, 63*(Suppl. 1), S557. https://doi.org/10.1016/s0924-9338(15)31398-5

Firth, J., Siddiqi, N., Koyanagi, A., Siskind, D., Rosenbaum, S., Galletly, C., Allan, L., Caneo, C., Carney, R., Catalan, A., Chatterton, M. L., Correll, C. U., Curtis, J., Gaughran, F., Heald, A., Hoare, E., Jackson, C., Kisely, S., Lovell, K., . . . Stubbs, B. (2020). The Lancet Psychiatry Commission: A blueprint for protecting physical health in people with mental illness. *The Lancet Psychiatry, 7*(8), 675–712. https://doi.org/10.1016/S2215-0366(19)30132-4[1]

Firth, J., Torous, J., Nicholas, J., Carney, R., Pratap, A., Rosenbaum, S., & Sarris, J. (2017a). The efficacy of smartphone-based mental health interventions for depressive symptoms: A meta-analysis of randomized controlled trials. *World Psychiatry, 16*(3), 287–298. https://doi.org/10.1002/wps.20472

Firth, J., Torous, J., Nicholas, J., Carney, R., Rosenbaum, S., & Sarris, J. (2017b). Can smartphone mental health interventions reduce symptoms of anxiety? A meta-analysis of randomized controlled trials. *Journal of Affective Disorders, 218,* 15–22. https://doi.org/10.1016/j.jad.2017.04.046

Fisher, J., Cabral de Mello, M., Patel, V., Rahman, A., Tran, T., Holton, S., & Holmes, W. (2020). Prevention of perinatal and postpartum depression: What is the evidence and where should investment go? *BJOG: An International Journal of Obstetrics & Gynaecology, 127*(6), 656–659. https://doi.org/10.1111/1471-0528.16119

Fisk, W. J., Eliseeva, E. A., & Mendell, M. J. (2010). Association of residential dampness and mould with respiratory tract infections and bronchitis: A meta-analysis. *Environmental Health, 9*(1), 72. https://doi.org/10.1186/1476-069X-9-72

Fitzpatrick, K. K., Darcy, A., & Vierhile, M. (2017). Delivering cognitive behavior therapy to young adults with symptoms of depression and anxiety using a fully automated conversational agent (Woebot): A randomized controlled trial. *JMIR Mental Health, 4*(2), e19. https://doi.org/10.2196/mental.7785

Food Foundation. (2020). *Demand for free school meals rises sharply as the economic impact of COVID-19 on families bites*. https://foodfoundation.org.uk/press-release/demand-free-school-meals-rises-sharply-economic-impact-covid-19-families-bites

Foresight Mental Capital & Wellbeing Project. (2008). *Final project report*. Government Office for Science.

Fortney JC, Yellowlees P, Flick L, et al. (2015). Telepsychiatry integration of mental health services into rural primary care settings. *International Review of Psychiatry.27*(6):525–539. https://doi.org/10.3109/09540261.2015.1085838

Fortune, S., & Hawton, K. (2018). Culture and mental disorders: Suicidal behaviour. In D. Bhugra & K. Bhui (Eds.), *Textbook of cultural psychiatry* (pp. 256–274). Cambridge University Press.

Fox, J. H., Burkle, F. M., Jr., Bass, J., Pia Vaccarezza, G., Epstein, J. L., & Markenson, D. (2012). The effectiveness of psychological first aid as a disaster intervention tool: Research analysis of peer-reviewed literature from 1990–2010. *Disaster Medicine and Public Health Preparedness, 6*(3), 247–252. https://doi.org/10.1001/dmp.2012.39

Frances, A. (2013). *Saving normal: An insider's revolt against out-of-control psychiatric diagnosis*. William Morrow.

Frankish, K., Ryan, C., & Harris, A. (2012). Psychiatry and online social media: Potential, pitfalls and ethical guidelines for psychiatrists and trainees. *Australasian Psychiatry, 20*(3), 1–7. https://doi.org/10.1177/1039856212447881

Freeman, D., Loe, B. S., Chadwick, A., Vaccari, C., Waite, F., Rosebrock, L., Jenner, L., Petit, A., Lewandowsky, S., Vanderslott, S., Innocenti, S., Larkin, M., Giubilini, A., Yu, L.-M., McShane, H., Pollard, A. J., & Lambe, S. (2022). COVID-19 vaccine hesitancy in the UK: The Oxford coronavirus explanations, attitudes, and narratives survey (Oceans) II. *Psychological Medicine, 52*(14), 3127–3141. https://doi.org/10.1017/S0033291720005188

Freudenberg, N., & Ruglis, J. (2007). Reframing school dropout as a public health issue. *Preventing Chronic Disease, 4*(4), A107. https://pubmed.ncbi.nlm.nih.gov/17875251/

Furber, G., Segal, L., Leach, M., Turnbull, C., Procter, N., Diamond, M., Miller, S., & McGorry, P. (2015). Preventing mental illness: Closing the evidence-practice gap through workforce and services planning. *BMC Health Services Research, 15*, 283. https://doi.org/10.1186/s12913-015-0954-

Gaffney, H., Ttofi, M. M., & Farrington, D. P. (2021). Effectiveness of school-based programs to reduce bullying perpetration and victimization: An updated systematic review and meta-analysis. *Campbell Systematic Reviews, 17*(2), e1143. https://doi.org/10.1002/cl2.1143

Gainsbury, S. M., Russell, A., Hing, N., Wood, R., Lubman, D., & Blaszczynski, A. (2015). How the Internet is changing gambling: Findings from an Australian prevalence survey. *Journal of Gambling Studies, 31*(1), 1–15. https://doi.org/10.1007/s10899-013-9404-7

Gale, C., O'Callaghan, F., Bredow, M., Martyn, C. N., & Avon Longitudinal Study of Parents and Children Study Team. (2006). The influence of head growth in fetal life, infancy and childhood on intelligence at the ages of 4 and 8 years. *Pediatrics, 118*(4), 1486–1492. https://doi.org/10.1542/peds.2005-2629

Galea, S., Tracy, M., Hoggatt, K. J., DiMaggio, C., & Karpati, A. (2011). Estimated deaths attributable to social factors in the United States. *American Journal of Public Health, 101*(8), 1456–1465. https://doi.org/10.2105/AJPH.2010.300086

Gardiner, C., Geldenhuys, G., & Gott, M. (2018). Interventions to reduce social isolation and loneliness among older people: An integrative review. *Health & Social Care in the Community, 26*(2), 147–157. https://doi.org/10.1111/hsc.12367

Garnham, L., & Rolfe, S. (2019). *Housing as a social determinant of health: Evidence from the housing through social enterprise study*. Glasgow Centre for Population Health.

Gautam, S., Jain, A., Chaudhary, J., Gautam, M., Gaur, M., & Grover, S. (2024). Concept of mental health and mental well-being, it's determinants and coping strategies. *Indian Journal of Psychiatry, 66*(Suppl 2), S231–S244. https://doi.org/10.4103/indianjpsychiatry.indianjpsychiatry_707_23

GBD 2016 Alcohol Collaborators. (2018). Alcohol use and burden for 195 countries and territories, 1990–2016: A systematic analysis for the Global Burden of Disease Study 2016. *The Lancet, 392*(10152), 1015–1035. https://doi.org/10.1016/S0140-6736(18)31310-2

GBD 2021 Suicide Collaborators. (2025). Global, regional, and national burden of suicide, 1990–2021: A systematic analysis for the Global Burden of Disease Study 2021. *The Lancet Public Health*. Advance online publication. https://doi.org/10.1016/S2468-2667(25)00006-4

Gelfand, M. J., Raver, J. L., Nishii, L., Leslie, L. M., Lun, J., Lim, B. C., Duan, L., Almaliach, A., Ang, S., Arnadottir, J., Aycan, Z., Boehnke, K., Boski, P., Cabecinhas, R., Chan, D., Chhokar, J., D'Amato, A., Subirats, F. M, . . . Yamaguchi, S. (2011). Differences between tight and loose cultures: A 33-nation study. *Science, 332*(6033), 1100–1104. https://doi.org/10.1126/science.1197754

Gemmill, A., Catalano, R., Casey, J. A., Karasek, D., Alcalá, H. E., Elser, H., & Torres, J. M. (2019). Association of preterm births among US Latina women with the 2016 presidential election. *JAMA Network Open, 2*(7), e197084. https://doi.org/10.1001/jamanetworkopen.2019.7084

Geoffroy, M. C., Gunnell, D., & Power, C. (2014). Prenatal and childhood antecedents of suicide: 50-year follow-up of the 1958 British birth cohort study. *Psychological Medicine, 44*(7), 1245–1256. https://doi.org/10.1017/S003329171300189X

Gillham, J. E., Reivich, K. J., Freres, D. R., Chaplin, T. M., Shatté, A. J., Samuels, B., Elkon, A. G. L., Litzinger, S., Lascher, M., Gallop, R., & Seligman, M. E. P. (2007). School-based prevention of depressive symptoms: A randomized controlled study of the effectiveness and specificity of the Penn Resiliency Program. *Journal of Consulting and Clinical Psychology, 75*(1), 9–19. doi:10.1037/0022-006X.75.1.9

Gilmour, H. (2019). Sexual orientation and complete mental health statistics. *Health Reports, 30*(3), 3–10. https://doi.org/10.25318/82-003-x201901100001-eng

Glantz, M. D., Moskelwicz, J., Caldar-de-Almeida, J. M., & Degenhardt, L. (2018). Alcohol use disorders. In K. M. Scott, P. de Jonge, D. J. Stein, & R. C. Kessler (Eds.), *Mental disorders around the world* (pp. 223–242). Cambridge University Press.

Gleason, J., Ross, W., Fossi, A., Blonsky, H., Tobias, J., & Stephens, M. (2021). The devastating impact of COVID-19 on individuals with intellectual disabilities in the United States. *NEJM Catalyst Innovations in Care Delivery, 2*(2). https://catalyst.nejm.org/doi/full/10.1056/CAT.21.0051

Global Agenda Council World Economic Forum. (2017). *Seven steps to build a mentally healthy workplace*. World Economic Forum. https://www.weforum.org/agenda/2017/04/7-steps-for-a-mentally-healthy-workplace/

Gloff, N. E., LeNoue, S. R., Novins, D. K., & Myers, K. (2015). Tele-mental health for children and adolescents. *International Review of Psychiatry, 27*(5), 513–524. https://doi.org/10.3109/09540261.2015.1086322

Goergen, R., & Ndonko, F. (2025). Trust in aunties: Testimony and counselling through teenage mothers. *Comminit*. https://www.comminit.com/africa/content/trust-aunties-testimony-and-counselling-through-teenage-mothers

Goetzel, R. Z., Roemer, E. C., Holingue, C., Fallin, M. D., McCleary, K., Eaton, W., Agnew, J., & Azocar, F. (2018). Mental health in the workplace: A call to action. *Journal of Occupational and Environmental Medicine, 60*(4), 322–330. https://doi.org/10.1097/JOM.0000000000001271

Goffman, E. (1963). *Stigma: Notes on the management of spoiled identity*. Touchstone.

Goldberg, J. M., Sklad, M., Elfrink, T. R., Schreurs, K. M., Bohlmeijer, E. T., & Clarke, A. M. (2019). Effectiveness of interventions adopting a whole school approach to enhancing social and emotional development: A meta-analysis. *European Journal of Psychology of Education, 34*(4), 755–782. https://doi.org/10.1007/s10212-018-0406-9

Goldstein, E., Chokshi, B., Melendez-Torres, G. J., Rios, A., Jelley, M., & Lewis-O'Connor, A. (2024). Effectiveness of trauma-informed care implementation in health care settings: Systematic review of reviews and realist synthesis. *The Permanente Journal, 28*(1), 135–150. https://doi.org/10.7812/TPP/23.127

Gopalkrishnan, N. (2019). Cultural diversity and mental health: Considerations for policy and practice. *Frontiers in Public Health, 6,* 179. https://doi.org/10.3389/fpubh.2018.00179

Gottesman, I. I., & Shields, J. (1967). A polygenic theory of schizophrenia. *Proceedings of the National Academy of Sciences, 58*(1), 199–205. https://doi.org/10.1073/pnas.58.1.199

Gough, J. W. (1936). *The social contract: A critical study of its development.* Clarendon Press.

Grant, C., Goodenough, T., Hine, C., & Harvey, I. (2000). A randomized controlled trial and economic evaluation of a referrals facilitator between primary care and the voluntary sector. *BMJ, 320*(7232), 419–423. https://doi.org/10.1136/bmj.320.7232.419

Green, J. G., McLaughlin, K. A., Berglund, P. A., Gruber, M. J., Sampson, N. A., Zaslavsky, A. M., & Kessler, R. C. (2010). Childhood adversities and adult psychiatric disorders in the National Comorbidity Survey Replication: Associations with first onset of DSM-IV disorders. *Archives of General Psychiatry, 67*(2), 113–123. https://doi.org/10.1001/archgenpsychiatry.2009.186

Greenberg, N., Docherty, M., Gnanapragasam, S., & Wessely, S. (2020). Managing mental health challenges faced by healthcare workers during covid-19 pandemic. *BMJ,* 369, m1211. https://doi.org/10.1136/bmj.m1211

Gunnell, D., Appleby, L., Arensman, E., Hawton, K., John, A., Kapur, N., Khan, M., O'Connor, R. C., Pirkis, J., & the COVID-19 Suicide Prevention Research Collaboration. (2020). Suicide risk and prevention during the COVID-19 pandemic. *The Lancet Psychiatry, 7*(6), 468–471. https://doi.org/10.1016/S2215-0366(20)30171-1.

Gutwinski, S., Schreiter, S., Deutscher, K., Fazel, S., & Schouler-Ocak, M. (2021). The prevalence of mental disorders among homeless people in high-income countries: An updated systematic review and meta-regression analysis. *PLOS Medicine, 18*(8), e1003750. https://doi.org/10.1371/journal.pmed.1003750

Gutierrez, G., Stephenson, C., Eadie, J., Asadpour, K., & Alavi, N. (2024). Examining the role of AI technology in online mental healthcare: Opportunities, challenges, and implications—a mixed-methods review. *Frontiers in Psychiatry, 15,* 1356773. https://doi.org/10.3389/fpsyt.2024.1356773

Haas, A. P., Eliason, M., Mays, V. M., Mathy, R. M., Cochran, S. D., D'Augelli, A. R., Silverman, M. E., Fisher, P. W., Hughes, T., Rosario, M., Russell, S. T., Malley, E., Reed, J., Litts, D. A., Haller, E., Sell, R. L., Remafedi, G., Bradford, J., Beautrais, A. L., . . . Clayton,

P. J. (2011). Suicide and suicide risk in lesbian, gay, bisexual, and transgender populations: Review and recommendations. *Journal of Homosexuality, 58*(1), 10–51. https://doi.org/10.1080/00918369.2011.534038

Hale, L., & Guan, S. (2015). Screen time and sleep among school-aged children and adolescents: A systematic literature review. *Sleep Medicine Reviews, 21*, 50–58. https://doi.org/10.1016/j.smrv.2014.07.007

Hall, W. J., Chapman, M. V., Lee, K. M., Merino, Y. M., Thomas, T. W., Payne, B. K., Eng, E., Day, S. H., & Coyne-Beasley, T. (2015). Implicit racial/ethnic bias among health care professionals and its influence on health care outcomes: A systematic review. *American Journal of Public Health, 105*(12), e60–e76. https://doi.org/10.2105/AJPH.2015.302903

Hampson, E., & Siegel, S. (2017). *Mental health and employers: The case for investment.* Deloitte Monitor. https://www.deloitte.com/uk/en/services/consulting/analysis/mental-health-and-employers-the-case-for-investment.html

Hamwaka, K. (2015). A peer mental health educator model in African schools. In S. Kutcher, Y. Wei, & M. D. Weist (Eds.), *School mental health: Global challenges and opportunities* (pp. 151–155). Cambridge University Press.

Haneberg, R., Fabelo, T., Osher, F., & Thompson, M. (2016). *Reducing the number of people with mental illnesses in jail: Draft report.* Stepping Up Initiative.

Hards, E., Loades, M. E., Higson-Sweeney, N., Shafran, R., Serafimova, T., Brigden, A., Reynolds, S., Crawley, E., Chatburn, E., Linney, C., McManus, M., & Borwick, C. (2022). Loneliness and mental health in children and adolescents with pre-existing mental health problems: A rapid systematic review. *The British Journal of Clinical Psychology, 61*(2), 313–334. https://doi.org/10.1111/bjc.12331

Hariman, K. (2022). Digital psychiatry. In D. Bhugra, D. Moussaoui, & T. Craig (Eds.), *Oxford textbook of social psychiatry* (pp. 567–574). Oxford University Press.

Hariman, K., Ventriglio, A., & Bhugra, D. (2019). Use of tele-psychiatry for the management of mental health problems in migrants. In D. Bhugra (Ed.), *Oxford textbook of migrant psychiatry* (pp. 633–642). Oxford University Press.

Harrington, J. R., & Gelfand, M. J. (2014). Tightness–looseness across the 50 United States. *Proceedings of the National Academy of Sciences, 111*(22), 7990–7995. https://doi.org/10.1073/pnas.1317937111

Harris, E. C., & Barraclough, B. (1998). Excess mortality of mental disorder. *British Journal of Psychiatry, 173*(1), 11–53. https://doi.org/10.1192/bjp.173.1.11

Harris, M., & Fallot, R. D. (2001). *Using trauma theory to design service systems.* Jossey-Bass.

Hart, L. M., Mason, R. J., Kelly, C. M., Cvetkovski, S., & Jorm, A. F. (2016). 'teen Mental Health First Aid': A description of the program and an initial evaluation. *International Journal of Mental Health Systems, 10*(3). https://doi.org/10.1186/s13033-016-0034-1

Harvey, S. B., Modini, M., Christensen, H., Glozier, N., & Mykletun, A. (2021). Can work make you mentally ill? A systematic meta-review of work-related risk factors for common mental disorders. *Occupational and Environmental Medicine, 78*(6), 430–436. https://doi.org/10.1136/oemed-2016-104015

Hashimoto, N., Suzuki, Y., Kato, T., Fujisawa, D., Sato, R., Aoyama-Uehara, K., & Otsuka, K. (2016). Effectiveness of suicide prevention gatekeeper-training for university administrative staff in Japan. *Psychiatry and Clinical Neurosciences, 70*(1), 62–70. https://doi.org/10.1111/pcn.12358

Hasin, D. S., Sarvet, A. L., Meyers, J. L., Saha, T. D., Ruan, W. J., Stohl, M., & Grant, B. F. (2018). Epidemiology of adult DSM-5 major depressive disorder and its specifiers in the United States. *JAMA Psychiatry, 75*(4), 336–346. https://doi.org/10.1001/jamapsychiatry.2017.4602

Haslam, N. (2016). Concept creep: Psychology's expanding concepts of harm and pathology. *Psychological Inquiry, 27*(1), 1–17. https://doi.org/10.1080/1047840X.2016.1082418

Haslam, N., Dakin, B. C., Fabiano, F., McGrath, M. J., Rhee, J., Vylomova, E., Weaving, M., & Wheeler, M. A. (2020). Harm inflation: Making sense of concept creep. *European Review of Social Psychology, 31*(1), 254–286. https://doi.org/10.1080/10463283.2020.1796080

Haslam, N., Tse, J. Y., & De Deyne, S. (2021). Concept creep and psychiatrization. *Frontiers in Sociology, 6*, Article 806147. https://doi.org/10.3389/fsoc.2021.806147

Hatzenbuehler, M., Keyes, K., & Hasin, D. (2009). State-level policies and psychiatric morbidity in lesbian, gay, and bisexual populations. *American Journal of Public Health, 99*(12), 2275–2281. https://doi.org/10.2105/AJPH.2008.153510

Hatzenbuehler, M. L., Lattanner, M. R., McKetta, S., & Pachankis, J. E. (2024). Structural stigma and LGBTQ+ health: A narrative review of quantitative studies. *The Lancet Public Health, 9*(2), e109–e127. https://doi.org/10.1016/S2468-2667(23)00312-2

Hatzenbuehler, M. L., McLaughlin, K. A., Keyes, K. M., & Hasin, D. S. (2010). The impact of institutional discrimination on psychiatric disorders in lesbian, gay, and bisexual populations: A prospective study. *American Journal of Public Health, 100*(3), 452–459. https://doi.org/10.2105/AJPH.2009.168815

Hatzenbuehler, M., O'Cleirigh, C., Grasso, C., Mayer, K., Safren, S., & Bradford, J. (2012). Effect of same-sex marriage laws on health care use and expenditures in sexual minority men: A quasi-natural experiment. *American Journal of Public Health, 102*(2), 285–291. https://doi.org/10.2105/AJPH.2011.300382

Hatzenbuehler, M. L. (2016). Advancing research on structural stigma and sexual orientation disparities in mental health among youth. *Journal of Clinical Child & Adolescent Psychology, 46*(3), 463–475. https://doi.org/10.1080/15374416.2016.1247360

Hawkley, L. C., & Capitanio, J. P. (2015). Perceived social isolation, evolutionary fitness, and health outcomes: A lifespan approach. *Philosophical Transactions of the Royal Society B: Biological Sciences, 370*(1669), Article 20140114. https://doi.org/10.1098/rstb.2014.0114

Hawryluck, L., Gold, W. L., Robinson, S., Pogorski, S., Galea, S., & Styra, R. (2004). SARS control and psychological effects of quarantine. *Emerging Infectious Diseases, 10*(7), 1206–1212. https://doi.org/10.3201/eid1007.030703

Heaton, M. M. (2018). The politics and practice of Thomas Adeoye Lambo: Towards a post-colonial history of transcultural psychiatry. *History of Psychiatry, 29*(3), 315–330. https://doi.org/10.1177/0957154X18765422

Hechanova, R., & Waelde, L. (2017). The influence of culture on disaster mental health and psychosocial support interventions in Southeast Asia. *Mental Health, Religion & Culture, 20*(1), 31–44. https://doi.org/10.1080/13674676.2017.1322048

Heinrich, C. J., Colomer, A., & Hieronimus, M. (2023). Minding the gap: Evidence, implementation and funding gaps in mental health services delivery for school-aged children. *Children and Youth Services Review, 150,* 107023. https://doi.org/10.1016/j.childyouth.2023.107023.

Henderson, C., Evans-Lacko, S., & Thornicroft, G. (2013). Mental illness stigma, help seeking, and public health programs. *American Journal of Public Health, 103*(5), 777–780. https://doi.org/10.2105/AJPH.2012.301056

Hermosilla, S., Forthal, S., Sadowska, K., Magill, E. B., & Watson, P, & Pike, K. M. (2023). We need to build the evidence: A systematic review of psychological first aid on mental health and well-being. *Journal of Traumatic Stress, 36*(1), 5–165. https://doi.org/10.1002/jts.22888

Hessel, F. (2008). Burden of disease. In W. Kirch (Ed.), *Encyclopedia of public health* (pp. 137–138). Springer. https://doi.org/10.1007/978-1-4020-5614-7_297

Hex, N., Bartlett, C., Wright, D., Taylor, M., & Varley, D. (2012). Estimating the current and future costs of Type 1 and Type 2 diabetes in the UK, including direct health costs and indirect societal and productivity costs. *Diabetic Medicine: A Journal of the British Diabetic Association, 29*(7), 855–862. https://doi.org/10.1111/j.1464-5491.2012.03698.x

Hickman, C. (2014). Cheerfulness and tranquility: Gardens in the Victorian asylum. *The Lancet Psychiatry, 1*(7), 506–507. https://doi.org/10.1016/S2215-0366(14)00098-4

Hilton, C. (2016). Parity of esteem for mental and physical healthcare in England: A hundred years war? *Journal of the Royal Society of Medicine, 109*(4), 133–136. https://doi.org/10.1177/0141076815616089

Hilty, D. M., Ferrer, D. C., Parish, M. B., Johnston, B., Callahan, E. J., & Yellowlees, P. M. (2013). The effectiveness of telemental health: A 2013 review. *Telemedicine and e-Health, 19*(6), 444–454. https://doi.org/10.1089/tmj.2013.0075

Hilty, D. M., Chan, S., Torous, J., Luo, J., & Boland, R. J. (2015). A competency-based framework for psych/behavioral health apps for trainees, faculty, programs and health systems. *Psychiatric Clinics of North America, 42,* 513–534. https://doi.org/10.1016/j.psc.2019.05.007.

Hiscock, R., Kearns, A., MacIntyre, S., & Ellaway, A. (2001). Ontological security and psychosocial benefits from the home: Qualitative evidence on issues of tenure. *Housing, Theory and Society, 18*(1–2), 50–66. ttps://doi.org/10.1080/140360901750424761

Hjelmeland, H. (2018). Cultural aspects of suicide. In D. Bhugra & K. Bhui (Eds.), *Textbook of cultural psychiatry* (pp. 482–492). Cambridge University Press.

Hobson, W. (1949). What is social medicine? *British Medical Journal, 2*(4619), 125–130. https://doi.org/10.1136/bmj.2.4619.125

Hofstede, G. (2001). *Culture's consequences: Comparing values, behaviors, institutions, and organizations across nations.* Sage.

Holmes, J. (2021). *Tackling obesity: The role of the NHS in a whole-system approach.* King's Fund.

Holmes, J. (2023). Scotland's minimum unit pricing of alcohol: Evaluating impacts on health and inequalities. *BMJ, 380,* Article e072465. https://doi.org/10.1111/add.16185

Holt-Lunstad, J., Smith, T. B., Baker, M., Harris, T., & Stephenson, D. (2015). Loneliness and social isolation as risk factors for mortality: A meta-analytic review. *Perspectives on Psychological Science, 10*(2), 227–237. https://doi.org/10.1177/1745691614568352

Holwerda, T. J., Deeg, D. J. H., Beekman, A. T. F., van Tilburg, T. G., Stek, M. L., Jonker, C., & Schoevers, R. A. (2014). Feelings of loneliness, but not social isolation, predict dementia onset: Results from the Amsterdam Study of the Elderly (AMSTEL). *Journal of Neurology, Neurosurgery & Psychiatry, 85*(2), 135–142. https://doi.org/10.1136/jnnp-2012-302755

Hood, B. J. (2024). Qualitative insights into mental health treatment through telemedicine during the COVID-19 crisis: A natural experiment in community mental health centers. *Health & Justice, 12*(1), Article 32. https://doi.org/10.1186/s40352-024-00282-9

Hopper, K., Harrison, G., Janca, A., & Sartorius, N. (2007). *Recovery from schizophrenia: An international perspective. A report from the WHO collaborative project, the International Study of Schizophrenia.* Oxford University Press.

Hossain, D., Gorman, D., Eley, R., & Coutts, J. (2010). Value of mental health first aid training of advisory and extension agents in supporting farmers in rural Queensland. *Rural and Remote Health, 10*(4), Article 1593. https://doi.org/10.22605/RRH1593

Huberty, J., Green, J., Glissmann, C., Larkey, L., Puzia, M., & Lee, C. (2019). Efficacy of the mindfulness meditation mobile app "Calm" to reduce stress among college students: Randomized controlled trial. *JMIR mHealth and uHealth, 7*(6), Article e14273. https://doi.org/10.2196/14273

Hubley, S., Lynch, S. B., Schneck, C., Thomas, M., & Shore, J. (2016). Review of key telepsychiatry outcomes. *World Journal of Psychiatry, 6*(2), 269–282. https://doi.org/10.5498/wjp.v6.i2.269

Huddleston-Casas, C., Charnigo, R., & Simmons, L. (2009). Food insecurity and maternal depression in rural low-income families: A longitudinal investigation. *Public Health Nutrition, 12*(8), 1133–1140. https://doi.org/10.1017/S1368980008003650

Huizink, A., Mulder, E., & Buitelaar, S. (2004). Prenatal stress and risk for psychopathology: Specific effects or induction of general susceptibility? *Psychological Bulletin, 130*(1), 115–142. https://doi.org/10.1037/0033-2909.130.1.115

Husk, K., Elston, J., Gradinger, F., Callaghan, L., & Asthana, S. (2019). Social prescribing: Where is the evidence? *British Journal of General Practice, 69*(678), 6–7. https://doi.org/10.3399/bjgp19X700325

Hutner, L. A., Catapano, L. A., Nagle-Yang, S. M., Williams, K. E., & Osborne, L. M. (Eds.). (2022). *Textbook of women's reproductive mental health.* American Psychiatric Association Publishing.

Hwang, W.-C., Myers, H. F., Abe-Kim, J., & Ting, J. Y. (2008). A conceptual paradigm for understanding culture's impact on mental health: The cultural influences on mental health (CIMH) model. *Clinical Psychology Review, 28*(2), 211–227. https://doi.org/10.1016/j.cpr.2007.05.001

Hyman, S., Chisholm, D., Kessler, R., Patel, V., & Whiteford, H. (2006). Mental disorders. In *Disease control priorities related to mental, neurological, developmental and substance abuse disorders* (pp. 1–20). World Health Organization.

Institute of Medicine Committee on Nervous System Disorders in Developing Countries. (2001). *Neurological, psychiatric, and developmental disorders: Meeting the challenges in the developing world.* National Academies Press.

Jablensky, A. (2018). Schizophrenia and related psychoses. In D. Bhugra, K. Bhui (Eds.), *Textbook of cultural psychiatry* (pp. 215–231). Cambridge University Press.

Jablensky, A., Sartorius, N., Ernberg, G., Anker, M., Korten, A., Cooper, J. E., Day, R., & Bertelsen, A. (1992). Schizophrenia: Manifestations, incidence and course in different cultures: A WHO ten-country study. *Psychological Medicine Monograph Supplement, 20,* 1–97. https://doi.org/10.1017/S0264180100000904

Jain, S., & Koon, A. D. (2022). Challenges in implementing task-sharing for mental health care: A global perspective. *Social Science & Medicine, 312*, Article 115489. https://doi.org/10.1016/j.socscimed.2022.115489

Jalloh, M. F., Li, W., Bunnell, R. E., Ethier, K. A., O'Leary, A., Hageman, K. M., Sengeh, P., Jalloh, M. B., Morgan, O., Hersey, S., Marston, B. J., Dafae, F., & Redd, J. T. (2018). Impact of Ebola experiences and risk perceptions on mental health in Sierra Leone, July 2015. *BMJ Global Health, 3*(2), Article e000471. https://doi.org/10.1136/bmjgh-2017-000471

Jani, A., & Gray, M. (2019). Making social prescriptions mainstream. *Journal of the Royal Society of Medicine, 112*(11), 459–461. https://doi.org/10.1177/0141076819848304

Jelleyman, T., & Spencer, N. (2008). Residential mobility in childhood and health outcomes: A systematic review. *Journal of Epidemiology and Community Health, 62*(7), 584–592. https://doi.org/10.1136/jech.2007.060103

Jeong, H., Yim, H. W., Song, Y.-J., Ki, M., Min, J.-A., Cho, J., & Chae, J.-H. (2016). Mental health status of people isolated due to Middle East Respiratory Syndrome. *Epidemiology and Health, 38*, Article e2016048. https://doi.org/10.4178/epih.e2016048

John, P., & Rajiv, K. J. S. (n.d.). *School mental health through empowering the education system*. Peejay's CGC.

Johnson, C., Noyes, J., Haines, A., Thomas, K., Stockport, C., Ribas, A. N., & Harris, M. (2013). Learning from the Brazilian community health worker model in North Wales. *Globalization and Health, 9*, Article 25. https://doi.org/10.1186/1744-8603-9-25

Jorm, A. F., Kitchener, B. A., & Reavley, N. J. (2023). Mental health first aid training: Lessons learned from the global spread of a community education program. *World Psychiatry, 22*(1), 114–115. https://doi.org/10.1002/wps.21023

Jorm, A. F., Kitchener, B. A., Sawyer, M. G., Scales, H., & Cvetkovski, S. (2010). Mental health first aid training for high school teachers: A cluster randomized trial. *BMC Psychiatry, 10*, Article 51. https://doi.org/10.1186/1471-244X-10-51

Kaiser Family Foundation (KFF). (2023). *Racial and ethnic disparities in mental health care: Findings from the KFF survey of racism, discrimination and health*. https://www.kff.org/racial-equity-and-health-policy/issue-brief/racial-and-ethnic-disparities-in-mental-health-care-findings-from-the-kff-survey-of-racism-discrimination-and-health/

Kapuściński, R. (2009). *The other*. Verso.

Kassew, T., Tarekegn, G. E., Alamneh, T. S., Kassa, S. F., Liyew, B., & Terefe, B. (2023). The prevalence and determinant factors of substance use among the youth in Ethiopia: A multilevel analysis of Ethiopian Demographic and Health Survey. *Frontiers in Psychiatry, 14*, 1096863. https://doi.org/10.3389/fpsyt.2023.1096863

Kataoka, A., Fukui, K., Sato, T., Kikuchi, H., Inoue, S., Kondo, N., Nakaya, T., & Ito, Y. (2021). Geographical socioeconomic inequalities in healthy life expectancy in Japan, 2010–2014: An ecological study. *The Lancet Regional Health—Western Pacific, 14*, Article 100204. https://doi.org/10.1016/j.lanwpc.2021.100204

Katschnig, H. (2010). Are psychiatrists an endangered species? Observations on external and internal challenges to the profession. *World Psychiatry, 9*(1), 21–28. https://doi.org/10.1002/j.2051-5545.2010.tb00257.x

Kawakami, N., & Tsutsumi, A. (2016). The Stress Check Program: A new national policy for monitoring and screening psychosocial stress in the workplace in Japan. *Journal of Occupational Health, 58*(1), 1–6. https://doi.org/10.1539/joh.15-0001-ER

Kaymaz, N., Drukker, M., Lieb, R., Wittchen, H.-U., Werbeloff, N., Weiser, M., Lataster, T., & van Os, J. (2012). Do subthreshold psychotic experiences predict clinical outcomes in unselected non-help-seeking population-based samples? A systematic review and meta-analysis, enriched with new results. *Psychological Medicine, 42*(11), 2239–2253. https://doi.org/10.1017/S0033291711002911

Kearns, A., Hiscock, R., Ellaway, A., & MacIntyre, S. (2000). Beyond four walls: The psychosocial benefits of home: Evidence from West Central Scotland. *Housing Studies, 15*(3), 387–410. https://doi.org/10.1080/02673030050009249

Keles, B., McCrae, N., & Grealish, A. (2020). A systematic review: The influence of social media on depression, anxiety, and psychological distress in adolescents. *International Journal of Adolescence and Youth, 25*(1), 79–93. https://doi.org/10.1080/02673843.2019.1590851

Kelly, D. (2007). *Applying quality management in healthcare*. Health Administration Press.

Kelly-Irving, M., Lepage, B., Dedieu, D., Bartley, M., Blane, D., Grosclaude, P., Lang, T., & Delpierre, C. (2013). Adverse childhood experiences and premature all-cause mortality. *European Journal of Epidemiology, 28*(9), 721–734. https://doi.org/10.1007/s10654-013-9832-9

Kendler, K. S., Gardner, C. O., & Prescott, C. A. (2003). Personality and the experience of environmental adversity. *Psychological Medicine, 33*(7), 1193–1202. https://doi.org/10.1017/s0033291703008298

Kenyan, C., Sandel, M., Silverstein, M., & Wasserman, R. (2007). Revisiting the social history for child health. *Pediatrics, 120*(3), e734–e738. https://doi.org/10.1542/peds.2006-2495

Kessler, R. C., Berglund, P., Demler, O., Jin, R., Merikangas, K. R., & Walters, E. E. (2005). Lifetime prevalence and age-of-onset distributions of DSM-IV disorders in the National Comorbidity Survey Replication. *Archives of General Psychiatry, 62*(6), 593–602. https://doi.org/10.1001/archpsyc.62.6.593

Kessler, R. C., Karam, E. G., Lee, S., Bunting, B., & Nierenberg, A. A. (2018). Bipolar spectrum disorder. In K. M. Scott, P. de Jonge, D. J. Stein, & R. C. Kessler (Eds.), *Mental disorders around the world: Facts and figures from the WHO World Mental Health Surveys* (pp. 57–78). Cambridge University Press.

Kessler, R. C., McLaughlin, K. A., Green, J. G., Gruber, M. J., Sampson, N. A., Zaslavsky, A. M., Aguilar-Gaxiola, S., Alhamzawi, A. O., Alonso, J., Angermeyer, M., Benjet, C., Bromet, E., Chatterji, S., de Girolamo, G., Demyttenaere, K., Fayyad, J., Florescu, S., Gal, G., Gureje, O., . . . Williams, D. R. (2010). Childhood adversities and adult psychopathology in the WHO World Mental Health Surveys. *British Journal of Psychiatry, 197*(5), 378–385. https://doi.org/10.1192/bjp.bp.110.080499

Kessler, R. C., & Üstün, T. B. (Eds.). (2008). *The WHO World Mental Health Surveys: Global Perspectives on the Epidemiology of Mental Disorders*. Cambridge University Press.

Khadija, A. B., Mukhtar, H. O., Adam, A. M., Abdalla, A. M., Abdelgadir, A. M. H. H., & Nooraldeen, N. J. (2024). War-related trauma and posttraumatic stress disorder in refugees and internally displaced people of Sudan. *BMC Psychiatry, 24*, Article 392. https://pmc.ncbi.nlm.nih.gov/articles/PMC11529004/

Kickbusch, J., Allen, L., & Franz, C. (2016). The commercial determinants of health. *Lancet Global Health, 4*(12), e895–e896. https://doi.org/10.1016/S2214-109X(16)30217-0

Kieling, C., Baker-Henningham, H., Belfer, M., Conti, G., Ertem, I., Omigbodun, O., Rohde, L. A., Srinath, S., Ulkuer, N., & Rahman, A. (2011). Child and adolescent mental health worldwide: Evidence for action. *The Lancet, 378*(9801), 1515–1525. https://doi.org/10.1016/s0140-6736(11)60827-1

Kilian, C., Lemp, J. M., Llamosas-Falcón, L., Carr, T., Ye, Y., Kerr, W. C., Mulia, N., Puka, K., Lasserre, A. M., Bright, S., Rehm, J., & Probst, C. (2023). Reducing alcohol use through alcohol control policies in the general population and population subgroups: A systematic review and meta-analysis. *eClinicalMedicine, 59*, Article 101996. https://doi.org/10.1016/j.eclinm.2023.101996

Kim, H., Sherman, D. K., & Taylor, S. E. (2021). Culture and social support. *Perspectives on Psychological Science, 16*(1), 74–89. https://doi.org/10.1037/0003-066x

Kim, T. W., Jeong, J. H., Kim, Y. H., Kim, Y., Seo, H. J., & Hong, S. C. (2015). Fifteen-month follow up of an assertive community treatment program for chronic patients with mental illness. *BMC Health Services Research, 15*(1). https://doi.org/10.1186/s12913-015-1058-y

Kimberlee, R. (2015). What is social prescribing? *Advances in Social Sciences Research Journal, 2*, 102–110. https://doi.org/10.14738/assrj.21.808

Kingston, S. (2013). Economic adversity and depressive symptoms in mothers: Do marital status and perceived social support matter? *American Journal of Community Psychology, 52*, 359–366. https://doi.org/10.1007/s10464-013-9601-7

Kirkbride, J. B., Anglin, D. M., Colman, I., Dykxhoorn, J., Jones, P. B., Patalay, P., Pitman, A., Soneson, E., Steare, T., Wright, T., & Griffiths, S. L. (2024). The social determinants of mental health and disorder: Evidence, prevention and recommendations. *World Psychiatry, 23*(1), 58–90. https://doi.org/10.1002/wps.21160

Kirmayer, L. J., Kronick, R., & Rousseau, C. (2018). Advocacy as key to structural competency in psychiatry. *JAMA Psychiatry, 75*(2), 119–120. https://doi.org/10.1001/jamapsychiatry.2017.3897

Kirmayer, L. J., & Ryder, A. G. (2018). Culture and psychopathology. *Current Opinion in Psychology, 19*, 113–118. https://doi.org/10.1016/j.copsyc.2015.10.020

Kitchener, B. A., & Jorm, A. F. (2008). Mental health first aid: An international programme for early intervention. *Early Intervention in Psychiatry, 2*(1), 55–61. https://doi.org/10.1111/j.1751-7893.2007.00056.x

Kleinman, A. (1987). Anthropology and psychiatry: The role of culture in cross-cultural research on illness. *The British Journal of Psychiatry, 151*(4), 447–454. https://doi.org/10.1192/bjp.151.4.447

Knai, C., & Savona, N. (2023). A systems perspective on the pathways of influence of commercial determinants of health. In N. Maani, M. Petticrew, & S. Galea (Eds.), *The commercial determinants of health* (pp. 7–16). Oxford University Press.

Knapp, M., McDaid, D., & Parsonage, M. (2011). *Mental health promotion and prevention: The economic case*. Personal Social Research Unit, London School of Economics and Political Science.

Knifton, L., & Quinn, N. (2013). *Public mental health-global perspectives*. Open University Press.

Knox, J., Hasin, D. S., Larson, F. R. R., & Kranzler, H. R. (2019). Prevention, screening, and treatment for heavy drinking and alcohol use disorder. *The Lancet Psychiatry, 6*(12), 1054–1067. https://doi.org/10.1016/s2215-0366(19)30213-5

Kohn, R. (2013). *Treatment gap in the Americas* [Technical document]. Pan American Health Organization. https://www.paho.org/hq/dmdocuments/2013/TGap-in-the-Americas-Final-Vesion.pdf

Kohn, R., Saxena, S., Levave, I., & Saraceno, B. (2004). The treatment gap in mental health care. *Bulletin of the World Health Organization, 82*, 858–866. https://pmc.ncbi.nlm.nih.gov/articles/PMC2623050/

Kohrt, B. A., Asher, L., Bhardwaj, A., Fazel, M., Jordans, M. J., Mutamba, B. B., Nadkarni, A., Pedersen, G. A., Singla, D. R., & Patel, V. (2018). The role of communities in mental health care in low- and middle-income countries: A meta-review of components and competencies. *International Journal of Environmental Research and Public Health, 15*(6), Article 1279. https://doi.org/10.3390/ijerph15061279

Kontoangelos, K., Economou, M., & Papageorgiou, C. (2020). Mental health effects of COVID-19 pandemia: A Review of clinical and psychological traits. *Psychiatry Investigation, 17*(6), 491–505. https://doi.org/10.30773/pi.2020.0161

Koplan, C., & Chard, A. (2015). Adverse early life experiences. In M. Compton & R. Shim (Eds.), *The social determinants of mental health* (pp. 47–75). American Psychiatric Association Publishing.

Kowalski, R. M., Giumetti, G. W., Schroeder, A. N., & Lattanner, M. R. (2014). Bullying in the digital age: A critical review and meta-analysis of cyberbullying research among youth. *Psychological Bulletin, 140*(4), 1073–1137. https://doi.org/10.1037/a0035618

Krabbendam, L., & van Os, J. (2005). Schizophrenia and urbanicity: A major environmental influence—conditional on genetic risk. *Schizophrenia Bulletin, 31*(4), 795–799. https://doi.org/10.1093/schbul/sbi060

Krieger, N. (2014). Discrimination and health inequities. *International Journal of Health Services, 44*(4), 643–710. https://doi.org/10.2190/hs.44.4.b

Krieger, N., Rehkopf, D., Chen, J., Waterman, P. D., Marcelli, E., & Kennedy, M. (2008). The fall and rise of US inequalities in premature mortality 1960–2002. *PLoS Medicine, 5*(2), Article e46. https://doi.org/10.1371/journal.pmed.0050046

Kruse, C., Betancourt, J. A., & Gonzales, M. (2022). Leveraging mobile health to manage mental health/behavioral health disorders: Systematic literature review. *JMIR mHealth and uHealth, 10*(11), e34677. https://doi.org/10.2196/42301

Kumar, D., Bharath, S., Hirisave, U., Agarwal, S., & Shah, H. (2015). School mental health programmes in India: Current status and future directions. In S. Kutcher, Y. Wei, & M. D. Weist (Eds.), *School mental health: Global challenges and opportunities* (pp. 95–104). Cambridge University Press.

Lacy-Nichols, J., de Lacy-Vawdon, C., & Moodie, R. (2023a). Defining the commercial determinants of health. In N. Maani, M. Petticrew, & S. Galea (Eds.), *The commercial determinants of health* (pp. 209–220). Oxford University Press.

Lacy-Nichols, J., Jones, A., & Buse, K. (2023b). Taking on the commercial determinants of health at the level of actors, practices and systems. *Frontiers in Public Health, 10*, Article 981039. https://doi.org/10.3389/fpubh.2022.981039

Lamothe, M., Rondeau, É., Malboeuf-Hurtubise, C., Duval, M., & Sultan, S. (2016). Outcomes of MBSR or MBSR-based interventions in health care providers: A systematic review with a focus on empathy and emotional competencies. *Complementary Therapies in Medicine, 24*, 19–28. https://doi.org/10.1016/j.ctim.2015.11.001

Lange, K. W. (2021). Task sharing in psychotherapy as a viable global mental health approach in resource-poor countries and also in high-resource settings. *Global Health Journal, 5*(3), 120–127. https://doi.org/10.1016/j.glohj.2021.07.001

Lavis, P., & Robson, C. (2015). *Promoting children and young people's mental health and wellbeing: A whole school and college approach.* Public Health England.

Lawrence, D., & Kisely, S. (2010). Inequalities in healthcare provision for people with severe mental illness. *Journal of Psychopharmacology, 24*(Suppl. 4), 61–68. https://doi.org/10.1177/1359786810382058

Lawson, M., Butt, A. P., Harvey, R., Sarosi, D., Coffey, C., Piaget, K., & Thekkudan, J. (2020). *Time to care: Unpaid and underpaid care work and the global inequality crisis.* Oxfam.

Layard, R. (2018). *Healthy minds: A four-year course in secondary schools.* Centre for Economic Performance & London School of Economics.

Lee, A., Smith-Millman, M., McDaniel, H., Flaspohler, P., Yalo, P., & Weist, M. D. (2015). Universal schooling and mental health: Towards school mental health in Northern Ghana. In S. Kutcher, Y. Wei, & M. D. Weist (Eds.), *School mental health: Global challenges and opportunities* (pp. 186–201). Cambridge University Press.

Lee, M. (2006). *Promoting mental health and well being in later life.* Age Concern and Mental Health Foundation.

Lee, Y., Muennig, P., Kawachi, I., Hatzenbuehler, M. L., Bradway, H., & Tsai, J. (2015). Effects of racial prejudice on the health of communities: A multilevel survival analysis. *American Journal of Public Health, 105*(11), 2349–2355. https://doi.org/10.2105/ajph.2015.302776

Leitner, J. B., Hehman, E., Ayduk, O., & Mendoza-Denton, R. (2016). Blacks' death rate due to circulatory diseases is positively related to Whites' explicit racial bias: A nationwide investigation using Project Implicit. *Psychological Science, 27*(10), 1299–1311. https://doi.org/10.1177/0956797616658450

Leslie, D. (2019). *Understanding artificial intelligence ethics and safety: A guide for the responsible design and implementation of AI systems in the public sector.* The Alan Turing Institute. https://doi.org/10.5281/zenodo.3240529

Levenson, J. C., Shensa, A., Sidani, J. E., Colditz, J. B., & Primack, B. A. (2017). The association between social media use and sleep disturbance among young adults. *Preventive Medicine, 85*, 36–41. https://doi.org/10.1016/j.ypmed.2016.01.001

Leventhal, T., & Brooks-Gunn, J. (2000). The neighborhoods they live in: The effects of neighborhood residence on child and adolescent outcomes. *Psychological Bulletin, 126*(2), 309–337. https://doi.org/10.1037/0033-2909.126.2.309

Levitsky, S., & Ziblatt, D. (2018). *How democracies die.* Crown Publishing.

Liddell, C., & Guiney, C. (2015). Living in a cold and damp home: Framework for understanding impacts on mental wellbeing. *Public Health, 129*(2), 191–199. https://doi.org/10.1016/j.puhe.2014.11.007

Liebrenz, M., Stohler, R., & Nordt, C. (2014). Ethnic- and gender-specific differences in the prevalence of HIV among patients in opioid maintenance treatment: A case register analysis. *Harm Reduction Journal, 11*, Article 23. https://doi.org/10.1186/1477-7517-11-23

Lindert, J., von Ehrenstein, O. S., Priebe, S., Mielck, A., & Brähler, E. (2009). Depression and anxiety in labor migrants and refugees: A systematic review and meta-analysis. *Social Science & Medicine, 67*(12), 1891–1904. https://doi.org/10.1016/j.socscimed.2009.04.032

Link, B. G., & Phelan, J. C. (2002). McKeown and the idea that social conditions are fundamental causes of disease. *American Journal of Public Health, 92*(5), 730–732. https://doi.org/10.2105/AJPH.92.5.730

Litz, B. T., Cummings, M. H., Grunthal, B., & McLean, C. L. (2021). A public health framework for preventing mental disorders in the context of pandemics. *Cognitive and Behavioral Practice, 28*(4), 519–531. https://doi.org/10.1016/j.cbpra.2020.11.004

Liu, J., Raine, A., Venables, P. H., Dalais, C., Mednick, S. A., & Sarnoff, A. (2020). Malnutrition at age 3 years and lower cognitive ability at age 11 years: Independence from psychosocial adversity. *Archives of Pediatrics & Adolescent Medicine, 158*(3), 212–218. https://doi.org/10.1001/archpedi.157.6.593

Liu, L., Wang, J., Rosenberg, D., Zhao, H., Lengyel, G., & Nadel, D. (2018). Fermented beverage and food storage in 13,000-year-old stone mortars at Raqefet Cave, Israel: Investigating Natufian ritual feasting. *Journal of Archaeological Science: Reports, 21*, 783–793. https://doi.org/10.1016/j.jasrep.2018.08.008

Liu, X., Kakade, M., Fuller, C., Fan, B., Fang, Y., Kong, J., Guan, Z., & Wu, P. (2012). Depression after exposure to stressful life events: Lessons learned from the SARS epidemic. *Comprehensive Psychiatry, 53*(1), 15–23. https://doi.org/10.1016/j.comppsych.2011.02.003

Livingston, G., Huntley, J., Sommerlad, A., Ames, D., Ballard, C., Banerjee, S., Brayne C., Burns A., Cohen-Mansfield, J., Cooper, C., Costafreda, S. G., Dias, A., Fox, N., Gitlin, L. N., Howard, R., Kales, H. C., Kivimäki, M., Larson, E. B., . . . Mukadam, N. (2020). Dementia prevention, intervention, and care: 2020 report of the Lancet Commission. *The Lancet, 396*(10248), 413–446. https://doi.org/10.1016/S0140-6736(20)30367-6

London School of Economics (LSE). (n.d.). *A four-year course in secondary schools: Healthy minds*. https://cep.lse.ac.uk/conference_papers/2018_11_30HealthyMinds_06.pdf

Lou, H. C., Hansen, D., Nordentoft, M., Pryds, O., Jensen, F., Nim, J., & Hemmingsen, R. (1994). Prenatal stressors of human life affect fetal brain development. *Developmental Medicine & Child Neurology, 36*(9), 826–832. https://doi.org/10.1111/j.1469-8749.1994.tb08192.x

Lown, M., Lewith, G., Simon, C., & Peters, D. (2015). Resilience: What is it, why do we need it and can it help us? *British Journal of General Practice, 65*(638), e708–e710. https://doi.org/10.3399/bjgp15x687133

Lu, J. G., Lee, J. J., Gino, F., & Galinsky, A. D. (2018). Polluted morality: Air pollution predicts criminal activity and unethical behavior. *Psychological Science, 29*(3), 340–355. https://doi.org/10.1177/0956797617735807

Lund, C., Breen, A., Flisher, A. J., Kakuma, R., Corrigall, J., Joska, J. A., Swartz, L., & Patel, V. (2010). Poverty and common mental disorders in low- and middle-income countries: A systematic review. *Social Science & Medicine, 71*(3), 517–528. https://doi.org/10.1016/j.socscimed.2010.04.027

Mao, K., Wu, Y., & Chen, J. (2023). A systematic review on automated clinical depression diagnosis. *npj Mental Health Research, 2*, 20. https://doi.org/10.1038/s44184-023-00040-z

Macinko, J., & Harris, M. (2015). Brazil's Family Health Strategy delivering community-based primary care in a universal system. *New England Journal of Medicine, 372*(23), 2177–2181. https://doi.org/10.1056/NEJMp1501140

MacIntyre, S. (2007). *Inequalities in health in Scotland*. MRC Social & Public Health Sciences Unit.

Maercker, A. (2001). Association of cross-cultural differences in psychiatric morbidity with cultural values: A secondary data analysis. *German Journal of Psychiatry, 4*, 17–23.

Magdol, L. (2002). Is moving gendered? The effects of residential mobility on the psychological well-being of men and women. *Sex Roles, 47*(9–10), 553–560. https://doi.org/10.1023/A:1022025905755

Mahase, E. (2020). Long Covid could be four different syndromes, review suggests. *BMJ, 371*, m3981. https://doi.org/10.1136/bmj.m3981

Maj, M. (2010). Are psychiatrists an endangered species? *World Psychiatry, 9*(1), 1–2. https://doi.org/10.1002/j.2051-5545.2010.tb00253.x

Mak, I. W. C., Chu, C. M., Pan, P. C., Yiu, M. G., & Chan, V. L. (2009). Long-term psychiatric morbidities among SARS survivors. *General Hospital Psychiatry, 31*(4), 318–326. https://doi.org/10.1016/j.genhosppsych.2009.03.001

Malhi, G., Bassett, D., Boyce, P., Bryant, R., Fitzgerald, P. B., Fritz, K., Hopwood, M., Lyndon, B., Mulder, R., Murray, G., Porter, R., & Singh, A. B. (2015). *RANZCP clinical practice guidelines for mood disorders*. The Australian and New Zealand College of Psychiatrists, *49*(12), 1087–1206. https://doi.org/10.1177/0004867415617657.

Malhi, G., & Byrow, Y. (2018). Affective disorder coloured by culture: Why the pigment of depression is more than skin deep. In D. Bhugra & K. Bhui (Eds.), *Textbook of cultural psychiatry* (pp. 232–243). Cambridge University Press.

Malhotra, S., Chakrabarti, S., Shah, R., Gupta, A., Mehta, A., Nithya, B., Kumar, V., & Sharma, M. (2014). Development of a novel diagnostic system for a telepsychiatric application: A pilot validation study. *BMC Research Notes, 7,* 508. https://doi.org/10.1186/1756-0500-7-508

Malhotra, S., Chakrabarti, S., Shah, R., Sharma, M., Sharma, K. P., Singh, H., et al. (2015). Diagnostic accuracy and feasibility of a net-based application for diagnosing common psychiatric disorders. *Psychiatry Research, 230*(2), 369–376. https://doi.org/10.1016/j.psychres.2015.09.020

Malhotra, S., Chakrabarti, S., Shah, R., Minali Sharma, K. P. Sharma, A. Malhotra, et al. (2017). Telepsychiatry clinical decision support system used by non-psychiatrists in remote areas: Validity & reliability of diagnostic module. *Indian Journal of Medical Research, 146*(2), 196–204. https://doi.org/10.4103/ijmr.IJMR_757_15

Malhotra, S., Chakrabarti, S., & Shah, R. (2019). A model for digital mental healthcare: Its usefulness and potential for service delivery in low- and middle-income countries. *Indian Journal of Psychiatry*, 61(1), 27–36. https://doi.org/10.4103/psychiatry.IndianJPsychiatry_350_18

Mani, A., Mullainathan, S., Shafir, E., & Zhao, J. (2013). Poverty impedes cognitive function. *Science, 319*(5862), 976–980. https://doi.org/10.1126/science.1238041

Manseau, M. (2015). Economic inequality, poverty, and neighbourhood deprivation. In M. T. Compton & R. Shim (Eds.), *The social determinants of mental health* (pp. 121–144). American Psychiatric Association Publishing.

Mansoor, M. A., & Ansari, K. H. (2024). Early detection of mental health crises through artificial-intelligence-powered social media analysis: A prospective observational study. *Journal of Personalized Medicine, 14*(9), 958. https://doi.org/10.3390/jpm14090958

Marlatt, G. A. (Ed.). (1998). *Harm reduction: Pragmatic strategies for managing high-risk behaviors.* Guilford Press.

Marmot, M. (2010). *Fair society, healthy lives: Strategic review of health inequalities in England post-2010.* UCL Marmot Review.

Marmot, M. (2014). *Review of social determinants and the health divide in the WHO European region.* World Health Organization.

Marmot, M. (2015). *The health gap: The challenges of an unequal world.* Bloomsbury.

Marmot, M. (2017). The Challenge of an Unequal World: The argument. *International Journal of Epidemiology, 46*(4),1312--1318. doi: 10.1093/ije/dyx163.

Mars, B., Burrows, S., Hjelmeland, H., & Gunnell, D. (2014). Suicidal behaviour across the African continent. *BMC Public Health, 14,* Article 606. https://doi.org/10.1186/1471-2458-14-606

Marsh, A., Gordon, D., Heslop, P., & Pantazis, C. (2000). Housing deprivation and health: A longitudinal analysis. *Housing Studies, 15*(3), 411–428. https://doi.org/10.1080/02673030050009258

Marshall, M., & Lockwood, A. (2000). Assertive community treatment for people with severe mental disorders. *Cochrane Database of Systematic Reviews* (2), CD001089. https://doi.org/10.1002/14651858.CD001089.

Martinotti, G., Santacroce, R., Pettorruso, M., Montemitro, C., Spano, M. C., Lorusso, M., di Giannantonio, M., & Lerner, A. G. (2018). Hallucinogen Persisting Perception Disorder: Etiology, Clinical Features, and Therapeutic Perspectives. *Brain sciences, 8*(3), 47. https://doi.org/10.3390/brainsci8030047

Mason, M., Cho, Y., Rayo, J., Gong, Y., Harris, M., & Jiang, Y. (2022). Technologies for Medication Adherence Monitoring and Technology Assessment Criteria: Narrative Review. *JMIR mHealth and uHealth, 10*(3), e35157. https://doi.org/10.2196/35157

Marx, K. (1990). *Capital: Vol. 1*. Penguin Classics.

Massey, J., Brooks, M., & Burrow, J. (2014). Evaluating the effectiveness of Mental Health First Aid training among student affairs staff at a Canadian university. *Journal of Student Affairs Research and Practice, 51*(3), 323–336. http://dx.doi.org/10.1515/jsarp-2014-0032

Mateen, F., & Dorji, C. (2009). Healthcare worker burnout and the mental health imperative. *The Lancet, 374*(9690), 595–597. https://doi.org/10.1016/S0140-6736(09)61483-5

Matte, B., Anselmi, L., Salum, G. A., Kieling, C., Gonçalves, H., Menezes, A., Grevet, E. H., & Rohde, L. A. (2015). ADHD in DSM-5: A field trial in a large, representative sample of 18- to 19-year-old adults. *Psychological Medicine, 45*(2), 361–373. https://doi.org/10.1017/s0033291714001470

Matthews, T., Danese, A., Caspi, A., Fisher, H. L., Goldman-Mellor, S., Kepa, A., Moffitt, T. E., & Arseneault, L. (2016). Lonely young adults in modern Britain: Findings from an epidemiological cohort study. *Psychological Medicine, 46*(13), 2771–2782. https://doi.org/10.1017/s0033291718000788

Mazar, N., & Aggarwal, P. (2011). Greasing the palm: Can collectivism promote bribery? *Psychological Science, 22*(7), 843–848. https://doi.org/10.1177/0956797611412389

McCabe, O. L., Everly, G. S., Jr., Brown, L. M., Wendelboe, A. M., Abd Hamid, N. H., Tallchief, V. L., & Links, J. M. (2014). Psychological first aid: A consensus-derived, empirically supported, competency-based training model. *American Journal of Public Health, 104*(4), 621–628. https://doi.org/10.2105/AJPH.2013.301219

McCartney, G., Hearty, W., Arnot, J., Popham, F., Cumbers, A., & McMaster, R. (2019). Impact of political economy on population health: A systematic review of reviews. *American Journal of Public Health, 109*(6), e1–e12. https://doi.org/10.2105/AJPH.2019.305001

McGeachan, C., & Philo, C. (2024). Geopsychiatry from below: Exploratory review and preliminary analysis. *International Journal of Social Psychiatry, 71*(5), 511–529. https://doi.org/10.1177/00207640251317017.

McGrath, J., Saha, S., Lim, C. C. W., Gureje, O., & Florescu, S. (2018). Psychotic experiences. In K. M. Scott, P. de Jonge, D. J. Stein, & R. C. Kessler (Eds.), *Mental disorders around the world: Facts and figures from the WHO World Mental Health Surveys* (pp. 286–296). Cambridge University Press.

McGregor, B., & Holden, K. (2015). Unemployment, underemployment, and job insecurity. In M. T. Compton & R. S. Shim (Eds.), *The social determinants of mental health* (pp. 99–119). American Psychiatric Association Publishing.

McKenzie, K., & Bhui, K. (2007). Institutional racism in mental health care. *BMJ, 334*(7595), 649–650. https://doi.org/10.1136/bmj.39163.395972.80

McKnight, J., & Russell, C. (2018). The four essential elements of an asset-based community development process. asset-based community development institute. https://www.nurturedevelopment.org/wp-content/uploads/2018/09/4_Essential_Elements_of_ABCD_Process.pdf

McLaughlin, K., Hatzenbuehler, M., & Keyes, K. (2010). Responses to discrimination and psychiatric disorders among Black, Hispanic, female, and lesbian, gay, and bisexual individuals. *American Journal of Public Health, 100*(8), 1477–1484. https://doi.org/10.2105/AJPH.2009.181586

McManus, S., Meltzer, H., Brugha, T., Bebbington, P., & Jenkins, R. (2009). *Adult psychiatric morbidity in England (2007).* NHS Information Centre for Health and Social Care.

Meadows, D. H. (2008). *Thinking in systems: A primer.* Chelsea Green Publishing.

Mealer, M., Conrad, D., Evans, J., Jooste, K., Solyntjes, J., Rothbaum, B., & Moss, M. (2014). Feasibility and acceptability of a resilience training program for intensive care unit nurses. *American Journal of Critical Care, 23*(6), e97–e105. https://doi.org/10.4037/ajcc2014747

Mellman, T., David, D., Kulick-Bell, R., Hebding, J., & Nolan, B. (1995). Sleep disturbance and its relationship to psychiatric morbidity after Hurricane Andrew. *American Journal of Psychiatry, 152*(11), 1659–1663. https://doi.org/10.1176/ajp.152.11.1659

Mental Health Foundation (MHF). (2008). *What works for you?* Mental Health Foundation.

Mental Health Foundation (MHF). (2015a). *A better understanding: Psychiatry's social contract.* Mental Health Foundation.

Mental Health Foundation (MHF). (2015b). *Fundamental facts about mental health.* Mental Health Foundation.

Mental Health Foundation (MHF). (2017). *Surviving or thriving? The state of the UK's mental health.* https://www.mentalhealth.org.uk/explore-mental-health/publications/surviving-or-thriving-state-uks-mental-health

Meyer, H., Dietrich, J., & Schwartz, S. (2007). Lifetime prevalence of mental disorders and suicide attempts in diverse lesbian, gay, and bisexual populations. *American Journal of Public Health, 97*(11), 9–11. https://doi.org/10.2105/AJPH.2006.096826

Meyer, I. H. (2003). Prejudice, social stress, and mental health in lesbian, gay, and bisexual populations: Conceptual issues and research evidence. *Psychological Bulletin, 129*(5), 674–697. https://doi.org/10.1037/0033-2909.129.5.674

MHFA International. (2022). *Research evidence.* https://www.mentalhealthfirstaid.org/about/research/

Miller, E., & Thabrew, H. (2024). Universal school-based e-health interventions for wellbeing, anxiety, and depression: A systematic review and meta-analysis. *Digital Health, 10.* https://doi.org/10.1177/20552076241302204

Miller, K., & Rasmussen, A. (2010). War exposure, daily stressors, and mental health in conflict and post-conflict settings: Bridging the divide between trauma-focused and psychosocial frameworks. *Social Science & Medicine, 70*(1), 7–16. https://doi.org/10.1016/j.socscimed.2009.09.029

Miller, S. (2023). *Migrants: The story of us all.* Abacus Books.

Milne, D., & Reiser, R. P. (2017). A systematic review and reformulation of outcome-based clinical supervision: Applying the fidelity framework to the supervision of healthcare workers. *Training and Education in Professional Psychology, 11*(4), 199–208.

Mind Wellbeing Index. (2016). Cited in Hampson, E., & Siegel, S. (2017). *Mental health and employers: The case for investment.* Deloitte Monitor. https://www.deloitte.com/uk/en/services/consulting/analysis/mental-health-and-employers-the-case-for-investment.html

Munoz, M., Crespo, M., & Pérez-Santos, E. (2005). Homelessness effects on men's and women's health. *International Journal of Mental Health, 34*(2), 47–61. https://doi.org/10.1080/00207411.2005.11043400

Miranda-Ojeda, R., Wickramasinghe, A., Ntolkeras, G., Castanho, I., & Yassin, W. (2025). The Neurodiversity Framework in Medicine: On the Spectrum. *Developmental neurobiology, 85*(1), e22960. https://doi.org/10.1002/dneu.22960.

Mishara, B. L., & Weisstub, D. N. (2016). The legal status of suicide: A global review. *International Journal of Law and Psychiatry, 44,* 54–74. https://doi.org/10.1016/j.ijlp.2015.08.032

Moffat, S., Steer, M., Lawson, S., Penn, L., & O'Brien, N. (2017). Link worker social prescribing to improve health and wellbeing for people with long-term conditions: Qualitative study of service user perceptions. *BMJ Open, 7*(7), Article e015203. https://doi.org/10.1136/bmjopen-2016-015203

Moffic, S., Levin, R., & Rouse, H. (2020). The history of burnout in society, medicine, and psychiatry. In S. LoboPrabhu, R. Summers, & S. Moffic (Eds.), *Combating physician burnout: A guide for psychiatrists* (pp. 3–26). American Psychiatric Association Publishing.

Moffitt, J., Bostock, J., & Cave, A. (2014). Promoting well-being and reducing stigma about mental health in the fire service. *Journal of Public Mental Health, 13*(2), 103–113. https://doi.org/10.1108/JPMH-01-2013-0004

Mohammed, A., Sheikh, T., Poggensee, G., Nguku, P., Olayinka, A., Ohuabunwo, C., & Eaton, J. (2015). Mental health in emergency response: Lessons from Ebola. *The Lancet Psychiatry, 2*(11), 955–957. https://doi.org/10.1016/S2215-0366(15)00451-4

Mohatt, N. V., Boeckmann, R., Winkel, N., Mohatt, D. F., & Shore, J. (2017). Military Mental Health First Aid: Development and preliminary efficacy of a community training for improving knowledge, attitudes, and helping behaviors. *Military Medicine, 182*(1), e1576–e1583. https://doi.org/10.7205/MILMED-D-16-00033.

Moleiro, C. (2018). Culture and psychopathology: New perspectives on research, practice, and clinical training in a globalized world. *Frontiers in Psychiatry, 9*, Article 366. https://doi.org/10.3389/fpsyt.2018.00366

Monteith, S., Glenn, T., Geddes, J. R., Whybrow, P. C., Achtyes, E. D., & Bauer, M. (2024). Implications of online self-diagnosis in psychiatry. *Pharmacopsychiatry, 57*(2), 45–52. https://doi.org/10.1055/a-2268-5441

Moodley, R., & Lee, E. (Eds.). (2020). *The Routledge international handbook of race, ethnicity and culture in mental health*. Routledge.

Moon, G. (2009). Health geography. In R. Kitchen & N. Thrift (Eds.), *International encyclopedia of human geography* (pp. 35–48). Elsevier Science. doi:10.1016/B978-008044910-4.00338-2).

Moreno, C., Wykes, T., Galderisi, S., Nordentoft, M., Crossley, N., Jones, N., Cannon, M., Correll, C. U., Byrne, L., Carr, S., Chen, E. Y. H., Gorwood, P., Johnson, S., Kärkkäinen, H., Krystal, J. H., Lee, J., Lieberman, J., López-Jaramillo, C., Männikkö, M., Phillips, M. R., . . . Arango, C. (2020). How mental health care should change as a consequence of the COVID-19 pandemic. *The Lancet. Psychiatry, 7*(9), 813–824. https://doi.org/10.1016/S2215-0366(20)30307-2

Morgan, O., & Majeed, A. (2005). Restricting paracetamol in the United Kingdom to reduce poisoning: A systematic review. *Journal of Public Health, 27*(1), 12–18. https://doi.org/10.1093/pubmed/fdh200.

Morgan, A. J., Ross, A., & Reavley, N. (2018). Systematic review and meta-analysis of Mental Health First Aid training: Effects on knowledge, stigma, and helping behaviour. *PLoS ONE, 13*(5), Article e0197102. https://doi.org/10.1371/journal.pone.0197102

Morganstein, J. C., & Ursano, R. J. (2020). Ecological disasters and mental health: Causes, consequences, and interventions. *Frontiers in Psychiatry, 11*, 1. https://doi.org/10.3389/fpsyt.2020.00001

Mori, R., Uchino, T., Mizuno, M., Yamaguchi, T., Katagiri, N., & Nemoto, T. (2022). Effectiveness of a comprehensive mental health literacy educational programme for junior high school students: A randomised controlled trial examining changes in their knowledge, attitudes, and behaviour. *Journal of Personalized Medicine, 12*(8), Article 1281. https://doi.org/10.3390/jpm12081281

Moriarty, D. G., Zack, M. M., Holt, J. B., Chapman, D. P., & Safran, M. A. (2009). Geographic patterns of frequent mental distress: US adults, 1993–2001 and 2003–2006. *American Journal of Preventive Medicine, 36*(6), 497–505. https://doi.org/10.1016/j.amepre.2009.01.038

Morland, L. A., Pozner, J. M., Williams, K. F., Masino, T., & Thorp, S. R. (2015). Home-based clinical video teleconferencing care: Clinical considerations and future directions. *International Review of Psychiatry, 27*(6), 504–512. https://doi.org/10.3109/09540261.2015.1082986

Morris, J. N. (2010). *Minimum income for healthy living (MIHL)*. London Centre for Life-course Studies, LSHTM.

Morrish, N., Choudhury, S., & Medina-Lara, A. (2023). What works in interventions targeting loneliness: A systematic review of intervention characteristics. *BMC Public Health, 23*, Article 2214. https://doi.org/10.1186/s12889-023-17097-2

Mothibe, M., & Sibanda, M. (2019). African traditional medicine: South African perspective. In C. Mordeniz (Ed). *Traditional and complementary medicine* (pp. 1–14). IntechOpen. https://doi.org/10.5772/intechopen.83790

Muntaner, C. (2018). Digital platforms, gig economy, precarious employment, and the invisible hand of social class. *International Journal of Health Services, 48*(4), 597–600. https://doi.org/10.1177/0020731418801413.

Murray, C. J. L., & Lopez, A. D. (Eds.). (1996a). Evidence-based health policies: Lessons from the Global Burden of Disease study. *Science, 274*(5288), 740–743. https://doi.org/10.1126/science.274.5288.740

Murray, C. J. L., & Lopez, A. D. (Eds.). (1996b). *The global burden of disease: A comprehensive assessment of mortality and disability from diseases, injuries, and risk factors in 1990 and projected to 2020*. Harvard School of Public Health on behalf of WHO and World Bank.

Murray, C. J. L., & Lopez, A. D. (Eds.). (1996c). *Global health statistics*. Harvard School of Public Health on behalf of WHO and World Bank.

Nagata, J. M., Al-Shoaibi, A. A. A., Leong, A. W., Zamora, G., Testa, A., Ganson, K. T., & Baker, F. C. (2024). Screen time and mental health: A prospective analysis of the

Adolescent Brain Cognitive Development (ABCD) Study. *BMC Public Health, 24*(1), 2686. https://doi.org/10.1186/s12889-024-20102-x.

Nardodkar, R., Pathare, S., Ventriglio, A., Castaldelli-Maia, J., Javate, K. R., Torales, J., & Bhugra, D. (2016). Legal protection of right to work and employment for people with mental health problems. *International Review of Psychiatry, 28*(4), 375–384. https://doi.org/10.1080/09540261.2016.1210575

Naslund, J. A., Bondre, A., Torous, J., & Aschbrenner, K. A. (2020). Social media and mental health: Benefits, risks, and opportunities for research and practice. *Journal of Technology in Behavioral Science, 5*(3), 245–257. https://doi.org/10.1007/s41347-020-00134-x

National Association for Social Prescribing (NASP). (2023). The future of social prescribing in England - National Academy for Social Prescribing. NASP. https://socialprescribingacademy.org.uk/resources/the-future-of-social-prescribing-in-england/.

NHS England. (2024). Social Prescribing. NHS England. https://www.england.nhs.uk/personalisedcare/social-prescribing/.

National Institute for Health and Care Research (NIHR). (2020, October 15). *Living with COVID-19: A dynamic review of the evidence around ongoing COVID-19 symptoms (often called Long COVID).* NIHR Themed Review. https://evidence.nihr.ac.uk/themedreview/living-with-covid19/

National Institute for Health and Care Research (NIHR). (2018). *Supported employment helps people with severe mental illness to obtain work.* NIHR Evidence. https://evidence.nihr.ac.uk/alert/supported-employment-helps-people-with-severe-mental-illness-to-obtain-work/

National Scientific Council on the Developing Child. (2015). *Supportive relationships and active skill building strengthen foundation of resilience* [Working Paper 13]. Harvard University.

NEF Consulting. (2019). *Project Smith evaluation: Executive summary.* NEF Consulting.

NEJM Catalyst. (2017). Social determinants of health (SDOH). *NEJM Catalyst Innovations in Care Delivery.* https://catalyst.nejm.org/doi/full/10.1056/CAT.17.0312

NHS Health Scotland. (2015). *Health inequalities: What are they? How do we reduce them?—briefing.* Scottish Government.

National Institute for Health and Care Excellence. (2011). *Common mental health disorders.* https://www.nice.org.uk/guidance/cg123

National Institute on Drug Abuse (NIDA). (2024). *Co-occurring disorders and health conditions.* https://nida.nih.gov/research-topics/co-occurring-disorders-health-conditions

Nishida, A., Sasaki, T., Nishimura, Y., Tanii, H., Hara, N., Inoue, K., Yamada, T., Takami, T., Shimodera, S., Itokawa, M., Asukai, N., & Okazaki, Y. (2010). Psychotic-like experiences are associated with suicidal feelings and deliberate self-harm behaviors in adolescents aged 12–15 years. *Acta Psychiatrica Scandinavica, 121*(4), 301–307. https://doi.org/10.1111/j.1600-0447.2009.01439.x

Nitz, J., Brack, F., Hertel, S., Krull, J., Stephan, H., Hennemann, T., & Hanisch, C. (2023). Multi-tiered systems of support with focus on behavioral modification in elementary schools: A systematic review. *Heliyon, 9*(6), e17506. https://doi.org/10.1016/j.heliyon.2023.e17506

Norman, R., Byambaa, M., De, R., Butchart, A., Scott, J., & Vos, T. (2012). The long-term health consequences of child physical abuse, emotional abuse, and neglect: A systematic review and meta-analysis. *PLoS Medicine, 9*(11), e1001349. https://doi.org/10.1371/journal.pmed.1001349

Nyanfor, S., & Xiao, S. (2020). The psychological impact of the Ebola epidemic among survivors in Liberia: A retrospective cohort study. *Health Economics & Outcomes Research.* https://doi.org/10.21203/rs.3.rs-18672/v1

Obermeyer, S., Powers, B., Vogeli, C., & Mullainathan, S. (2019). Dissecting racial bias in an algorithm used to manage the health of populations. *Science, 366*(6464), 447–453. https://doi.org/10.1126/science.aax2342

O'Connell, J. (2005). *Premature mortality in homeless populations: A review of the literature.* National Healthcare for the Homeless Council.

Oken, B. S., Fonareva, I., Haas, M., Wahbeh, H., Lane, J. B., Zajdel, D., & Amen, A. (2010). Pilot controlled trial of mindfulness meditation and education for dementia caregivers. *Journal of Alternative and Complementary Medicine, 16*(10), 1031–1038. https://doi.org/10.1089/acm.2009.0733

O'Leary, A., Jalloh, M. F., & Neria, Y. (2018). Fear and culture: Contextualising mental health impacts of the 2014–2018 Ebola epidemic in West Africa. *BMJ Global Health, 3*(3), e000924. https://doi.org/10.1136/bmjgh-2018-000924

Office for Health Improvement and Disparities. (2023). *Premature mortality in adults with serious mental illness.* https://www.gov.uk/government/publications/premature-mortality-in-adults-with-severe-mental-illness/premature-mortality-in-adults-with-severe-mental-illness-smi

Office for National Statistics (ONS). (2015). *Relationship between wealth, income and personal wellbeing, July 2011–June 2012.* ONS.

Office for National Statistics (ONS). (2017). *Common mental disorders: Gov UK facts and figures.* https://www.ethnicity-facts-figures.service.gov.uk/health/mental-health/adults-experiencing-common-mental-disorders/latest/

Oishi, S., Cha, Y., Komiya, A., & Ono, H. (2022). Money and happiness: The income-happiness correlation is higher when income inequality is higher. *PNAS Nexus, 1*(5), pgac224. https://doi.org/10.1093/pnasnexus/pgac224

Ojio, Y., Ohnuma, K., Miki, T., & Sasaki, T. (2015). Development of a mental health literacy programme for secondary school students in Japan. In S. Kutcher, Y. Wei, & M. D. Weist (Eds.), *School mental health: Global challenges and opportunities* (pp. 139–150). Cambridge University Press.

Oladeji, B. D., & Gureje, O. (2016). Brain drain: A challenge to global mental health. *BJPsych International, 13*(3), 61–63. https://doi.org/10.1192/s2056474000001240

Oliver, A., Chandler, E., & Gillard, J. A. (2024). Impact of digital inclusion initiative to facilitate access to mental health services: Service user interview study. *JMIR Mental Health, 11*, e51315. https://doi.org/10.2196/51315

Oram, S., Khalifeh, H., & Howard, L. M. (2017). Violence against women and mental health. *The Lancet Psychiatry, 4*(2), 159–170. https://doi.org/10.1016/S2215-0366(16)30261-9

O'Reilly, C. L., Bell, J. S., Kelly, P. J., & Chen, T. F. (2011). Impact of mental health first aid training on pharmacy students' knowledge, attitudes and self-reported behaviour: A controlled trial. *Australian and New Zealand Journal of Psychiatry, 45*(7), 549–557. https://doi.org/10.3109/00048674.2011.585454

Organization of American States. (1948). *American declaration on the rights and duties of man.* Retrieved October 23, 2019, from https://www.ohchr.org/EN/Issues/Education/Training/Compilation/Pages/2AmericanDeclarationoftheRightsandDutiesofMan(1948).aspx

Overholt, L., Wohl, D. A., Fischer, W. A., 2nd, Westreich, D., Tozay, S., Reeves, E., Pewu, K., Adjasso, D., Hoover, D., Merenbloom, C., Johnson, H., Williams, G., Conneh, T., Diggs, J., Buller, A., McMillian, D., Hawks, D., Dube, K., & Brown, J. (2018). Stigma and Ebola survivorship in Liberia: Results from a longitudinal cohort study. *PloS one, 13*(11), e0206595. https://doi.org/10.1371/journal.pone.0206595

Ozier, E. M., Taylor, V. J., & Murphy, M. C. (2019). The cognitive effects of experiencing and observing subtle racial discrimination. *Journal of Social Issues, 75*(4), 1087–1115. https://doi.org/10.1111/josi.12349

Padgett, D. K., Henwood, B. F., & Tsemberis, S. J. (2016). *Housing first: Ending homelessness, transforming systems, and changing lives.* Oxford University Press.

Pallesen, S., Andreassen, C. S., Griffiths, M. D., Gjertsen, S. R., Krossbakken, E., Kvam, S., & Torsheim, T. (2012). Development of a Facebook addiction scale. *Psychological Reports, 110*(2), 501–517. https://doi.org/10.2466/02.09.18.PR0.110.2.501-517

Pan American Health Organization. (2014). *53rd Directing Council. 66th session of the regional committee of WHO for the Americas.* PAHO.

Park, C., Majeed, A., Gill, H., Tamura, J., Ho, R. C., Mansur, R. B., Nasri, F., Lee, Y., Rosenblat, J. D., Wong, E., & McIntyre, R. S. (2020). The effect of loneliness on distinct health outcomes: A comprehensive review and meta-analysis. *Psychiatry Research, 294,* 113514. https://doi.org/10.1016/j.psychres.2020.113514

Parsapoor, M., Koudys, J. W., & Rudzicz, F. (2023). Suicide risk detection using artificial intelligence: The promise of creating a benchmark dataset for research on the detection of suicide risk. *Frontiers in Psychiatry, 14,* 1186569. https://doi.org/10.3389/fpsyt.2023.1186569

Patalay, P., & Fitzsimons, E. (2016). Correlates of mental illness and wellbeing in children: Are they the same? Results from the UK millennium cohort study. *Journal of the American Academy of Child & Adolescent Psychiatry, 55*(9), 771–783. https://doi.org/10.1016/j.jaac.2016.05.019

Patel, V., Saxena, S., Lund, C., Thornicroft, G., Baingana, F., Bolton, P., Chisholm, D., Collins, P. Y., Cooper, J. L., Eaton, J., Herrman, H., Herzallah, M. M., Huang, Y., Jordans, M. J. D., Kleinman, A., Medina-Mora, M. E., Morgan, E., Niaz, U., Omigbodun, O., . . . UnÜtzer, J. (2018). The Lancet Commission on global mental health and sustainable development. *The Lancet, 392*(10157), 1553–1598. https://doi.org/10.1016/S0140-6736(18)31612-X

Pathare, S., Nardodkar, R., Shields, L., Bunders, J. F., & Sagade, J. (2015). Gender, mental illness and the Hindu Marriage Act, 1955. *Indian Journal of Medical Ethics, 12*(1), 7–13. https://doi.org/10.20529/IJME.2015.003

Pathare, S., Ventriglio, A., Dantas, R., & Bhugra, D. (2017). Discrimination in urban settings. In D. Bhugra (Ed.), *Mental Health and Illness in the City* (pp. 191–203). Springer. http://dx.doi.org/10.1007/978-981-10-0752-1_8-1

Patnaik, I., Sane, R., Shah, A., & Subramanian, S. V. (2023). Distribution of self-reported health in India: The role of income and geography. *PLOS ONE, 18*(1), e0279999. https://doi.org/10.1371/journal.pone.0279999

Paul, D. P., Washington, B., Robinson, A., Tonnie, M., & Coustasse, A. (2018). Telepsychiatry: Access in rural areas. In *Northeast Business & Economics Association Proceedings* (pp. 245–252). Northeast Business & Economics Association, Galloway, NJ.

Paul, K. I., & Moser, K. (2009). Unemployment impairs mental health: Meta-analyses. *Journal of Vocational Behavior, 74*(3), 264–282. https://doi.org/10.1016/j.jvb.2009.01.001

Pearce, J., Rafiq, S., Simpson, J., & Varese, F. (2019). Perceived discrimination and psychosis: A systematic review of the literature. *Social Psychiatry and Psychiatric Epidemiology, 54*(9), 1023–1044. https://doi.org/10.1007/s00127-019-01729-3

Pearson, M., Metcalfe, C., Jayamanne, S., Gunnell, D., Weerasinghe, M., Pieris, R., Priyadarshana, C., Knipe, D. W., Hawton, K., Dawson, A. H., Bandara, P., de Silva, D., Gawarammana, I., Eddleston, M., & Konradsen, F. (2017). Effectiveness of household lockable pesticide storage to reduce pesticide self-poisoning in rural Asia: A community-based, cluster-randomised controlled trial. *The Lancet, 390*(10105), 1863–1872. https://doi.org/10.1016/S0140-6736(17)31961-X

Perry, Y., Petrie, K., Buckley, H., Cavanagh, L., Clarke, D., Winslade, M., Hadzi-Pavlovic, D., Manicavasagar, V., & Christensen, H. (2014). Effects of a classroom-based educational resource on adolescent mental health literacy: A cluster randomized controlled trial. *Journal of Adolescence, 37*(7), 1143–1151. https://doi.org/10.1016/j.adolescence.2014.08.001

Persaud, A., Day, G., Bhugra, D., Castaldelli-Maia, J. M., Torales, J., Valsraj, K., Bhavsar, V., Watson, C., Clissold, E., & Ventriglio, A. (2021). CAPE Vulnerability Index. *International Review of Psychiatry,* 33(1-2), 43-55. https://doi.org/10.1080/09540261.2020.1738093.

Persaud, A., & Ventriglio, A. (2023). Why we need geopsychiatry. *International Journal of Social Psychiatry*. https://doi.org/10.1177/00207640231203529

Pescheny, J., Randhawa, G., & Pappas, Y. (2018b). Patient uptake and adherence to social prescribing: A qualitative study. *BJGP Open, 2*(3).1–12. https://doi.org/10.3399/bjgpopen18x101598

Petera, L., Rajda, T., & Ho, K.-A. (2021). Peer support programs in the fields of medicine and nursing. *Cureus, 13*(6), e15944. https://pubmed.ncbi.nlm.nih.gov/34249197/.

Pfefferbaum, B., & North, C. S. (2020). Mental health and the Covid-19 pandemic. *New England Journal of Medicine, 383*(6), 510–512.

Pinals, D. A., Hovermale, L., Mauch, D., & Anacker, L. (2022a). Persons With Intellectual and Developmental Disabilities in the Mental Health System: Part 1. Clinical Considerations. *Psychiatric Services (Washington, D.C.), 73*(3), 313–320. https://doi.org/10.1176/appi.ps.201900504.

Pinals, D. A., Hovermale, L., Mauch, D., & Anacker, L. (2022b). Persons With Intellectual and Developmental Disabilities in the Mental Health System: Part 2. Policy and Systems Considerations. *Psychiatric Services 73*(3), 321–328. https://doi.org/10.1176/appi.ps.201900505.

Public Health England (PHE). (2019). *Social prescribing: Applying all our health*. Public Health England. https://www.gov.uk/government/publications/social-prescribing-applying-all-our-health

Public Health England (PHE). (2020). *Beyond the data: Understanding the impact of COVID-19 on BAME communities*. Public Health England. https://assets.publishing

.service.gov.uk/media/5ee761fce90e070435f5a9dd/COVID_stakeholder_engagement_synthesis_beyond_the_data.pdf

Public Health England (PHE). (n.d.). *A toolkit for schools and colleges*. Public Health England. Retrieved June 13, 2020, from https://www.gov.uk

Pierce, D., Liaw, S. T., Dobell, J., & Anderson, R. (2010). Australian rural football club leaders as mental health advocates: An investigation of the impact of the Coach the Coach project. *International Journal of Mental Health Systems, 4*(10). https://doi.org/10.1186/1752-4458-4-10

Pierce, G. L., & Cleary, P. F. (2024). The persistent educational digital divide and its impact on societal inequality. *PLOS ONE, 19*(4), e0286795. https://doi.org/10.1371/journal.pone.0286795

Pierce, M. E., Mirabito, G., & Verhaeghen, P. (2024). Mind the app: More time spent on Headspace leads to beneficial day-to-day changes in mindfulness, depression, anxiety, and stress in college students. *Cogent Mental Health, 3*(1), Article 2400878. https://doi.org/10.1080/28324765.2024.2400878

Pigoni, A., Delvecchio, G., Turtulici, N., Madonna, D., Pietrini, P., Cecchetti, L., & Brambilla, P. (2024). Machine learning and the prediction of suicide in psychiatric populations: A systematic review. *Translational Psychiatry, 14*(1), 140. https://doi.org/10.1038/s41398-024-02852-9

Pinquart, M., & Sörensen, S. (2003). Differences between caregivers and noncaregivers in psychological and physical health: A meta-analysis. *Psychology and Aging, 18*(2), 250–267. https://doi.org/10.1037/0882-7974.18.2.250

Pinto, R., Ashworth, M., & Jones, R. (2008). Schizophrenia in Black Caribbeans living in the UK: An exploration of underlying causes of high incidence rate. *British Journal of General Practice, 58*(549), 429–434. https://doi.org/10.3399/bjgp08X299254

Place, S., Blanch-Hartigan, D., Rubin, C., Gorrostieta, C., Mead, C., & Kane, J. (2017). Behavioral indicators on a mobile sensing platform predict clinically validated psychiatric symptoms of mood and anxiety disorders. *Journal of Medical Internet Research, 19*(3), e75. https://doi.org/10.2196/jmir.6678

Polanczyk, G. V., Salum, G. A., Sugaya, L. S., Caye, A., & Rohde, L. A. (2015). Annual research review: A meta-analysis of the worldwide prevalence of mental disorders in children and adolescents. *Journal of Child Psychology and Psychiatry, 56*(3), 345–365. https://doi.org/10.1111/jcpp.12381

Polley, M., Bertotti, M., Kimberlee, R., Pilkington, K., & Refsum, C. (2017a). *Review of evidence assessing impact of social prescribing on healthcare demand and cost implications.* Westminster University. Retrieved from: https://www.westminster.ac.uk/file/107671/download

Polley, M., Fleming, J., Anfilogoff, T., & Carpenter, A. (2017b). *Making sense of social prescribing* [Technical Report]. University of Westminster. Retrieved from: https://westminsterresearch.westminster.ac.uk/download/f3cf4b949511304f762bdec1378442 51031072697ae511a462eac9150d6ba8e0/1340196/Making-sense-of-social-prescribing %202017.pdf

Porter, A. (2012). *Mobile pastoralism and the foundation of Near Eastern civilizations.* Cambridge University Press.

Porter, C., Favara, M., Sánchez, A., & Scott, D. (2021). The impact of COVID-19 lockdowns on physical domestic violence: Evidence from a list randomization experiment. *SSM - Population Health, 14,* 100792. https://ncbi.nlm.nih.gov/pmc/articles/PMC8080075/

Powers, R. (2015). Poor education. In M. T. Compton & R. Shim (Eds.), *The social determinants of mental health* (pp. 77–98). American Psychiatric Association Publishing.

Pressman, S. D., & Cohen, S. (2005). Does positive affect influence mental health? *Psychological Bulletin, 131*(6), 925–971. https://doi.org/10.1037/0033-2909.131.6.925

Priebe, S., Giacco, D., & El-Nagib, R. (2016). Public health aspects of mental health among migrants and refugees: A review of the evidence on mental health care for refugees, asylum seekers, and irregular migrants in the WHO European Region. WHO Regional Office for Europe.

Prince, M., Albanese, E., Guerchet, M., & Prina, M. (2014). *World Alzheimer's Report: Dementia and risk reduction.* Alzheimer's Disease International. Retrieved from: https://www.alzint.org/u/WorldAlzheimerReport2014.pdf

Prince, M., Patel, V., Saxena, S., Maj, M., Maselko, J., Phillips, M. R., & Rahman, A. (2007). No health without mental health. *The Lancet, 370*(9590), 859–877. https://doi.org/10.1016/S0140-6736(07)61238-0

Qin, X., & Hsieh, C.-R. (2020). Understanding and addressing the treatment gap in mental healthcare: Economic perspectives and evidence from China. *INQUIRY: The Journal of Health Care Organization, Provision, and Financing, 57.* https://doi.org/10.1177/0046958020950566

Qu, D., Wen, X., Cheng, X., Zhu, A., Wu, Z., Che, L., & Chen, R. (2024). School mental health prevention and intervention strategies in China: A scoping review. *The Lancet Regional Health—Western Pacific,* 53. https://doi.org/10.1016/j.lanwpc.2024.101243

Rabie, S., Poudyal, A., King, A., Ndwandwa, E. S., Marais, A., Andersen, L., Joska, J. A., & Sikkema, K. J. (2023). A supervision framework for task-shared mental health workers: Implications for clinical trials and beyond. *Global Health: Science and Practice, 11*(6), e2300092. https://doi.org/10.9745/GHSP-D-23-00092

Radparvar, S. (2023). The clinical assessment and treatment of inhalant abuse. *The Permanente Journal, 27*(2), 99–109. https://doi.org/10.7812/TPP/22.164

Rafferty, J., Abelson, J., Bryant, K., & Vachs, J. (2015). Discrimination. In M. T. Compton & R. S. Shim (Eds.), *The social determinants of mental health* (pp. 23–45). American Psychiatric Association Publishing.

Rahman, A., Malik, A., Sikander, S., Roberts, C., & Creed, F. (2008). Cognitive behaviour therapy-based intervention by community health workers for mothers with depression and their infants in rural Pakistan: A cluster-randomised controlled trial. *The Lancet, 372*(9642), 902–909. https://doi.org/10.1016/S0140-6736(08)61400-2

Rahman, A., Riaz, N., Dawson, K. S., Usman Hamdani, S., Chiumento, A., Sijbrandij, M., Bryant, R. A., & van Ommeren, M. (2016). Problem Management Plus (PM+): Pilot trial of a WHO transdiagnostic psychological intervention in conflict-affected Pakistan. *World Psychiatry, 15*(2), 182–183. https://doi.org/10.1002/wps.20312

Ramsetty, A., & Adams, C. (2020). Impact of the digital divide in the age of COVID-19. *Journal of the American Medical Informatics Association, 27*(7), 1147–1148. https://doi .org/10.1093/jamia/ocaa078

Rao, A. U., Mahendran, N., & Gopalakrishnan, C. (1989). One hundred female burn cases: A study in suicidology. *Indian Journal of Psychiatry, 31*(4), 330–333.

Reece, A. G., & Danforth, C. M. (2017). Instagram photos reveal predictive markers of depression. *EPJ Data Science, 6*, Article 15. https://doi.org/10.1140/epjds/s13688-017 -0110-z

Rêgo, X., Oliveira, M. J., Lameira, C., & Cruz, O. S. (2021). 20 years of Portuguese drug policy—developments, challenges and the quest for human rights. *Substance Abuse Treatment, Prevention, and Policy, 16*(1), 59. https://doi.org/10.1186/s13011-021 -00394-7

Rehm, J., & Shield, K. D. (2019). Global burden of disease and the impact of mental and addictive disorders. *Current Psychiatry Reports, 21*, Article 10. https://doi.org/10 .1007/s11920-019-0997-0

Reibling, N., Beckfield, J., Huijts, T., Schmidt-Catran, A. W., Thomson, K. H., & Wendt, C. (2017). Depressed during the depression: Has the economic crisis affected mental health inequalities in Europe? *European Journal of Public Health, 27*(Suppl. 1), 47–54. https://doi.org/10.1093/eurpub/ckw225

Reid, S. (2019). The rural determinants of health: Using critical realism as a theoretical framework. *Rural and Remote Health, 19*, 5184. https://doi.org/10.22605/RRH5184

Reiss, F. (2013). Socioeconomic inequalities and mental health problems in children and adolescents: A systematic review. *Social Science & Medicine, 90*, 24–31. https://doi .org/10.1016/j.socscimed.2013.04.026

Rentfrow, P. J. (2010). Statewide differences in personality: Toward a psychological geography of the United States. *American Psychologist, 65*(6), 548–558. https://doi.org/10.1037/a0018194

Rentfrow, P. J., Gosling, S. D., Jokela, M., Stillwell, D. J., Kosinski, M., & Potter, J. (2013). Divided we stand: Three psychological regions of the United States and their political, economic, social, and health correlates. *Journal of Personality and Social Psychology, 105*(6), 996–1012. https://doi.org/10.1037/a0034434

Rentfrow, P. J., Gosling, S. D., & Potter, J. (2008). A theory of the emergence, persistence, and expression of geographic variation in psychological characteristics. *Perspectives on Psychological Science, 3*(5), 339–369. https://doi.org/10.1111/j.1745-6924.2008.00084.x

Rentfrow, P. J., Jokela, M., & Lamb, M. E. (2015). Regional personality differences in Great Britain. *PLoS ONE, 10*(3), e0122245. https://doi.org/10.1371/journal.pone.0122245

Rentfrow, P. J., Mellander, C., & Florida, R. (2009). Happy states of America: A state-level analysis of psychological, economic, and social well-being. *Journal of Research in Personality, 43*(6), 1073–1082. https://doi.org/10.1016/j.jrp.2009.08.005

Repper, J., & Carter, T. (2011). A review of the impact of peer support programs on mental health service users. *Journal of Mental Health, 20*(4), 392–411. https://doi.org/10.3109/09638237.2011.583947

Ricci-Cabello, I., Meneses-Echávez, J. F., Serrano-Ripoll, M. J., Fraile-Navarro, D., Fiol-deRoque, M. A., Moreno, G. P., Castro, A., Ruiz-Pérez, I., Campos, R. Z., & Gonçalves-Bradley, D. (2020). Impact of viral epidemic outbreaks on mental health of healthcare workers: A rapid systematic review and meta-analysis. *Journal of Affective Disorders, 277*, 347–357. https://doi.org/10.1016/j.jad.2020.08.034

Richardson, T., Elliott, P., & Roberts, R. (2013). The relationship between personal unsecured debt and mental and physical health: A systematic review and meta-analysis. *Clinical Psychology Review, 33*(8), 1148–1162. https://doi.org/10.1016/j.cpr.2013.08.009.

Richardson, M., Jones, O., Wallace, C., & Williams, S. (2017). Universities and third sector working in partnership to co-deliver accredited, community mental health training. *Widening Participation & Lifelong Learning, 19*(1), 77–94. https://doi.org/10.5456/WPLL.19.1.77

Rickwood, D., Thomas, K., & Bradford, S. (2005). Help-seeking for mental health problems by young people: A review of the literature. *Medical Journal of Australia, 203*(11), 436–440. https://doi.org/10.5694/mja15.00576.

Robertson, M. B., & Walter, G. (2011). Psychiatric ethics and "new professionalism." In D. Bhugra, A. Malik, & G. Ikkos (Eds.), *Psychiatry's contract with society* (pp. 221–239). Oxford University Press.

Roest, A. M., de Jonge, P., Lim, C. C. W., Stein, D. J., Medina-Mora, M. E., & Scott, K. M. (2018). Agoraphobia. In K. M. Scott, P. de Jonge, D. J. Stein, & R. C. Kessler (Eds.), *Mental disorders around the world: Facts and figures from the WHO World Mental Health Surveys* (pp. 106–119). Cambridge University Press.

Rogers, J. P., Chesney, E., Oliver, D., Pollak, T. A., McGuire, P., Fusar-Poli, P., Zandi, M. S., Lewis, G., & David, A. S. (2020). Psychiatric and neuropsychiatric presentations associated with severe coronavirus infections: A systematic review and meta-analysis with comparison to the COVID-19 pandemic. *The Lancet Psychiatry, 7*(7), 611–627. https://doi.org/10.1016/S2215-0366(20)30203-0

Romano, G. V. S., Bazán, P. R., Sato, J. R., da Cruz, N. V. C. J., Pacifico, E. D. S., Lacerda, S. S., Kolchraiber, F. C., Frazier, T., & Kozasa, E. H. (2025). Mental health outcomes following a four week online training on social emotional and ethical learning for public school teachers. *Scientific reports, 15*(1), 9179. https://doi.org/10.1038/s41598-025-91967-0

Rose, T., Leitch, J., Collins, K. S., Frey, J. J., & Osteen, P. J. (2017). Effectiveness of Youth Mental Health First Aid USA for social work students. *Research on Social Work Practice, 29*(3), 291–302. https://doi.org/10.1177/1049731517729039

Ross, L. E., Salway, T., Tarasoff, L. A., MacKay, J. M., Hawkins, B. W., & Fehr, C. P. (2018). Prevalence of depression and anxiety among bisexual people compared to gay, lesbian, and heterosexual individuals: A systematic review and meta-analysis. *Journal of Sex Research, 55*(4–5), 435–456. https://doi.org/10.1080/00224499.2017.1387755

Rowling, L., & Mason, J. (2005). A case study of multimethod evaluation of complex school mental health promotion and prevention: The MindMatters Evaluation Suite. *Australian Journal of Guidance and Counselling, 15*(2), 125–136. https://doi.org/10.1375/ajgc.15.2.125

Royal College of General Practitioners (RCGP). (2017). *Mental health in primary care.* RCGP: London. https://www.rcgp.org.uk/representing-you/policy-areas/mental-health-in-primary-care

Royal College of General Practitioners (RCGP). (2018). *RCGP calls on government to facilitate social prescribing for all practices.* RCPG: London. https://www.rcgp.org.uk/about-us/news/2018/may/rcgp-calls-on-government-to-facilitate-social-prescribing-for-all-practices.aspx

Royal College of Physicians and Surgeons of Canada. (2015). *The CanMEDS physician competency framework.* https://www.royalcollege.ca/content/dam/document/standards-and-accreditation/2015-canmeds-framework-reduced-e.pdf

Royal College of Psychiatrists. (2017). *Core values for psychiatrists.* RCPsych Publications.

Ruiz, L., & Strain, E. (Eds.). (2021). *Lowinson and Ruiz's substance abuse: A comprehensive textbook* (6th ed.). Wolters Kluwer.

Ruscio, A. M., Hallion, L. S., Demyttenaere, K., Lee, S., & Lim, C. C. W. (2018). Generalized anxiety disorder. In K. M. Scott, P. de Jonge, D. J. Stein, & R. C. Kessler (Eds.), *Mental disorders around the world: Facts and figures from the WHO World Mental Health Surveys* (pp. 79–92). Cambridge University Press.

Russell, S. T., & Fish, J. N. (2016). Mental health in lesbian, gay, bisexual, and transgender (LGBT) youth. *Annual Review of Clinical Psychology, 12*, 465–487. https://doi.org/10.1146/annurev-clinpsy-021815-093153

Ryff, C. D. (1989). Happiness is everything, or is it? Explorations on the meaning of psychological well-being. *Journal of Personality and Social Psychology, 57*(6), 1069–1081. https://doi.org/10.1037/0022-3514.57.6.1069

Ryu, S., & Fan, L. (2023). The relationship between financial worries and psychological distress among US adults. *Journal of Preventive Medicine and Public Health, 55*(1), 58–67 . https://www.ncbi.nlm.nih.gov/pmc/articles/PMC8806009/

Sabin, J. E., & Skimming, K. (2015). A framework of ethics for telepsychiatry practice. *International Review of Psychiatry, 27*(6), 490–495. https://doi.org/10.3109/09540261.2015.1094034

Sagar, R., Pattanayak, R. D., Chandrasekaran, R., & Chaudhury, P. K. (2017). Twelve-month prevalence and treatment gap for common mental disorders: Findings from a large-scale epidemiological survey in India. *Indian Journal of Psychiatry, 59*(1), 46–55. https://doi.org/10.4103/psychiatry.IndianJPsychiatry_333_16

Saha, S., Scott, J., Varghese, D., & McGrath, J. (2011b). The association between physical health and delusionlike experiences: A general population study. *PLOS ONE, 6*(4), e18566. https://doi.org/10.1371/journal.pone.0018566

Saha, S., Scott, J., Varghese, D., McGrath, J., & Fonseca, L. (2011a). The association between delusion-like experiences and suicidal thoughts and behaviours. *Schizophrenia Research, 132*(2–3), 197–202. https://doi.org/10.1016/j.schres.2011.07.012

Saha, S., Varghese, D., Slade, T., Degenhardt, L., Mills, K., McGrath, J., & Scott, J. (2011c). The association between trauma and delusional-like experiences. *Psychiatry Research, 189*(2), 259–264. https://doi.org/10.1016/j.psychres.2011.03.019

Said, E. (1978). *Orientalism*. Pantheon Books.

Salmoiraghi, A., & Hussain, S. (2015). A systematic review of the use of telepsychiatry in acute settings. *Journal of Psychiatric Practice*, 21(5), 389–393. https://doi.org/10.1097/PRA.0000000000000103

Sanchez, A. L., Cornacchio, D., Poznanski, B., Golik, A. M., Chou, T., & Comer, J. (2018). The effectiveness of school-based mental health services for elementary-aged children: A meta-analysis. *Journal of the American Academy of Child & Adolescent Psychiatry, 57*(3), 153–165. https://doi.org/10.1016/j.jaac.2017.11.022

Sanders, M. R. (1999). Triple P-Positive Parenting Program: Towards an empirically validated multilevel parenting and family support strategy for the prevention of behavior and emotional problems in children. *Clinical Child and Family Psychology Review, 2*(2), 71–90. https://doi.org/10.1023/A:1021843613840

Sangraula, M., Turner, E. L., Luitel, N. P., van't Hof, E., Shrestha, P., Ghimire, R., Bryant, R. A., Kohrt, B. A., & Jordans, M. J. D. (2021). Feasibility of Group Problem Management Plus (PM+) to improve mental health and functioning of adults in earthquake-affected communities in Nepal. *Epidemiology and Psychiatric Sciences, 30*, e15. https://doi.org/10.1017/S2045796020001189

Santiago, C. D., Sosa, S., Raviv, T., Flores, R., Donis, A., Jolie, S., Bustos, Y., Elahi, S., Ford-Paz, R., Ramos, B., Cicchetti, C., Torres, S., Zarzour, H., & Kang, S. (2025). Supporting Transition Resilience Among Newcomer Groups (STRONG): Examining effectiveness and acceptability in urban public schools. *American Journal of Community Psychology*. 75: 237–251. https://doi.org/10.1002/ajcp.12777

Santini, Z. I., Jose, P. E., Cornwell, E. Y., Koyanagi, A., Nielsen, L., Hinrichsen, C., Meilstrup, C., Madsen, K. R., & Koushede, V. (2020). Social disconnectedness, perceived isolation, and symptoms of depression and anxiety among older Europeans. *Social Psychiatry and Psychiatric Epidemiology, 55*(7), 973–985. https://doi.org/10.1007/s00127-020-01848-9

Sareen, J., Afifi, T., McMillan, K., & Asmundson, G. (2011). Relationship between household income and mental disorders: Findings from a population-based longitudinal study. *Archives of General Psychiatry, 68*(4), 419–427. https://doi.org/10.1001/archgenpsychiatry.2011.15

Sartorius, N. (2002). *Fighting for mental health.* Cambridge University Press.

Sartorius, N., Jablensky, A., Gulbinat, W., & Ernberg, G. (1980). WHO collaborative study: Assessment of depressive disorders. *Psychological Medicine, 10*(4), 743–749. https://doi.org/10.1017/S0033291700055033

Sartorius, N., Shapiro, R., & Jablensky, A. (1974). The International Pilot Study of Schizophrenia. *Schizophrenia Bulletin,* 1(11), 21–34. https://doi.org/10.1093/schbul/1.11.21.

Sarvet, B., Gold, J., & Straus, J.H. (2011). Bridging the divide between child psychiatry and primary care: The use of telephone consultation within a population-based collaborative system. *Child and Adolescent Psychiatric Clinics of North America, 20*(1), 41–53. https://doi.org/10.1016/j.chc.2010.08.009

Schifano, F., Napoletano, F., Chiappini, S., Guirguis, A., Corkery, J. M., Bonaccorso, S., Ricciardi, A., Scherbaum, N., & Vento, A. (2021). New/emerging psychoactive substances and associated psychopathological consequences. *Psychological Medicine, 51*(1), 30–42. https://doi.org/10.1017/S0033291719001727

Schmeck, K., Schlüter-Müller, S., Foelsch, P. A., & Doering, S. (2013). The role of identity in the DSM-5 classification of personality disorders. *Child and Adolescent Psychiatry and Mental Health, 7*(1), 27. https://doi.org/10.1186/1753-2000-7-27

Schmeckenbecher, J., Kapusta, N. D., Krausz, R. M., & Emilian, C. A. (2024). Autopsy rates and the misclassification of suicide and accident deaths. *European Journal of Epidemiology, 39*(10), 1109–1126. https://doi.org/10.1007/s10654-024-011142-4

Schulz, R., & Sherwood, P. R. (2008). Physical and mental health effects of family caregiving. *American Journal of Nursing, 108*(Suppl. 9), 23–27https://doi.org/10.1097/01.NAJ.0000336406.45248.4c

Schuster, M., McGlynn, E., Pham, C., Spar, M., & Brook, R. (2001). The quality of healthcare in the US: A review of articles. In Institute of Medicine, *Crossing the quality chasm: A new health system for the 21st century (Chapter 2).* Washington (DC): National Academies Press. https://doi.org/10.17226/10027.

Schwartz, R. C., & Blankenship, D. M. (2014). Racial disparities in psychotic disorder diagnosis: A review of empirical literature. *World Journal of Psychiatry, 4*(4), 133–140. https://doi.org/10.5498/wjp.v4.i4.133

Schweinhart, L., Montie, J., Xiang, Z., Barnett, W. S., Belfield, C. R., & Nores, M. (2005). *The High/Scope Perry Preschool study through age 40: Summary, conclusions and FAQs.* HighScope Educational Research Foundation.

Scott, K. M., Stein, D. J., de Jonge, P., & Kessler, R. C. (2018). Discussion. In K. M. Scott, P. De Jonge, D. J. Stein, & R. C. Kessler (Eds.), *Mental disorders around the world* (pp. 324–336). Cambridge University Press.

Scott, S., Sylva, K., Doolan, M., Price, J., Jacobs, B., Crook, C., & Landau, S. (2010). Randomised controlled trial of parent groups for child antisocial behaviour targeting multiple risk factors: The SPOKES project. *Journal of Child Psychology & Psychiatry, 51*(1), 48–57. https://doi.org/10.1111/j.1469-7610.2009.02127.x

Secor, A., Macauley, R., Stan, L., Kagone, M., Sidibe, S., Sow, S., Aronovich, D., Litvin, K., Davis, N., Alva, S., & Sanderson, J. (2020). Mental health among Ebola survivors in Liberia, Sierra Leone and Guinea: Results from a cross-sectional study. *BMJ Open, 10*(5), e035217. https://doi.org/10.1136/bmjopen-2019-035217

Seedat, S., Scott, K. M., Angermeyer, M. C., Berglund, P., Bromet, E. J., Brugha, T. S., Demyttenaere, K., de Girolamo, G., Haro, J. M., Jin, R., Karam, E. G., Kovess-Masfety, V., Levinson, D., Medina Mora, M. E., Ono, Y., Ormel, J., Pennell, B. E., Posada-Villa, J., Sampson, N. A., . . . Kessler, R. C. (2009). Cross-national associations between gender and mental disorders in the WHO World Mental Health Surveys. *Archives of General Psychiatry, 66*(7), 785–795. https://doi.org/10.1001/archgenpsychiatry.2009.36

Seiferth, C., Vogel, L., Aas, B., Aas, E., Bäcke, J., Boorsma, C., Bredenoord, A. L., Cuijpers, P., De Gier, B., Hoogendijk, W. J. G., Holtmann, M., Koch, S., Peetoom, K., Schuurmans, J., & Schaub, M. P. (2023). How to e-mental health: A guideline for researchers and practitioners using digital technology in the context of mental health. *Nature Mental Health, 1*, 542–554. https://doi.org/10.1038/s44220-023-00085-1

Semlyen, J., King, M., Varney, J., & Hagger-Johnson, G. (2016). Sexual orientation and symptoms of common mental disorder or low wellbeing: Combined meta-analysis of 12 UK population health surveys. *BMC Psychiatry, 16*(1), 67. https://doi.org/10.1186/s12888-016-0767-z

Seresinhe, C. I., Preis, T., MacKerron, G., & Moat, H. S. (2019). Happiness is greater in more scenic locations. *Scientific Reports, 9*, 4498. https://doi.org/10.1038/s41598-019-40854-6

Shaw, M. (2004). Housing and public health. *Annual Review of Public Health, 25*, 397–418. https://doi.org/10.1146/annurev.publhealth.25.101802.123036

Shea, T., Sripipatana, A., & Shin, P. (2022). Racial and ethnic inequities in inpatient psychiatric civil commitment. *Psychiatric Services, 73*(12), 1322–1329. https://doi.org/10.1176/appi.ps.202100342

Sher, L. (2020). The impact of the COVID-19 pandemic on suicide rates. *QJM: An International Journal of Medicine, 113*(10), 707–712. https://doi.org/10.1093/qjmed/hcaa202

Shereen, M. A., Khan, S., Kazmi, A., Bashir, N., & Siddique, R. (2020). COVID-19 infection: Origin, transmission, and characteristics of human coronaviruses. *Journal of Advanced Research, 24*, 91–98. https://doi.org/10.1016/j.jare.2020.03.005

Shields, L., Chauhan, P., Bakre, R., Hamlai, M., Lynch, D., & Bunders, J. (2016). How can mental health and faith-based practitioners work together? A case study of collaborative mental health in Gujarat, India. *Transcultural Psychiatry, 53*(3), 368–391. https://doi.org/10.1177/1363461516649835

Shifrin, N. V., & Michel, J. S. (2021). Flexible work arrangements and employee health: A meta-analytic review. *Work & Stress, 36*(1), 60–85. https://doi.org/10.1080/02678373.2021.1936287

Shim, R., Compton, M., Mauseau, M., Koplan, C., Langheim, F., & Powers, R. (2015). Overview of the social determinants of mental health. In M. T. Compton & R. Shim (Eds.), *The social determinants of mental health*. American Psychiatric Association Publishing.

Shim, R. S., & Vinson, S. Y. (2021). *Social (in)justice and mental health*. American Psychiatric Association Publishing.

Shinde, S., Weiss, H. A., Varghese, B., Khandeparkar, P., Pereira, B., Sharma, A., Gupta, R., Ross, D. A., Patton, G., & Patel, V. (2018). Promoting school climate and health outcomes with the SEHER multi-component secondary school intervention in Bihar, India: A cluster-randomised controlled trial. *The Lancet, 392*(10163), 2465–2477. https://doi.org/10.1016/S0140-6736(18)31615-5

Shore, J. H. (2015a). The technological transformation of psychiatric care—Telepsychiatry comes of age. *International Review of Psychiatry, 27*(6), 467–468. https://doi.org/10.3109/09540261.2015.1120008

Shore, J. H. (2015b). The evolution and history of telepsychiatry and its impact on psychiatric care: Current implications for psychiatrists and psychiatric organizations. *International Review of Psychiatry, 27*(6), 469–475. https://doi.org/10.3109/09540261.2015.1072086

Shultz, J., Baingana, F., & Neria, Y. (2014). The 2014 Ebola outbreak and mental health: Current status and recommended response. *JAMA, 313*(6), 576–568. https://doi.org/10.1001/jama.2014.17934

Shultz, J., Cooper, J., Baingana, F., Oquendo, M. A., Espinel, Z., Althouse, B. M., Marcelin, L. H., Towers, S., Espinola, M., McCarten, J. M., N'zi, I., Musani, S., Rechkemmer, A., Mazur, L., & Reifels, L. (2016). The role of fear-related behaviors in the 2013–2016 West Africa Ebola virus disease outbreak. *Current Psychiatry Reports, 18*(11), Article 104. https://doi.org/10.1007/s11920-016-0741-y

Shultz, J. M., & Forbes, D. (2014). Psychological first aid: Rapid proliferation and the search for evidence. *Disaster Health, 2*(1), 3–12. https://doi.org/10.4161/dish.26006

Silove, D., Ventevogel, P., & Rees, S. (2017). The contemporary refugee crisis: An overview of mental health challenges. *World Psychiatry, 16*(2), 130–139. https://doi.org/10.1002/wps.20438

Simms, L., Ottman, K. E., Griffith, J. L., Knight, M. G., Norris, L., Karakcheyeva, V., & Kohrt, B. A. (2023). Psychosocial peer support to address mental health and burnout of health care workers affected by COVID-19: A qualitative evaluation. *International Journal of Environmental Research and Public Health*, 20(5), 4536. https://doi.org/10.3390/ijerph20054536.

Simmons, L., Braun, B., Charnigo, R., Havens, J. R., & Crosby, R. A. (2008). Depression and poverty among rural women: A relationship of social causation or social selection? *Journal of Rural Health, 24*(3), 292–298. https://doi.org/10.1111/j.1748-0361.2008.00171.x

Sisto, A., Vicinanza, F., Campanozzi, L. L., Ricci, G., Tartaglini, D., & Tambone, V. (2019). Towards a transversal definition of psychological resilience: A literature review. *Medicina, 55*(11), Article 745. https://doi.org/10.3390/medicina55110745

Skaalvik, E. M., & Skaalvik, S. (2016). Teacher stress and teacher self-efficacy as predictors of engagement, emotional exhaustion, and motivation to leave the teaching profession. *Creative Education, 8*(12), 1997–2005. https://doi.org/10.4236/ce.2016.713182

Smith, G. L., Banting, L., Eime, R., O'Sullivan, G., & van Uffelen, J. G. Z. (2017). The association between social support and physical activity in older adults: A systematic review. *International Journal of Behavioral Nutrition and Physical Activity, 14,* Article 56. https://doi.org/10.1186/s12966-017-0509-8

Smith, P. B., Fischer, R., & Vignoles, V. L. (2018). *Understanding social psychology across cultures: Engaging with others in a changing world.* Sage.

Smith, P. J., & Merwin, R. M. (2021). The role of exercise in management of mental health disorders: An integrative review. *Annual Review of Medicine, 72,* 45–62. https://doi.org/10.1146/annurev-med-060619-022943

Smokowski, P. R., Cotter, K. L., Robertson, C. I. B., & Guo, S. (2013). Anxiety and aggression in rural youth: Baseline results from the Rural Adaptation Project. *Child Psychiatry & Human Development, 44*(4), 479–492. https://doi.org/10.1007/s10578-012-0342-x

Sollberger, D. (2013). On identity: From a philosophical point of view. *Child and Adolescent Psychiatry and Mental Health, 7,* Article 29. https://doi.org/10.1186/1753-2000-7-29

Sourander, A., Jensen, P., Rönning, J. A., Niemelä, S., Helenius, H., Sillanmäki, L., Kumpulainen, K., Piha, J., Tamminen, T., Moilanen, I., & Almqvist, F. (2007). What is the early adulthood outcome of boys who bully or are bullied in childhood? The Finnish "From a Boy to a Man" study. *Pediatrics, 120*(2), 397–404. https://doi.org/10.1542/peds.2006-2704

South, J., Higgins, T. J., Woodall, J., & White, S. M. (2008). Can social prescribing provide the missing link? *Primary Health Care Research & Development, 9*(4), 310–318. https://doi.org/10.1017/S146342360800087X

Southwick, S. M., & Charney, D. S. (2012). The science of resilience: Implications for the prevention and treatment of depression. *Science, 338*(6103), 79–82. https://doi.org/10.1126/science.1222942

Sow, S., Desclaux, A., Taverne, B., Ndawinz, J. D. A., Faye, S. L., Diop, M., Diallo, P. D., Doukouré, M., Setbon, M., Dieng, A. B., Traoré, M., Cissokho, S., Sarr, F., & Msellati, P. (2016). Ebola in Guinea: Experience of stigma among health professional survivors. *Bulletin de la Société de Pathologie Exotique, 109*(5), 309–313. https://doi.org/10.1007/s13149-016-0510-5

Stack, S., & Kposowa, A. J. (2011). Religion and suicide acceptability: A cross-national analysis. *Journal for the Scientific Study of Religion, 50*(2), 289–306. https://doi.org/10.1111/j.1468-5906.2011.01568.x

Staszak, J.-F. (2009). Other/otherness. In R. Kitchin & N. Thrift (Eds.), *International encyclopedia of human geography* (pp. 43–47). Elsevier Science. https://doi.org/10.1016/B978-008044910-4.00980-9

Statista. (2022). *Number of mHapps available in the Google Play Store from 1st quarter 2015 to third quarter 2022.* https://www.statista.com/statistics/779919/health-apps-available-google-play-worldwide/

Stein, D. J., Kawakami, N., de Girolamo, G., & Lepine, J. P. (2018). Social anxiety disorder. In K. M. Scott, P. de Jonge, D. J. Stein, & R. C. Kessler (Eds.), *Mental disorders around the world* (pp. 120–133). Cambridge University Press. https://doi.org/10.1017/9781316336168.009

Stewart-Brown, S. (2005). Interpersonal relationships and the origins of mental health. *Journal of Public Mental Health, 4*(1), 26–30. https://doi.org/10.1108/17465729200500007

Stickley, A., Oh, H., Sumiyoshi, T., Narita, Z., DeVylder, J., Jacob, L., Waldman, K., & Koyanagi, A. (2019). Perceived discrimination and psychotic experiences in the English general population. *European Psychiatry, 62*, 50–57. https://doi.org/10.1016/j.eurpsy.2019.08.004

Stoicea, N., Costa, A., Periel, L., Uribe, A., Weaver, T., & Bergese, S. D. (2019). Current perspectives on the opioid crisis in the US healthcare system: A comprehensive literature review. *Medicine, 98*(20), Article e15425. https://doi.org/10.1097/MD.0000000000015425

Stormshak, E. A., & Dishion, T. J. (2009). A school-based, family-centered intervention to prevent substance use: The Family Check-Up. *American Journal of Drug and Alcohol Abuse, 35*(4), 227–232. https://doi.org/10.1080/00952990903005908

Strauss, A. (2017). *Mirrors and masks: The search for identity*. Routledge. https://doi.org/10.4324/9781315124582

Stuckler, D., & Basu, S. (2013). *The body economic: Why austerity kills*. Basic Books.

Subedi, P., Li, C., Gurung, A., Bizune, D., Dogbey, M. C., Johnson, C. C., & Yun, K. (2015). Mental health first aid training for the Bhutanese refugee community in the United States. *International Journal of Mental Health Systems, 9*, Article 20. https://doi.org/10.1186/s13033-015-0012-z

Substance Abuse and Mental Health Services Administration (SAMHSA). (2021). *Treatment for stimulant use disorders: Updated 2021*. US Department of Health and Human Services.

Sudhinaraset, M., Wigglesworth, C., & Takeuchi, D. T. (2016). Social and cultural contexts of alcohol use: Influences in a social–ecological framework. *Alcohol Research: Current Reviews, 38*(1), 35–45. PMID: 27159810.

Suglia, S. F., Chambers, E. C., & Sandel, M. T. (2015). Poor housing quality and housing instability. In M. T. Compton & R. S. Shim (Eds.), *The social determinants of mental health* (pp. 171–192). American Psychiatric Association Publishing.

Suijkerbuijk, Y. B., Schaafsma, F. G., Krupa, T., Regeer, B. J., van Mechelen, W., & Anema, J. R. (2017). Interventions for obtaining and maintaining employment in adults with severe mental illness: A network meta-analysis. *Cochrane Database of Systematic Reviews, (9),* Article CD011867. https://doi.org/10.1002/14651858.CD011867.pub2

Sunderji, N., Crawford, A., & Jovanovic, M. (2015). Telepsychiatry in graduate medical education: A narrative review. *Academic Psychiatry, 39*(1), 55–62. https://doi.org/10.1007/s40596-014-0176-x

Sze, S., Pan, D., Nevill, C. R., Gray, L. J., Martin, C. A., Nazareth, J., Minhas, J. S., Divall, P., Khunti, K., Abrams, K. R., Nellums, L. B., & Pareek, M. (2020). Ethnicity and clinical outcomes in COVID-19: A systematic review and meta-analysis. *eClinicalMedicine, 29–30,* Article 100630. https://doi.org/10.1016/j.eclinm.2020.100630

Taleban, R., Zamani, A., Moafi, M., Jiryaee, N., & Khadivi, R. (2016). Applications of text messaging and bibliotherapy for treatment of patients affected by depressive symptoms. *International Journal of Preventive Medicine, 7,* Article 46. https://doi.org/10.4103/2008-7802.177889

Talge, N. M., Neal, C., & Glover, V. (2007). Antenatal maternal stress and long-term effects on child neurodevelopment: How and why? *Journal of Child Psychology and Psychiatry, 48*(3–4), 245–261. https://doi.org/10.1111/j.1469-7610.2006.01714.x

Teicher, M. H., & Samson, J. A. (2016). Annual research review: Enduring neurobiological effects of childhood abuse and neglect. *Journal of Child Psychology and Psychiatry, 57*(3), 241–266. https://doi.org/10.1111/jcpp.12507

Thara, R., Kamath, S., & Kumar, S. (2003a). Women with schizophrenia and broken marriages: Doubly disadvantaged? Part II: Family perspective. *International Journal of Social Psychiatry, 49*(3), 233–240. https://doi.org/10.1177/00207640030493009

Thara, R., Kamath, S., & Kumar, S. (2003b). Women with schizophrenia and broken marriages—Doubly disadvantaged? Part I: Patient perspective. *International Journal of Social Psychiatry, 49*(3), 225–232. https://doi.org/10.1177/00207640030493008

Thara, R., Padmavati, R., & Srinivasan, T. N. (2004). Focus on psychiatry in India. *British Journal of Psychiatry, 184*(4), 366–373. https://doi.org/10.1192/bjp.184.4.366

Thara, R., & Patel, V. (2010). Role of non-governmental organizations in mental health in India. *Indian Journal of Psychiatry, 52*(Suppl. 1), S389–S395. https://doi.org/10.4103/0019-5545.69276

Thirunavurakasu, M., Thirunavukarasu, P., & Bhugra, D. (2013). Concepts of mental health: definitions and challenges. *International Journal of Social Psychiatry, 59*(3), 197–198. https://doi.org/10.1177/0020764011422006.

Thomas, B., Dorling, D., & Davey Smith, G. (2010). Inequalities in premature mortality in Britain: Observational study from 1921–2007. *BMJ, 341,* Article c3639. https://doi.org/10.1136/bmj.c3639

Thomeer, M. B., Moody, M. D., & Yahirun, J. (2023). Racial and ethnic disparities in mental health and mental health care during the COVID-19 pandemic. *Journal of Racial and Ethnic Health Disparities, 10*(2), 961–976. https://doi.org/10.1007/s40615-022-01284-9

Thomson, H., Thomas, S., Sellström, E., & Petticrew, M. (2013). Housing improvements for health and associated socio-economic outcomes. *Cochrane Database of Systematic Reviews, 28*(2), Article CD008657. https://doi.org/10.1002/14651858.CD008657.pub2

Thornicroft, G. (2011). Physical health disparities and mental illness: the scandal of premature mortality. *British Journal of Psychiatry, 199*(6), 441–442. https://doi.org/10.1192/bjp.bp.111.092718

Thorson, A., Formenty, P., Lofthouse, C., & Broutet, N. (2016). Systematic review of the literature on viral persistence and sexual transmission from recovered Ebola survivors: Evidence and recommendations. *BMJ Open, 6*(1), Article e008859. https://doi.org/10.1136/bmjopen-2015-008859

Tidy, C. (2015). *Occupational burnout.* Patient.info. Retrieved October 23, 2020, from http://patient.info/doctor/occupational-burnout#ref3

Tkacz, J., & Brady, B. (2021). Increasing rate of diagnosed childhood mental illness in the United States: Incidence, prevalence and costs. *Public Health in Practice, 2,* Article 100204. https://doi.org/10.1016/j.puhip.2021.100204

Todman, L. C., & Holliday, C. (2015). Adverse features of built environment. In M. T. Compton & R. S. Shim (Eds.), *The social determinants of mental health* (pp. 193–212). American Psychiatric Association Publishing.

Tol, W. A., Barbui, C., Galappatti, A., Silove, D., Betancourt, T. S., Souza, R., Golaz, A., & van Ommeren, M. (2011). Mental health and psychosocial support in humanitarian settings: Linking practice and research. *The Lancet, 378*(9802), 1581–1591. https://doi.org/10.1016/S0140-6736(11)61094-5

Tompson, A. C., Mulrenan, C., Hartwell, G., Petticrew, M., & van Schalkwyk, M. C. I. (2022). Commercial determinants of health. *BMJ, 378,* Article o2034. https://doi.org/10.1136/bmj.o2034

Tønnesen, I. (2016). Social prescribing could help alleviate pressure on GPs. *BMJ, 352,* Article i1436. https://doi.org/10.1136/bmj.i1436

Torrents, E. G., & Björkdahl, A. (2024). Alternatives to coercion. In N. Hallett, R. Whittington, D. Richter, & E. Eneje (Eds.), *Coercion and violence in mental health settings* (pp. 189–206). Springer.

Totsika, V., Liew, A., Absoud, M., Adnams, C., & Emerson, E. (2022). Mental health problems in children with intellectual disability. *The Lancet Child & Adolescent Health, 6*(6), 432–444. https://doi.org/10.1016/S2352-4642(22)00067-0

Triandis, H. C., & Gelfand, M. J. (2012). A theory of individualism and collectivism. In P. A. M. Van Lange, A. W. Kruglanski, & E. T. Higgins (Eds.), *Handbook of theories of social psychology* (Vol. 2, pp. 498–520). Sage. https://doi.org/10.4135/9781446249222.n51

Tribe, R., & Bhugra, D. (2025). *Social justice, social discrimination and mental health: Theory, practice and professional issues*. Routledge.

Turvey, C. L., & Roberts, L. J. (2015). Recent developments in the use of online resources and mobile technologies to support mental health care. *International Review of Psychiatry, 27*(6), 547–557. https://doi.org/10.3109/09540261.2015.1087975

Twenge, J. M., & Campbell, W. K. (2018). *The narcissism epidemic: Living in the age of entitlement*. Atria Books.

Ungvari, G. S., Caroff, S. N., Csihi, L., & Gazdag, G. (2023). Catatonia: "Fluctuat nec mergitur." *World Journal of Psychiatry, 13*(5), 131–137. https://doi.org/10.5498/wjp.v13.i5.131

UNFPA. (2012). *Ageing in the twenty-first century: A celebration and a challenge*. United Nations Population Fund (UNFPA) & HelpAge International.

UNICEF. (2021). The State of the World's Children 2021. Www.unicef.org; UNICEF. https://www.unicef.org/reports/state-worlds-children-2021

UNICEF. (2023, October 10). *Mental health a human right, but only 1 psychiatrist per 1,000,000 people in sub-Saharan Africa—UNICEF/WHO*. https://www.unicef.org/esa/press-releases/mental-health-a-human-right

United Nations. (1948). Universal Declaration of Human Rights. General Assembly Resolution 217 A (III). https://www.un.org/en/about-us/universal-declaration-of-human-rights

United Nations. (1966). *International Covenant on Economic, Social and Cultural Rights*. Treaty Series, 993, 3–19. https://www.ohchr.org/en/instruments-mechanisms/instruments/international-covenant-economic-social-and-cultural-rights

United Nations. (1966). *International Covenant on Civil and Political Rights*. Treaty Series, 999, 171–186. https://www.ohchr.org/en/instruments-mechanisms/instruments/international-covenant-civil-and-political-rights

United Nations. (1976). *International Covenant on Economic, Social and Cultural Rights*. Treaty Series, 993, 3–19. https://www.ohchr.org/en/instruments-mechanisms/instruments/international-covenant-economic-social-and-cultural-rights

United Nations. (2006). *Convention on the rights of persons with disabilities*. Treaty Series, 2515, 3. https://www.un.org/development/desa/disabilities/convention-on-the-rights-of-persons-with-disabilities.html

United Nations. (2007). Convention on the Rights of Persons with Disabilities. Treaty Series, 2515, 3–46. https://www.un.org/disabilities/documents/convention/convoptprot-e.pdf

United Nations. (2020, April). *UN COVID-19 Response and Recovery Fund.* https://unsdg.un.org/sites/default/files/2020-04/COVID19-Response-Recovery-Fund-Document.pdf

United Nations Office on Drugs and Crime (UNODC). (2013). *World drug report 2013.* United Nations. https://www.unodc.org/unodc/secured/wdr/wdr2013/World_Drug_Report_2013.pdf

United Nations Office on Drugs and Crime (UNODC). (2023). *World drug report 2023.* United Nations. https://www.unodc.org/unodc/en/data-and-analysis/world-drug-report-2023.html

United Nations Office on Drugs and Crime (UNODC). (2024). *World drug report 2024.* United Nations. https://www.unodc.org/unodc/en/data-and-analysis/world-drug-report-2024.html

van Bortel, T., Basnayake, A., Wurie, F., Jambai, M., Koroma, A. S., Muana, A. T., Hann, K., Eaton, J., Martin, S., & Nellums, L. B. (2016). Psychosocial effects of an Ebola outbreak at individual, community and international levels. *Bulletin of the World Health Organization, 94*(3), 210–214. https://doi.org/10.2471/BLT.15.158543

Van Os, J., & Kapur, S. (2009). Schizophrenia. *The Lancet, 374*(9690), 635–645.

van Voren, R., & Keukens, R. (2014). The role of non-governmental organizations. In S. O. Okpaku (Ed.), *Essentials of global mental health* (pp. 346–355). Cambridge University Press.

Vandello, J. A., & Cohen, D. (1999). Patterns of individualism and collectivism across the United States. *Journal of Personality and Social Psychology, 77*(2), 279–292. https://doi.org/10.1037/0022-3514.77.2.279

Veling, W., Hoek, H. W., & Mackenbach, J. P. (2008). Perceived discrimination and the risk of schizophrenia: A case-control study. *Social Psychiatry and Psychiatric Epidemiology, 43*(12), 953–958. https://doi.org/10.1007/s00127-008-0381-6

Victor, C. R., Mansfield, L., Kay, T., Daykin, N., Lane, J., Grigsby-Duffy, L., & Meads, C. (2018). *An overview of reviews: The effectiveness of interventions to address loneliness at all stages of the life-course.* What Works Wellbeing.

Vijayakumar, L., John, S., Pirkis, J., & Whiteford, H. (2005). Suicide in developing countries. *Crisis, 26*(3), 112–119. https://doi.org/10.1027/0227-5910.26.3.112

Vindegaard, N., & Benros, M. E. (2020). COVID-19 pandemic and mental health consequences: Systematic review of the current evidence. *Brain, Behavior, and Immunity, 89*, 531–542. https://doi.org/10.1016/j.bbi.2020.05.048

Votaw, V. R., Geyer, R., Rieselbach, M. M., & McHugh, R. K. (2019). The epidemiology of benzodiazepine misuse: A systematic review. *Drug and Alcohol Dependence, 200*, 95–114. https://doi.org/10.1016/j.drugalcdep.2019.02.033

Wachter, M., Ventriglio, A., & Bhugra, D. (2015). Micro-identities, adjustment and stigma. *International Journal of Social Psychiatry, 61*(5), 436–437. https://doi.org/10.1177/0020764015590080

Wahlbeck, K., Cresswell-Smith, J., Haaramo, P., & Parkkonen, J. (2017). Interventions to mitigate the effects of poverty and inequality on mental health. *Social Psychiatry and Psychiatric Epidemiology, 52*(5), 505–514. https://doi.org/10.1007/s00127-017-1370-4

Walker, E. R., McGee, R. E., & Druss, B. G. (2015). Mortality in mental disorders and global disease burden implications: A systematic review and meta-analysis. *JAMA Psychiatry, 72*(4), 334–341. https://doi.org/10.1001/jamapsychiatry.2014.2502

Walter, H. J., Kaye, A. J., Dennery, K. M., & DeMaso, D. R. (2019). Three-year outcomes of a school-hospital partnership providing multitiered mental health services in urban schools. *Journal of School Health, 89*(8), 643–652. https://doi.org/10.1111/josh.12792

Wang, F., Gao, Y., Han, Z., Yu, Y., Long, Z., Jiang, X., Wu, Y., Pei, B., Cao, Y., Ye, J., Wang, M., Zhao, Y. (2023). A systematic review and meta-analysis of 90 cohort studies of social isolation, loneliness and mortality. *Nature Human Behaviour, 7*(8), 1307–1319. https://doi.org/10.1038/s41562-023-01617-6

Wang, Y., & Zeng, Y. (2024). Relationship between loneliness and internet addiction: A meta-analysis. *BMC Public Health, 24*, Article 858. https://doi.org/10.1186/6s12889-024-18366-4Wardenaar, K. J., Benjet, C., Viana, M. C., & de Jonge, P. (2018). Specific phobias. In K. M. Scott, P. de Jonge, D. J. Stein, & R. C. Kessler (Eds.), *Mental disorders around the world: Facts and figures from the WHO World Mental Health Surveys* (pp. 134–152). Cambridge University Press.

Watson, P. (2022). Stress, PTSD, and COVID-19: The utility of disaster mental health interventions during the COVID-19 pandemic. *Current Treatment Options in Psychiatry, 9*(1), 14–40. https://doi.org/10.1007/s40501-021-00253-z

Weare, K., & Nind, M. (2011). Mental health promotion and problem prevention in schools: What does the evidence say? *Health Promotion International, 26*(Suppl. 1), i29–i69. https://doi.org/10.1093/heapro/dar075

Weaver, L., Karasz, A., Muralidhar, K., Jaykrishna, P., Krupp, C., & Madhavan, P. (2023). Will increasing access to mental health treatment close India's mental health gap? *SSM—Mental Health, 3*, Article 100184. https://doi.org/10.1016/j.ssmmh.2022.100184

Weaver, L. J., & Hadley, C. (2009). Moving beyond hunger and nutrition: A systematic review of the evidence linking food insecurity and mental health in developing countries. *Ecology of Food and Nutrition, 48*(4), 263–284. https://doi.org/10.1080/03670240903001167

Wei, Y., Kutcher, S., Blackwood, A., Glover, D., Weaver, C., MacKay, M., & McGrath, P. (2015). A collaborative and sustainable approach to address mental health promotion and early identification in schools in the Canadian province of Nova Scotia and beyond. In S. Kutcher, Y. Wei, & M. D. Weist (Eds.), *School mental health: Global challenges and opportunities* (pp. 30–45). Cambridge University Press.

Weissman, M. M., Bland, R. C., Canino, G. J., Faravelli, C., Greenwald, S., Hwu, H.-G., Joyce, P. R., Karam, E. G., Lee, C.-K., Lellouch, J., Lépine, J.-P., Newman, S. C., Rubio-Stipec, M., Wells, J. E., Wickramaratne, P. J., Wittchen, H.-U., & Yeh, E.-K. (1996). Cross-national epidemiology of major depression and bipolar disorder. *JAMA, 276*(4), 293–299. https://doi.org/10.1001/jama.1996.03540040037030

Wheeler, P. H., Patten, C. A., Wi, C. I., Bublitz, J. T., Ryu, E., Ristagno, E. H., & Juhn, Y. J. (2022). Role of geographic risk factors and social determinants of health in COVID-19 epidemiology: Longitudinal geospatial analysis in a Midwest rural region. *Journal of Clinical and Translational Science, 6*(1), Article e51. https://doi.org/10.1017/cts.2021.885

Whitaker, R. C., Phillips, S. M., & Orzol, S. M. (2006). Food insecurity and the risks of depression and anxiety in mothers and behavioral problems in their preschool-aged children. *Pediatrics, 118*(3), e859–e868. https://doi.org/10.1542/peds.2006-0239

Whitney, D. G., & Peterson, M. D. (2019). US national and state-level prevalence of mental health disorders and disparities of mental health care use in children. *JAMA Pediatrics, 173*(4), 389–391. https://doi.org/10.1001/jamapediatrics.2018.5399

WHO. (n.d.). *Thailand's 1 million village health volunteers—"unsung heroes"—are helping guard communities nationwide from COVID-19*. World Health Organization. https://www.who.int/thailand/news/feature-stories/detail/thailands-1-million-village-health-volunteers-unsung-heroes-are-helping-guard-communities-nationwide-from-covid-19

WHO. (1946). *WHO constitution*. World Health Organization. https://www.who.int/about/governance/constitution

WHO. (1973). *Report of the international pilot study of schizophrenia*. World Health Organization.

WHO. (1975). *Organisation of mental health services in developing countries: Sixteenth report of the WHO Expert Committee on Mental Health* [Technical Report Series 564]. World Health Organization.

WHO. (1979). *Schizophrenia: An international follow-up*. World Health Organization.

WHO. (1988). *Ottawa charter for health promotion*. World Health Organization.

WHO. (1993). *ICD-10: The international classification of diseases*. World Health Organization.

WHO. (2004). *Promoting mental health: Concepts, emerging evidence, practice*. World Health Organization. https://www.who.int/publications/i/item/9241562943

WHO. (2006). *Disease control priorities related to mental, neurological, developmental and substance abuse disorders*. World Health Organization.

WHO. (2008a). *Closing the gap in a generation: Final report of the Commission on Social Determinants of Health*. World Health Organization.

WHO. (2008b). *Global burden of disease: 2004 update*. World Health Organization. https://apps.who.int/iris/bitstream/handle/10665/43942/9789241563710_eng.pdf

WHO. (2013a). *Comprehensive mental health action plan 2013–2020*. World Health Organization.

WHO. (2013b). *Investing in mental health: Evidence for action*. World Health Organization.

WHO. (2014a). *Global status report on alcohol and health*. World Health Organization.

WHO. (2014b). *Preventing suicide: A global imperative*. World Health Organization.

WHO. (2014c). *Social determinants of mental health*. World Health Organization. https://www.who.int/publications/i/item/9789241506809

WHO. (2017). *Stress at workplace*. World Health Organization.

WHO. (2018). *SAFER—Pricing policies*. World Health Organization. https://www.who.int/initiatives/SAFER/pricing-policies

WHO. (2019). *WHO global report on traditional and complementary medicine 2019*. World Health Organization. https://www.who.int/traditional-complementary-integrative-medicine/en/

WHO. (2020a). *Mental health and psychosocial considerations during the COVID-19 outbreak, 18 March 2020*. World Health Organization. https://apps.who.int/iris/handle/10665/331490

WHO. (2020b). *Mental health atlas*. World Health Organization. https://www.who.int/publications/i/item/9789240036703

WHO. (2021a). *Mental health action plan 2013–2030*. World Health Organization. https://www.who.int/publications

WHO. (2021b). *Mental health of adolescents*. World Health Organization. https://www.who.int/news-room/fact-sheets/detail/adolescent-mental-health

WHO. (2021c). *Task-shifting to improve access to mental health care: WHO guidelines and best practices* [WHO Technical Report Series]. World Health Organization.

WHO. (2021d). *Tobacco.* World Health Organization. https://www.who.int/news-room/fact-sheets/detail/tobacco

WHO. (2022a). *Child and adolescent mental and brain health.* World Health Organization. https://www.who.int/activities/improving-the-mental-and-brain-health-of-children-and-adolescents

WHO. (2022b). *Commercial determinants of health.* World Health Organization. https://www.who.int/health-topics/commercial-determinants-of-health#tab=tab_1

WHO. (2022c). *Gender and mental health.* World Health Organization. https://iris.who.int/handle/10665/68884

WHO. (2022d). *Health inequities and their causes.* World Health Organization. https://www.who.int/news-room/fact-sheets/detail/health-inequities-and-their-causes

WHO. (2022e). *Preventing intimate partner violence improves mental health.* World Health Organization. https://www.who.int/news/item/06-10-2022-preventing-intimate-partner-violence-improves-mental-health

WHO. (2022f). *Mental disorders.* World Health Organization. https://www.who.int/news-room/fact-sheets/detail/mental-disorders

WHO. (2022g). *Task shifting for mental health care in low-resource settings* (WHO Policy Brief). World Health Organization.

WHO. (2022h). *WHO guidelines on mental health at work.* World Health Organization. https://www.who.int/publications/i/item/9789240053052

WHO. (2022i). *World mental health report: Transforming mental health for all.* World Health Organization. https://www.who.int/publications/i/item/9789240049338

WHO. (2023). *No level of alcohol consumption is safe for our health.* World Health Organization. https://www.who.int/europe/news/item/04-01-2023-no-level-of-alcohol-consumption-is-safe-for-our-health

WHO. (2024). *Suicide.* World Health Organization. https://www.who.int/news-room/fact-sheets/detail/suicide

WHO Collaborative Study on Standardized Assessment of Depressive Disorders., & Sartorius, N. (1983). *Depressive disorders in different cultures: report on the WHO Collaborative Study on Standardized Assessment of Depressive Disorders.* World Health Organization.

WHO, War Trauma Foundation & World Vision International. (2011). *Psychological first aid: Guide for field workers.* World Health Organization. https://www.who.int/publications/i/item/9789241548205

Wig, N. N., Menon, D. K., Bedi, H., Leff, J., Kuipers, L., Ghosh, A., Day, R., Korten, A., Ernberg, G., Sartorius, N., & Jablensky, A. (1987). Expressed emotion and schizophrenia in North India. *British Journal of Psychiatry, 151*(2), 156–160. https://doi.org/10.1192/bjp.151.2.156

Wilkinson, R., & Pickett, K. (2006). Income inequality and population health: A review and explanation of the evidence. *Social Science & Medicine, 62*(7), 1768–1784. https://doi.org/10.1016/j.socscimed.2005.08.036

Wilkinson, R., & Pickett, K. (2009). *The spirit level: Why more equal societies almost always do better*. Allen Lane.

Williams, D. R., & Mohammed, S. A. (2009). Discrimination and racial disparities in health: Evidence and needed research. *Journal of Behavioral Medicine, 32*(1), 20–47. https://doi.org/10.1007/s10865-008-9185-0

Williams, D. R. (2018). Stress and the mental health of populations of color: Advancing our understanding of race-related stressors. *Journal of Health and Social Behavior, 59*(4), 466–485. https://doi.org/10.1177/0022146518814251

Williams, E., Buck, D., Babalola, G., & Maguire, D. (2022). *What are health inequalities?* The King's Fund. https://www.kingsfund.org.uk/insight-and-analysis/long-reads/what-are-health-inequalities

Wilson, C., & Cariola, L. A. (2020). LGBTQI+youth and mental health: A systematic review of qualitative research. *Adolescent Research Review, 5*(2), 187–211. https://doi.org/10.1007/s40894-019-00118-w

Wilson, J., & Read, J. (2001). What prevents GPs from using outside resources for women experiencing depression? A New Zealand study. *Journal of Family Practice, 18*(1), 84–86. https://doi.org/10.1093/fampra/18.1.84

Winkler, P., Formanek, T., Mlada, K., Kagstrom, A., Mohrova, Z., Mohr, P., & Csemy, L. (2020). Increase in prevalence of current mental disorders in the context of COVID-19: Analysis of repeated nationwide cross-sectional surveys. *Epidemiology and Psychiatric Sciences, 29*, Article e173. https://doi.org/10.1017/S2045796020000888

Witteveen, A. B., Young, S., Cuijpers, P., Ayuso-Mateos, J. L., Barbui, C., Bertolini, F., Cabello, M., Cadorin, C., Downes, N., Franzoi, D., Gasior, M., John, A., Melchior, M., McDaid, D., Palantza, C., Purgato, M., van der Waerden, J., Wang, S., & Sijbrandij, M. (2022). Remote mental health care interventions during the COVID-19 pandemic: An umbrella review. *Behaviour Research and Therapy, 159*, Article 104226. https://doi.org/10.1016/j.brat.2022.104226

Wittgens, C., Fischer, M. M., Buspavanich, P., Theobald, S., Schweizer, K., & Trautmann, S. (2022). Mental health in people with minority sexual orientations: A meta-analysis of population-based studies. *Acta Psychiatrica Scandinavica, 145*(4), 357–372. https://doi.org/10.1111/acps.13405

World Bank. (1993). *World development report 1993: Investing in health*. Oxford University Press.

World Economic Forum, Global Agenda Council on Mental Health. (2016, May 26). Seven steps towards a mentally healthy organisation. http://rialnet.org/sites/default/files/presentation_vanbortel.pdf

World Psychiatric Association. (2017). *Good Psychiatric Practice* [Position Statement]. World Psychiatric Association. https://www.researchgate.net/publication/320160893_World_Psychiatric_Association_Position_Statement_on_Good_Psychiatric_Practice

World Psychiatric Association (WPA). (2019a). *Public mental health.* https://www.wpanet.org/public-mental-health

World Psychiatric Association (WPA). (2019b). *Roles and Responsibilities of the Psychiatrist of the Twenty-First Century* [Position Statement]. World Psychiatric Association. https://psikiyatri.org.tr/userfiles/file/WPA24.pdf

Wu, P., Liu, X., Fang, Y., Fan, B., Fuller, C. J., Guan, Z., Yao, Z., Kong, J., Lu, J., & Litvak, I. J. (2008). Alcohol abuse/dependence symptoms among hospital employees exposed to a SARS outbreak. *Alcohol and Alcoholism, 43*(6), 706–712. https://doi.org/10.1093/alcalc/agn073

Wu, Y., Wang, L., Tao, M., Cao, H., Yuan, H., Ye, M., Chen, X., Wang, K., & Zhu, C. (2023). Changing trends in the global burden of mental disorders from 1990 to 2019 and predicted levels in 25 years. *Epidemiology and Psychiatric Sciences, 32,* Article e63. https://doi.org/10.1017/S2045796023000756

Wyman, P. A., Brown, C. H., LoMurray, M., Schmeelk-Cone, K., Petrova, M., Yu, Q., Walsh, E., Tu, X., & Wang, W. (2010). An outcome evaluation of the Sources of Strength suicide prevention program delivered by adolescent peer leaders in high schools. *American Journal of Public Health, 100*(9), 1653–1661. https://doi.org/10.2105/AJPH.2009.190025

Xie, Y., Boom, J., Sin, W. H., & Fung, D. (2015). A Singapore model—REACH. In S. Kutcher, Y. Wei, & M. D. Weist (Eds.), *School mental health: Global challenges and opportunities* (pp. 202–217). Cambridge University Press.

Xiong, J., Lipsitz, O., Nasri, F., Lui, L. M. W., Gill, H., Phan, L., Chen-Li, D., Iacobucci, M., Ho, R., Majeed, A., & McIntyre, R. S. (2020). Impact of COVID-19 pandemic on mental health in the general population: A systematic review. *Journal of Affective Disorders, 277,* 55–64. https://doi.org/10.1016/j.jad.2020.08.001

Yamaguchi, S., Wu, S.-I., Biswas, M., Yate, M., Aoki, Y., Barley, E. A., & Thornicroft, G. (2013). Effects of short-term interventions to reduce mental health–related stigma in university or college students: A systematic review. *Journal of Nervous and Mental Disease, 201*(6), 490–503. https://doi.org/10.1097/NMD.0b013e31829480df

Yamasaki, S., Ando, S., Shimodera, S., Endo, K., Okazaki, Y., Asukai, N., Usami, S., Nishida, A., & Sasaki, T. (2016). The recognition of mental illness, schizophrenia identification, and help-seeking from friends in late adolescence. *PLoS ONE, 11*(3), Article e0151298. https://doi.org/10.1371/journal.pone.0151298

Yang, G. H., Phillips, M. R., Zhou, M. G., Wang, L. J., Zhang, Y. P., & Xu, D. (2005). Understanding the unique characteristics of suicide in China: National psychological autopsy study. *Biomedical and Environmental Sciences, 18*(6), 379–389.

Yang, X., & Mak, W. W. S. (2020). Addressing socio-political determinants of mental health: An emerging challenge in Hong Kong. *The Lancet,* 395(10220), 249–250. https://doi.org/10.1016/S0140-6736(20)30057-X

Yang, X., She, R., Lau, M. M. C., & Lau, J. T. F. (2020). Anticipated socio-political developments and related personal responses as structural determinants of mental health problems: A population-based study. *International Journal of Social Psychiatry, 66*(1), 58–66. https://doi.org/10.1177/0020764019879948

Yang, Y. (2018, November 19). *Ping An Good Doctor blazes trail in developing unstaffed, AI-assisted clinics in China*. South China Morning Post. https://www.scmp.com/tech/enterprises/article/2173657/ping-good-doctor-blazes-trail-developing-unstaffed-ai-assisted

Yao, H., Chen, J.-H., & Xu, Y.-F. (2020). Patients with mental health disorders in the COVID-19 epidemic. *The Lancet Psychiatry, 7*(4), e21. https://doi.org/10.1016/S2215-0366(20)30090-0

Yap, P. M. (1951). Mental diseases peculiar to certain cultures: A survey of comparative psychiatry. *British Journal of Psychiatry, Journal of Mental Science, 97*(408), 313–327. https://doi.org/10.1192/bjp.97.407.313

Yazgan, Y., & Karacau, S. (2015). Improving mental health via schools. In S. Kutcher, Y. Wei, & M. D. Weist (Eds.), *School mental health: Global challenges and opportunities* (pp. 218–238). Cambridge University Press.

Ye, J., Shim, R., Lukaszewski, T., Yun, K., Kim, S. H., & Ruth, G. (2012). Telepsychiatry services for Korean immigrants. *Telemedicine and e-Health, 18*(10), 797–802. https://doi.org/10.1089/tmj.2012.0041

Yellowlees, P., Chan, S. C., & Parish, M. B. (2015). The hybrid doctor-patient relationship in the age of technology: Telepsychiatry consultations and the use of virtual space. *International Review of Psychiatry, 27*(6), 476–489. https://doi.org/10.3109/09540261.2015.1082987

Yellowlees, P. M., Odor, A., Iosif, A.-M., Parish, M. B., Nafiz, N., Patrice, K., Xiong, G., McCaron, R., Sanchez, R., Ochoa, E., & Hilty, D. (2013). Transcultural psychiatry made simple—asynchronous telepsychiatry as an approach to providing culturally relevant care. *Telemedicine and e-Health, 19*(4), 259–264. https://doi.org/10.1089/tmj.2012.0077

Yeung, A., Johnson, D. P., Trinh, N.-H., Weng, W.-C. C., Kvedar, J., & Fava, M. (2009). Feasibility and effectiveness of telepsychiatry services for Chinese immigrants in a nursing home. *Telemedicine and e-Health, 15*(4), 336–341. https://doi.org/10.1089/tmj.2008.0138

Yeung, A., Martinson, M. A., Baer, L., Chen, J., Clain, A., Williams, A., Chang, T. E., Trinh, N.-H., Alpert, J. E., & Fava, M. (2016). The effectiveness of telepsychiatry-based culturally sensitive collaborative treatment for depressed Chinese American immigrants: A randomized controlled trial. *Journal of Clinical Psychiatry, 77*(8), e996–e1002. https://doi.org/10.4088/JCP.15m09952

Younan, H.-C., Junghans, C., Harris, M., Majeed, A., & Gnani, S. (2020). Maximising the impact of social prescribing on population health in the era of COVID-19. *Journal of the Royal Society of Medicine, 113*(10), 377–382. https://doi.org/10.1177/0141076820947057

Zevallos, Z. (2011, October 11). What is otherness? *The Other Sociologist.* https://othersociologist.com/otherness-resources/

Zhabenko, N., & Zhabenko, O. (2015). School and community mental health promotion strategies for youth in Ukraine. In S. Kutcher, Y. Wei, & M. D. Weist (Eds.), *School mental health: Global challenges and opportunities* (pp. 239–251). Cambridge University Press.

Zhang, J., Sun, L., Liu, Y., & Zhang, J. (2014). The change in suicide rates between 2002 and 2011 in China. *Suicide and Life-Threatening Behavior, 44*(5), 560–568. https://doi.org/10.1111/sltb.12090

Zhang, J., Xiao, S., & Zhou, L. (2010). Mental disorders and suicide among young rural Chinese: A case-control psychological autopsy study. *American Journal of Psychiatry, 167*(7), 773–781. https://doi.org/10.1176/appi.ajp.2010.09101476

Zhang, X., Chen, X., & Zhang, X. (2018). The impact of exposure to air pollution on cognitive performance. *Proceedings of the National Academy of Sciences, 115*(37), 9193–9197. https://doi.org/10.1073/pnas.1809474115

Zhen, R., Quan, L., & Zhou, X. (2018). Fear, negative cognition, and depression mediate the relationship between traumatic exposure and sleep problems among flood victims in China. *Psychological Trauma: Theory, Research, Practice, and Policy, 10*(6), 602–609. https://doi.org/10.1037/tra0000331.

Ziol-Guest, K. M., & McKenna, C. C. (2014). Early childhood housing instability and school readiness. *Child Development, 85*(1), 103–113. https://doi.org/10.1111/cdev.12105

Zisman-Ilani, Y. (2022). The mental health crisis of individuals with intellectual and developmental disabilities. *Psychiatric Services, 73*(3), 245–246. https://doi.org/10.1176/appi.ps.202200022

Index

Publisher contact:
The MIT Press
Massachusetts Institute of Technology
77 Massachusetts Avenue, Cambridge, MA 02139
mitpress.mit.edu

EU Authorised Representative:
Easy Access System Europe, Mustamäe tee 50,
10621 Tallinn, Estonia
gpsr.requests@easproject.com

Printed by Integrated Books International,
United States of America